Caregiver
a Role We Least
Expected

Tips and Tidbits to Help in Your Role

Peggy A. Rossi, BSN, MPA Retired RN
and Case Manager and Case Management
Administrator Certified

NEWMAN SPRINGS PUBLISHING
320 Broad Street
Red Bank, NJ 07701

First originally published by Newman Springs Publishing 2024

ISBN 979-8-89061-322-6 (Paperback)
ISBN 979-8-89061-323-3 (Digital)

Printed in the United States of America

Unfortunately, as weblinks change so frequently and they might be outdated even before this book is published, I have not included any weblinks. However, it is critical you know as much as you can as this will help you in your role, and the Internet is one way to learn as much as you can. Thus, I have given you key words to use as you conduct your Internet search which hopefully will allow you to go directly to a site where you can find the information that may be of help. As you do your research, I always advise the patients I worked with to use primarily the state or federal government or the national disease-specific agencies—this gives you unbiased information on a topic.

This book is dedicated to all caregivers, past and present. My hat goes off to all of you. You will be taking on tasks and situations that most of us never encounter. You must also learn to do many tasks quickly. Yet they are ones that we as nurses had to learn in school, often over an extended period.

It, more specifically, is dedicated to my sister Vikki and her husband, Thomas. Vikki was initially Mom's on-call caregiver when she resided in a local assisted living facility, often getting thirty phone calls per day. When Mom's money ran out, we decided to not place her in a memory care facility, as Vikki and Thomas agreed it was best if she moved in with them. Vikki did a stellar job, and while we expected Mom to slip into her eternal sleep at any time, she lived an added three years, with her physician still able to certify her for ongoing hospice care.

Her hospice team was a wonderful addition, and they—or at least the nurse—and the chaplain became close friends. Despite the overwhelming caregiving tasks, Vikki and Thomas kept their home a calm and happy place. In fact, often, the nurse or the chaplain would stop by just for coffee or a visit, as they wanted to not see doom and gloom.

Contents

Acknowledgments

I WANT TO acknowledge the following people who helped me make my dream come true. Without their time and expertise, the book may not have been possible.

Luis A. Torres and I have been colleagues for several years, and I needed his expertise in dealing with emotions and psychological issues and expertise on therapy tips for self-care and other topics. He is a licensed family and marriage counselor and, like me, is a strong proponent of taking care of our self.

Janet Rogers and I have been colleagues for many, many years, and we have seen multiple changes in health care in the Sacramento Valley area. Janet's career includes a wide variety of health care settings—director of nurses for Option Care, a large infusion company; manager of utilization and case management for Hill Physicians Medical Group, a large physician group in Sacramento; and then manager of the Sacramento County Medically Indigent Services Program. In addition, she worked for years as a hospice nurse. Thus, her expertise in the review and her added comments were invaluable as she helped me validate what is written.

I also want to thank three key reviewers from Alta California Regional Center (ACRC), who helped me tremendously, as each of them is literally a walking textbook on diagnoses and services needed for the intellectually and developmentally disabled (IDD) population: Camelia Houston, MS, director of intake and clinical services, Alta California Regional Center; Jennifer Bloom, MA, director of clinical services, Alta California Regional Center; and Amy McCreary, MS, BCBA, clinical services manager, Alta California Regional Center, with expertise on autism spectrum disorder (ASD) and clients with challenging behaviors.

ACRC is one of twenty-one nonprofit agencies that contracts with the California Department of Developmental Services (DDS) to serve the IDD population in California.

Introduction

WRITING THIS BOOK has been a dream after my many years of working—sixty-two years—as a nurse, a public health nurse, with the last fifty-five years spent primarily in nursing management, serving as a director or consultant of either hospital discharge planning or for health plan insurers as the director of their medical management programs (utilization management, case management, and quality management).

As such, I have also been responsible for writing the utilization and case management programs for a start-up independent physician association (IPA) and a new health maintenance organization (HMO) in California, Western Health Advantage, and then writing for Foundation Health after their award from the Department of Defense for a program called the CHAMPUS Reform Imitative (CRI), which is now TRICARE.

For all these, I have written each of the programs in their entirety, including all the policies and procedure, as well as teaching nurses in various regions what and how to do case management. This means I have written thousands of policies and procedures, as well as multiple proposals, as my company sought new lines of business. I have also written multiple monthly news columns for each business entity, trying to educate members of community resources that may help to augment any health plan benefits.

Added to all this, I have also written three nursing textbooks on case management, two of which have been used in many schools of nursing across the US and abroad, with my second edition winning the *American Journal of Nursing* award for best nursing management book of 2003. My third text focuses strictly on hospital discharge planning and case management, designed to specifically assist new discharge planners of all they need to know. Much of what is written in this book will be from either training nurses what to do or, equally as important, the tips and suggestions I have made to the families I have worked with as they begin their journey of being a caregiver and accessing community resources.

Caregiving can certainly take on many meanings and for many—not only those with medical or mental health care needs but also those with developmental or intellectual disabilities, any one of whom can require a wide variety of care but many of whom can live fairly independently. However, this book is intended more for those caregivers who must assume total care of a loved one, regardless of age and diagnosis. Despite all my experience in teaching caregiving, the last months of my husband's life and my own experience as a caregiver was a real eye-opener, to say the least.

I will be honest with you. Being a caregiver, especially for one who is total care either physically, mentally, or both, is the hardest role you can assume. It is exhausting both mentally and physically, and the key is, you must remember the following:

- Take care of yourself—mentally, emotionally, and physically.
- If people or friends offer to help, accept it.
- Learn to say no and yes when appropriate.
- Learn to have those hard or difficult or those nitty-gritty conversations when a difficult or hard decision must be made.
- Keep a notebook or your cell phone handy so you can write down questions as they arise, and then make notes of whom you spoke with when and what might be the answer. This will assist you as you do your own research of what might be right for you and your situation.
- Learn to ask questions, and as necessary, request a full explanation of details if you do not understand what is said.
- Keep current copies of any annual health plan handbooks (called Evidence of Coverage), as this will teach you what

your annual deductible and co-payments will be and also what will be a benefit versus not and if care is limited or excluded. This booklet will also explain how to appeal when something that might be medically necessary is denied.

○ By all means, call your loved one's health plan and request that a case manager be assigned. This will help you if you need any care or services authorized.

○ Because many persons who are total care often have many medical conditions, thus, many treating physicians, who might be prescribing a variety of medications, make every attempt to use the same pharmacy. This will give you an advantage, as you can ask the pharmacist to do a periodic review of all the medications. This will help ensure all the medications are working as they should, and this will help avoid any adverse reactions should one drug react differently from how it should.

○ Join a local or online or telephonic support group. Here you can then learn firsthand what they have found works versus what does not. Additionally, they may have suggestions as to what community resources are available to help with the specific illness or injury. Equally as important, they may offer tips on how to take care of yourself.

○ By all means, in today's world of technology, get yourself a smartphone, and take advantage of appropriate apps. If you cannot afford one, check into the one offered by the federal government. By having a cell phone, this will allow you to have basically a computer at your fingertips. You can find information by typing in the web browser "Lifeline—Federal Communications Commission."

○ Make use of one of the best resources to explore local community resources that might be available. The best way to explore will be to use the United Way telephone number: 2-1-1. It is an online resource established by the Federal Communications in 2000 to help consumers locate local health care and other services within a local region.

My book will give you some tips not only on what I learned as I counseled others as they were to assume the role at discharge. But it was the struggles my sister endured when she became the 24-7 caregiver for our mom, who had end-stage Alzheimer's, that really opened my eyes. It is also from now witnessing what my niece is going through as I give her tips on resources to explore and as we struggle to get the help my sister, her mom, needs.

To assist me, I also interviewed other caregivers, especially parents who have been a caregiver for a severely developmentally disabled individual and another who was a caregiver of a severely intellectually disabled child. So my goal is, again, to give you all as many tips as I can in my attempts to educate you of things you may want to do to make your role a little easier.

My husband became physically disabled at a young age (fifty-two), and so we experienced role reversal—I took on any financial responsibilities and did tasks he previously did—early on and then the financial struggle that ensued due to limited income. While we had income, we fell in that gray area—too much to qualify for Medicaid or any pharmaceutical programs to help pay the high co-pays we had to pay since most of his medications were brand drugs. This meant I had to work not only a full-time job but also a part-time one as well.

To make matters even worse, we lived in a county that did not offer any managed care plans. This meant that initially, my husband only had his employer's fee-for-service or indemnity health insurance to cover medical costs. Then once eligible for Medicare, he had traditional or original Medicare, which again is basically a fee-for-service or indemnity health plan. This meant even with two insurances, we were faced with an extra outlay of money due to balance billing.

But two of our biggest yearly outlays of money were not only the co-payments for his medications. Because he was on so many drugs, his teeth were slowly deteriorating; and as he, at that point, didn't have cancer, health plans would pay for dental care in prep for radiation therapy. Thus, one of our biggest outlays of money each year was for dental care, as costs were far over and above what most dental plans covered, which was basically about $1,500 yearly.

Disclaimer: I have mentioned agencies or websites, and they are merely so you can conduct your own research. This does not mean, in no way, that I or the publisher endorse such. Listen to your loved one's physician or health care team or any legal counsel you use for advice. I have included them in this book merely to assist you as you conduct your own research and learn what might or might not help in your situation.

These are some basic keys for caregiving:

- Do your research.
- Educate yourself on your loved one's diagnosis and potential treatment options.
- Make notes so you can remember to ask the right questions or use as you do your own research.
- Learn to say no if the situation calls for it, but equally as important, learn to say yes if friends or family offer to help.

The biggest key? Learn to take care of yourself, both mentally and physically. If you don't, you will burn out with the end result not being what your intent was when you started your role: allowing your loved one to remain at home.

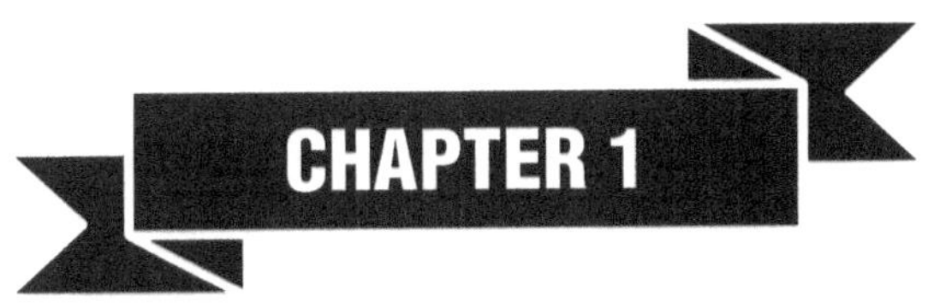

CHAPTER 1

Hospitals—Often, Your Role Starts Here

THE START OF your new role as a caregiver often starts with your loved one's reason for hospitalization, whether it is from a birth defect or birth injury, a multiple-trauma accident or injury, a stroke or other major illness, or a change in a previous illness that has now taken a turn for the worse. Often, it also may be from a continued decline in their mental and/or physical condition, with the decline now affecting their abilities for self-care, reasoning, and even common sense. Despite the cause, this chapter will be devoted to the hospitalization and consequent discharge.

During your loved one's hospital stay, the following are key pointers and actions you will possibly want to take into account and use. Remember, you are now possibly the eyes, ears, and voice of your loved one. Due to some of the overwhelming events that may occur, I always suggest to families I work with to keep a notebook—the spiral kind so pages are all kept together—handy. But now we have the advent of a new product, a cell phone, so learn to use it.

Whether you use a notebook or a cell phone, the key will be to jot down or record notes or information on topics you may wish other information on. Doing this will allow you to keep on top of all, especially since if your loved one is hospitalized, you will be under undue stress, often spending sleepless nights in your vigil to be there.

Do this especially if you want to ask questions when the physicians or other health care professionals make rounds or perform your loved one's treatments. Your notes can also be used as well as you do any research on the topic.

As you begin your journey as the caregiver, it is critical to also start planning for how you will take care of yourself—not only physically but, equally as important, mentally and emotionally. Sadly, many caregivers or family members may feel they cannot leave the bedside or step away for a while. This is not true; it is going to be okay to do so. Your loved one will be cared for, and the time you are away and doing such allows you to take care of yourself.

Before we get into preparing for your role as a caregiver, we need to discuss some key pointers and facts or information that may be helpful or trigger stuff you may wish to explore. Definitely for some, you will want to ensure they are in place before the discharge occurs.

Hospitalists

During your loved one's hospital stay, he will be cared for by a wide variety of health care professionals. But the biggest difference in today's hospital care—maybe the only exception is a small rural or community hospital—will be that your loved one's care will no longer be coordinated by his primary care physician (PCP) but by a team of physicians, who are called hospitalists. A hospitalist is a doctor with some of the same medical degrees as a community physician. However, they specialize in providing hospital care, focusing on diagnosing and treating a wide variety of illnesses. They basically do the same work the PCP does, but they only practice in a hospital setting. I can honestly say, I have met many hospitalists over the past many years, and everyone is top-notch in my books.

Hospitalists are a team of physicians employed by the hospital. This means, if your loved one has a prolonged hospital stay, they will be seen by any number of the doctors who make up the hospitalist team. This is due to the fact that as a rule, the team has a rotational schedule so that all shifts are covered 24-7. This means they then work a shift seven days on and then seven days off with a reporting session of whom the team sees and what has been done during the past seven days. So do not be surprised if during the stay you deal with more than one hospitalist. These physicians will be in addition to any specialty physicians your loved one may require.

You will certainly want to ask the doctor about any medical issues, but two (2) hospital professionals you will want to link up with as soon as possible after admission will be the hospital discharge planner / case manager and the social worker. This is necessary, as in most large hospitals, the discharge planner / case manager will be there to help you plan the discharge and help set up the final plan(s), and the social worker will help you emotionally deal with situations or feelings as they arise.

Even if your loved one may be in an intensive care unit (ICU) bed, the Centers for Medicare and Medicaid Services (CMS) has standards in place called conditions of participation (CoPs), which sets the conditions all entities that provide health care for beneficiaries must follow. One of the CoPs is designed for hospital care. This CoP requires all hospitals to ensure a discharge plan is started as early as possible in the stay. Consequently, do not be surprised if you are approached about what may your plans be for the discharge, as the standard set for hospitals and discharge planning reads thus:

> The hospital must have an effective discharge planning process that focuses on the patient's goals and treatment preferences and includes the patient and his or her caregivers / support person(s) as active partners in the discharge planning for post-discharge care. The discharge planning process and the discharge plan must start early in the hospital stay and must be consistent with the patient's goals for care and his or her treatment preferences, ensure an effective transition of the patient from hospital to post-discharge care, and reduce the factors leading to preventable hospital readmissions.

CMS does not specify in the CoPs when to perform the initial discharge planning evaluation, best practice calls for it to be completed on the day of admission whenever possible with the plan typically developed by registered nurses or social work case managers. The CoPs also says other personnel can complete the assessment, but they must work under the supervision of the nurse or social worker. (For information on the conditions of participation for discharge planning type in your web browser, "discharge planning COPs")

The hospital social worker will also be one you may wish to work with if your loved one is hospitalized, and especially if hospitalized in a large hospital, called a tertiary hospital, you will have not only a discharge planner / case manager but also a social worker. A tertiary hospital is a large medical hospital that offers highly specialized care in specific areas, and unfortunately, they are often located in larger cities, possibly away from your loved one's home. Examples of tertiary care hospitals include specialist cancer management, neurosurgery, cardiac surgery, transplant services, plastic surgery, treatment for severe burns, advanced neonatology services, and palliative and other complex medical and surgical interventions.

If your loved one is hospitalized in a tertiary care center, this means you most often will need a place to stay. If this is the case, the hospital social worker can link you to possibly any hotels or motels the hospital has contracted with to allow you to receive a discounted rate for your room. The social worker may also be able to obtain bus passes and food vouchers that can assist with keeping your own costs as low as possible.

Advance Directive and Financial Power of Attorney

The most common types of advance directives are the living will and the durable power of attorney for health care (sometimes known as the medical power of attorney). In recent years, a new form of a directive has surfaced and is referred to as the Physician Orders for Life Sustaining Treatment (POLST); in some states, it is called Medical Orders for Life Sustaining Treatment (MOLST). A POLST or MOLST form also helps describe a person's wishes for health care, but it is not an advance directive. A POLST or MOLST form has a set of specific medical orders that a seriously ill person can fill in and ask their health care provider to sign. A POLST or MOLST form addresses the person's wishes in an emergency, such as whether to use CPR (cardiopulmonary resuscitation) in an emergency or whether to go to a hospital in an emergency and be put on a breathing machine or have a feeding tube inserted if necessary or whether they should stay where they are and be made comfortable.

If your loved one has a living will or an advance directive or a POLST or MOLST complete, one of your first duties will be to ensure the hospital has a copy of such on file. If not and your loved one maintains decision-making capacity, you should take two (2) steps.

Have your loved one discuss with the attending physician his wishes.

This may be one of the first of many hard or difficult conversations that may have to occur now and possibly sometime later if your loved one can communicate. However, it is critical to have these conversations take place, and your loved one's goals and wishes can be documented in their chart. This does not take the place of a hard copy of a formally written and witnessed advance directive. So make every effort to get one formally completed and signed as soon as possible.

For an advance directive, many hospitals will have the state-specific form you must use, and it is often available in the hospital admissions or business office. If not, you can download one from the internet using the American Association of Retired Persons (AARP) weblink listed as "Free Advance Directive forms by state from AARP." This website also has information on a variety of caregiver topics that may assist you as you start your planning.

States have different requirements for what is acceptable and not, so ask before you act on getting all in order, and check what your loved one's state requires. The advance directive form you need is basically an amazingly simple form that does not require an attorney to draw it up. However, six states (Iowa, Kansas, Missouri, Montana, North Carolina, and West Virginia) do not allow witnesses on the form but require the form to be notarized. If this is the case, you will have to secure a public notary. If you are in a state that allows it, you can have two (2) nonfamily members to witness it. Unfortunately, hospitals do not allow their staff to serve as witnesses to such documents. This means you may need to bring or find two (2) witnesses who are present when the form is signed.

To have the form witnessed, it is critical your loved one has the mental abilities or what is termed decision-making capacity. Otherwise, your only other option might be to file for conservatorship.

If there is no advance directive, now what? If there is not an advance directive or health care power of attorney or financial power of attorney or any conservatorship documents on file and your loved one is not in a coma or in the late stages of dementia but lacks the mental capacity to make an appropriate and informed decision regarding what they want and, more importantly, what might realistically be needed, the end result can result in disastrous consequences.

Why? Laws require health care providers to honor what the patient wants. This means, if there is nothing on file that represents the patient's wishes and he has not appointed a person to act as their agent or proxy for health care or financial decisions, the health care team must honor what the patient wants. Possibly worse yet, you will not have access to funds to pay for any ongoing bills or upcoming bills for care and services. Such an event leads to the hospital having no other choice but to do any of the following:

- To protect both the hospital and treating physician, the patient will be discharged, but he will be required to sign an against medical advice (AMA) letter. The AMA designation is used in part to help legally shield the doctor and hospital from liability if a patient gets ill or dies because of the premature discharge.

- This action then triggers another task, especially if the health care team has major concerns regarding the fact that the patient is then considered at risk of being a danger to themselves. So not only is an AMA letter on file, but also either the discharge planner / case manager or social worker will notify Adult Protective Services (APS) for a follow-up visit to further investigate competency and take other actions if required.

- The second alternative will be that you will need to file for conservatorship. Anytime a conservator is required, a physician or mental health professional must evaluate your loved one for competency and decision-making capacity.

- Conservatorship can only be created by a court order and is handled in probate court in the county where the adult in question resides. The standard under which a person is deemed to require a conservator or guardian differs from state to state, and it also depends on care versus financial matters. For example, Governor Newsom in California just signed into law a recent legislation (Assembly Bill 1663) known as the Probate Conservatorship Reform and Supported Decision-Making Act. This new law makes changes to probate conservatorship laws and creates a law that defines supported decision-making. Changes to the conservatorship law include who may be a conservator, selection of a conservator, inclusion of least restrictive alternatives attempted in a conservatorship petition, and investigation and reporting duties of court investigators. The new law also establishes a conservatorship alternative program, defines supported decision-making, and creates a process for entering a supported decision-making agreement. For more information on conservatorship-supported decision making and the new law, see The ARC of California website.

- If a conservator is required, this can be a long and complicated process, especially if you do not have the money to pay privately to hire an attorney. This means you must then work with the local county's conservator's office, which often has a huge backlog of cases. If you have the funds to afford an attorney, the process can be much shorter. However, if questions arise, call your local state or county conservator office.

Ensure a financial power of attorney form is available.

This is another legal document that grants a trusted agent—someone named to make decisions—the power to make and execute financial decisions when one is incapacitated or unable to make rational decisions about their finances. Remember, your loved one might be sick and unable to make decisions, but household and other bills continue. So on top of all the hard or difficult decisions you may now be making and the stress you are under, the last thing you need is more stress as you are being harassed by credit collectors.

What if there is no financial power of attorney? Financial power of attorney forms can be accessed from an online weblink. However, from experience, this may not be a wise choice. Why? The form may not be accepted by many banks or financial institutions. In fact, state laws vary; and unfortunately, there is no uniform power of attorney form that can be used anywhere. The critical things to do will be the following:

- Do your homework for what will be accepted from your loved one's financial institution.
- Ensure if your loved one has decision-making capacity and if your financial institution can assist with getting the document completed and notarized. If not, what or who do they recommend helping with this process?
- Start the conservatorship process if your loved one is in a coma or mentally unable to make any decisions. This is going to be your only recourse.

Who Pays for the Stay

Who pays for the stay is critical, especially since health care is so expensive, and there are often many limitations or exclusions to many health plans. As I write this book, I feel it important to include a few highlights in this section, but they will be discussed in more detail in another chapter.

If your loved one has their own health care insurance, whether the plan is paid by their own employer, privately, or they are covered as a dependent under your health plan, the stay, except for deductibles or other costs you might be charged, should be paid for. However, one of your best tools will be to keep any health care plan handbooks handy. These booklets are often referred to as Evidence of Coverage, or most often referred to as the EOC. You can either request a copy directly from the health plan, or you can also download an electronic copy from the health plan's website.

If your loved one must retire due to this new injury or illness, his health plan coverage, under most conditions, will terminate. This means no further coverage by that health plan unless you and he have decided to elect to move coverage and benefits to a COBRA (the Consolidated Omnibus Budget Reconciliation Act of 1985) plan. However, a word to the wise: COBRA is expensive, and you and your loved one may now be on a very limited budget, so this may not be a wise choice for coverage. This means you may want to research and purchase other insurance or even apply for your loved one's state Medicaid plan. The US Department of Labor has a great handbook online that describes COBRA which you can find online at the Department of Labor (dol.gov) website. The booklet is called *An Employee's Guide to Health Benefits Under COBRA.*

If your loved one's insurance is Medicare, you can either print out the current annual version or sign up for the e-handbook by accessing the Medicare web link and then search for the booklet *Medicare and You.* Once you get access to this booklet, it will keep you informed of any out-of-pocket (OOP) costs to expect and, more importantly, if there are exclusions or limitations. The only time Medicare will not cover a hospital stay is if your loved one has the original Medicare program as their health plan, but they have exhausted the inpatient days, including their bank of lifetime reserve days. For full information on Medicare and the many topics you may wish information on, one of your best resources will be to go to the Centers for Medicare and Medicaid website (CMS.gov) and do a search.

Other coverage for inpatient hospitalizations might be from the following:

- There is Medicaid (or in California Medi-Cal or in Arizona, Arizona Health Care Cost Containment System [AHCCCS]). Persons can also have other insurance or Medicare as well as Medicaid, but if they also have Medicaid, Medicaid is always second.
- If your loved one is age eighteen or younger, they might have their health care covered under a program called the Children's Health Insurance Program (CHIP). CHIP is a program for children without health insurance whose families earn too much to qualify for Medicaid but cannot afford health insurance.
- For more information on the Children's Health Insurance Program (CHIP), go to the Centers for Medicare and Medicaid (CMS.gov) website, and on the top bar, you will be allowed to search for the CHIP information, if you double click on Medicaid/CHIP. This site will also provide a map which will allow you to view what is available for children in the state in which they live.
- For general information on Medicaid, see the Centers for Medicare and Medicaid website at CMS.gov. While California, Texas, and Arizona have a different name for their Medicaid program and may offer some varied benefits than others, you can still access the programs by using the CMS web link to find what is offered.
- If your loved one's illness or injury is work related, then coverage and costs for care will then be covered under the

employer's workers' compensation plan, if it is determined the illness or injury is work related.

- If your loved one's injury is due to a fall in a business or someone's home or from an auto or other vehicle accident or possibly a sporting event, during the review of the claims submitted for care, it is discovered the costs for care are not the legal responsibility of your loved one's health plan; costs for the care will be shifted to the other payer if that entity has insurance. This means your loved one's health plan will not be responsible for payment, as it will be shifted to what is called a third-party payer, which may be a business or possibly a friend's homeowners insurance.

- If your loved one is on active duty with any branch of the United States and the military defense system, their coverage will be from TRICARE. If retired, they may have their coverage provided by TRICARE for Life or from the Veterans Administration.

- If your loved one is a newborn with birth defects or injuries and ongoing care will be needed after you, as the mother, are discharged, coverage by your health plan is limited to thirty days after your discharge. So it will be necessary to enroll your baby in either your or your spouse's health plan or, if not that, your state's Medicaid program. Regardless, signing them up must be done as soon as possible.

- If your loved one is a newborn with birth defects or injuries, it is critical you work with the hospital's social worker or financial counselor and ensure a referral is made immediately to your state's Title V (formerly called Crippled Children's Services). If eligible, the program can assist with coordination of benefits if your child is a dependent under a parent's health plan or if they are also eligible for your state's Medicaid program. To find your state's program, you can type in your child's state name and then the special health care needs program in your web browser, and this should bring up information you can use.

- If your loved one has a developmental or intellectual delay and is getting services from his state's Department of Developmental Services (DDS), this program does not pay for any inpatient care, as the services provided are designed to allow the individual to live in their own community. This means your loved one's inpatient care must be paid for by your state's Medicaid program or as a dependent under other health plan coverage.

- If your loved one is a dependent under a parent's or grandparent's health plan, they are often only eligible for coverage until age twenty-six, married or not. But some states allow coverage beyond that age. If unfamiliar with your loved one's eligibility, you can validate such information by calling the state insurance department. Some basic information on this topic can be found on either the *Forbes Advisor* health insurance website and an article on this topic. You can also find a wealth of information on health insurance on the insure.com website. If your loved one is a dependent on your or your spouse's health plan and they are eligible for your state's DDS program, as their disability has been established before the state's age they designate for potential eligibility (often this is age eighteen), they serve eligible clients from birth to end of life.

- If your loved one is not a US citizen or is undocumented, he might qualify for a program called permanent residence under color of law (PRUCOL). PRUCOL is administered by Social Security, and if eligible, they will have full Medicaid benefits.

- If your loved one is Native American or Alaskan Indian or Native, coverage can be provided through Indian Health Services (IHS). IHS provides a full range of health care services, and if you are unfamiliar with what type of care and services are available in your loved one's region, you can find information on health services for Native Americans or Alaskan Indian or Native, on the IHS website.

- If your loved one is a dependent under your or your spouse's health plan and is pregnant and the plan is to keep the baby, you must verify coverage with that health plan. This is necessary, as while the health plan may cover the prenatal care, many health plans offer no coverage for the delivery or any ongoing care. This means you must enroll them into a health plan or into your state's Medicaid program.

- If your loved one's injury is due to the fact that he or she was a victim of a violent crime, a program you will want to inquire about will be his state's victims of violent crimes. You can do your research on the US Office of Justice and their search link will take you to information on "Victims of Violent Crimes." Under the tab Overview, if you click there, it will allow you to search for info on your loved one's state.

Utilization Reviews and How It Might
Impact the Stay and Who Pays

If a provider is to participate and offer services for either Medicare or Medicaid beneficiaries—all health care plans require providers to participate in at least Medicare if they are to be considered part of the health plan's network of providers—CMS requires standards be in place (we briefly discussed this earlier). Any health entity, like hospitals, home health companies, and a myriad of other types of health care providers, is to have an effective utilization review (UR) program in place. This means most or all care, whether it

1. is yet to be given, referred to as prospective review, or prior authorization (PA) for a soon-to-be-scheduled event (this is to ensure that what is requested is medically necessary and will be provided in the right care setting);
2. is happening now (this review is called concurrent review, as reviews occur during the time care is being provided, and this is to ensure the patient is at the right level of care

(LOC) and that care is being ordered appropriately and care occurs as ordered); and

3. has already occurred (this review is called retrospective review, and this occurs before the provider's claim and must prove the care and services provided are medically necessary and given in the right place for the illness or injury).

If for any reason the facts UR uncovers as the review is conducted do not support approval, a denial will be issued. If care is denied, you will receive a written notice of non-coverage, including why the denial is issued and, if you disagree, the steps to follow if you wish to file an appeal.

Utilization reviews are a necessary process to help ensure hospitals and various health care providers provide appropriate patient care, and insurance companies cover the costs they are required to. Some health plans and other review agencies may use their own tools they have developed for reviews. Most reviewers or review companies conduct UR using one (1) of two (2) nationally recognized evidence-based review tools developed. These are those developed by MCG (Milliman Care Guidelines) Health or Change Healthcare.

Care must also be medically necessary and administered via proven methods (nationally or regionally recognized by standards of care). The process should result in high-quality care administered as economically as possible and in accordance with current evidence-based care guidelines.

Using the criteria the health plan has selected for its reviews, most UR is performed by nurses. They can perform the review, but they can never be the entity that issues a denial. If the facts discovered in the review do not meet the criteria used, the nurse must forward the case on to a physician for the final coverage decision. The physician reviewer is then able to use his own medical expertise or review the case details with a specialist from the same medical specialty treating the patient, as the final coverage determination is made to either approve or deny the case.

The goals of UR are to make sure patients get

- care that is medically necessary, meaning the care is reasonable and necessary;
- care that is based on evidence-based, clinical standards of care (this simply means that practitioners across the health care profession review and assess the most current, highest-quality research to keep informed and current with the delivery of care for their area of medical practice);
- care that is given in the right place (inpatient or outpatient);
- care that is given at the right time and as ordered;
- care that is given at the right level (ICU versus medical/surgical bed or, in some cases, a community hospital versus a tertiary hospital); and
- the right type of care by the right physicians and other health care team providers.

Most health plans no longer perform their own UR during any time one of their members or beneficiaries is hospitalized. They have contracted or delegated this task to the hospital. Why? Historically, charting was not electronic, as it is now. This meant the health plan had to hire staff to go to each hospital it had in its network. Now such review is no longer necessary, as charting is now done electronically, and on-site review by the health plan is not needed. To help with cost containment, health plans now delegate review to the hospital.

This is not to say the health plan has no say-so. It does. In fact, as director of UR for many of the health plans I worked for, patients or families would call when they needed help. The health plan also keeps close tabs through at least annual audits of the delegated tasks, a reviewing of policies and procedures, and performing their own review of the review done to see if they agree with the coverage determination issued.

Let us hope all is going well, and criteria are met. However, if for some reason your loved one's care is denied, you will be issued a letter of denial. In this letter, it will inform you, if you should disagree with the decision, on how to file the appeal with the health plan. If your loved one has the original Medicare or their health plan is provided by an insurer who offers a Medicare Advantage plan, the Quality Improvement Organization (QIO) that has been assigned by CMS will review the appeal. If the denial occurs during a hospitalization and your loved one has been formally admitted by a physician's written order, this appeal will be called an expedited appeal, meaning the health plan, or QIO, must render its coverage determination—agree with the hospital's denial or your reason for the appeal—within seventy-two hours of receipt of the request for appeal.

We will discuss briefly the appeals process later in this book, but your best source for what may be needed will be found in your loved one's Evidence of Coverage (EOC) booklet, or you may want to visit a website or two to read more on the topic. The web links you may want to review to help you with your appeal might be to merely type in your web browser "How to appeal and health insurance denial." This will bring up a variety of web links that will give you the help and guidance you might need.

Hospice versus Palliative Care

When describing hospice or palliative care, there is often confusion, even when it comes to answers given by some health care professionals. This is especially true as they try to describe what is meant and what services are provided for what groups of patients when the words *palliative care* or *hospice* are mentioned. It is common to hear both terms used interchangeably, and there are some similarities in the programs, but they are not the same. Similarly, we will discuss palliative and hospice care in more detail in another section in this book.

Palliative care is for anyone who has a chronic medical condition, and in contrast, hospice care is for anyone who is at the end of life. Deciding to pursue palliative care for your loved one will be easier than choosing to enter hospice care, because this means your loved one will continue to receive treatments for their medical condition, and their medical condition and overall health are likely to improve from the added services. Unfortunately, if hospice is elected, all treatment related to the terminal diagnosis will be discontinued, as death is expected.

Eligibility for palliative care depends on your loved one's health plan coverage. If you do not have a current copy of the EOC, it is important that you reach out to your loved one's health plan, whether it is Member Services or your loved one's assigned case manager. This is critical, as health plans vary with the medical conditions they cover in the palliative care benefit plan they offer.

Most health plans cover hospice, but eligibility for hospice care has some very stringent rules that must be followed. The major ones are the following:

- A physician must certify that your loved one has a terminal illness.
- Your loved one is not expected to live more than six months.
- It is agreed by you if you are your loved one's appointed agent for health care decisions—if not, they must have decision-making capacity—that curative treatment will not be sought for the medical treatment that qualifies them for hospice.
- It is agreed, your loved one's care will focus on managing their symptoms as end of life approaches, as plan for hospice care and services will focus more on comfort and quality than quantity of life.

One thing in common is that both programs are medical specialties aimed at supporting people of all ages with serious medical and long-term illnesses. Some illnesses may be but are not limited to

- cancer,
- chronic obstructive pulmonary disease (COPD),
- dementia,
- heart failure,
- Huntington's disease,
- kidney disease,
- liver disease,

- organ failure,
- Parkinson's disease,
- stroke.

Regardless of your loved one's illness or medical condition, the ultimate goal of both programs will be to

- improve quality of life,
- increase overall comfort,
- provide emotional support for you and your loved one,
- help you make important decisions about your loved one's medical treatment

Both programs work in collaboration with your loved one's primary doctor to coordinate and manage his or her care.

Setting Up Your Team

We previously discussed that the two (2) main hospital staff you must work closely with will be the discharge planner / case manager and the social worker. It is important to note that if for some reason you are unhappy with either one, you can contact their manager and discuss your concerns, and a change can be made.

As you prepare for your role, it will be key to add others to your team as well. Development of your own team will not only allow you to become an informed consumer, but it will also allow you to have their input as information is gathered or as they train you in the ongoing care that will be needed.

Believe me, the whole hospital experience can often be overwhelming. However, one of your first considerations will be where the money is going to come from. Many times, your loved one worked and was possibly the breadwinner. Or you were, and now roles are reversed, and income is possibly limited. Some of the first steps to take will be the following:

1. Double-check how the hospital bill will be paid. One key representative to meet with as soon as possible will be someone from the hospital business office, often referred to as a financial counselor. Here they can help you get started on possible linkage to other alternative programs that may help cover costs. In most cases, the primary program they will discuss with you will be for you to apply for your state's Medicaid program. If your loved one is under the age of twenty-one, you will want to explore possibly your state's Title V program, which is designed to help children with special health care needs.

2. If you apply for your loved one's state Medicaid program, you may also be able to apply for the Supplemental Nutrition Assistance Program (SNAP), formerly referred to as food stamps, your state offers.

3. Another key person to link with, if not already established, will be your loved one's health plan, and request that a case manager be assigned to his case. This professional should now become part of the hospital health care team you will be working with and should be included in any major case conferences, where the intensity and severity of the injury or illness and plans for ongoing care will be discussed.

In your case, as caregiving for your loved one will be long-term, the health plan case manager may not be working with you only during the period of time your loved one is hospitalized. If not already assigned, you will want to call your loved one's health plan and request one. You will want them to stay involved as long as they can and throughout your caregiver journey, if possible. It is important to have a health plan case manager assigned to your loved one. (If you find you do not get along with the assigned case manager, you can request a change to another.) But key is to have someone at the health plan help you and help represent any issues that could cause a potential utilization review or discharge planning problems.

Outside the hospital, you will want to ensure either or both of your employers are notified of the event. This will allow you to work with your loved one's human resources department to ensure they are signed up for sick leave or what other income benefits he may be entitled to. For you, you will want to call your employer's human resources department and start any paperwork you may need. This may be any Family and Medical Leave Act (FMLA) paperwork, as well as any other applications you will need to complete for any employee benefits you might be entitled to.

If your loved one was employed before his or her illness or injury through another program, you will want to apply for State Disability Insurance (SDI). Unfortunately, only five (5) states and one (1) US territory offer an SDI program. This application is important, as if your loved one is deemed eligible and is hospitalized, the income check will be retroactive; benefits are paid for the first day hospitalized. This also means, if they were employed and had any sick or vacation benefits, this amount can be combined and coordinated, allowing income to be slightly greater. If you are a new mother, check with your state's SDI program, as for example in California, the SDI program covers pregnant mommies; and if you are off from work on maternity leave, this extra income can be used to supplement any vacation or sick time pay you may get.

Proper nutrition plays a key role in all our lives. Another health care professional you will want and need on your team will be the hospital dietitian. Dietitians are experts on how to better use food and nutrition to promote the health or the management of disease for a patient or client. A dietician will offer advice on what to eat so one can lead a healthier lifestyle or to attain a set of health-related goals, including weight loss or, at times, even weight gain. They are also key in helping with the management of diabetes, the reduction of high blood pressure, and proper nutrition for persons with kidney disease or other major medical conditions where diet is critical. While they may give you some tips on menus and other ideas for food, if you and your loved one will rely on also using some ready prepared foods, they will give you advice on what brands you may wish to consider, ones that will not only be nourishing but also with less sodium or other unnatural flavorings or seasonings.

Dependent upon your loved one's medical diagnosis, illness or injury, and the unit they may be getting their care from (ICU, medical/surgical unit, neonatal ICU), other team members you may want to include on your team may be any nurse or disease-specific coordinator. This may include but is not limited to such staff as

a. the stroke coordinator;
b. the end-stage renal disease (ESRD) or dialysis nurse;
c. if in a transplant center, the transplant coordinator;
d. the diabetic nurse educator;
e. the wound care nurse;
f. the ostomy nurse;
g. the palliative care coordinator;
h. the hospital chaplain.

If your loved one's condition is determined to be terminal, then you will want to consider the hospice nurse as part of the team as well. A hospital or even outpatient professional often not included in a team will be the pharmacist. A pharmacist is critical when there is a need for medication review to help determine if they are interacting as they should with other medications your loved one may be taking.

Other Factors to Deal With

As scary as it is to think about the seriousness of your loved one's injury or illness, you must make time to take care of yourself; this means both your mental and physical health. Far too often, I have seen family members dreadfully neglect their own needs of sleep, proper nutrition, and even proper hygiene. If this is you, you are not doing yourself or your loved one or the team any good. Too often, unnecessary anger arises; and worse yet, sound decision-making is lacking.

Also, make every attempt to educate yourself, and do research on any topic you are unfamiliar with; or if you see or hear things that concern you, write them down so you can take appropriate actions. I have always advised families to keep a notebook handy (the spiral kind so that all pages are connected, and you cannot lose a page), as because many of us have fuzzy brains when we are tired or stressed. This then allows you to ask questions when either the team makes their daily rounds or when care is rendered for a specific health care issue (for example: wound care or rehabilitation therapy). It also will help as you conduct your own research on a topic.

As I write this book, I may suggest a resource or suggestion. This by no means implies that I endorse it. What you decide will be based off the research you do and then making the best decision that fits best for you and your situation. Also, remember the following:

- Do not be afraid to ask questions. As you ask questions, be clear and direct; instead of hinting around or beating around the bush, be straightforward about what questions you want to ask.
- If necessary and you have a hard time understanding, tell the team member you are asking the questions to, to tell you what is meant by using simple medical terms or even pictures or drawings to help you better understand.
- If the health care team uses or writes a *funny* or *confusing* word or a bunch of letters, such as *tid*, which means three times per day, request that they tell you in simple terms what it means. In my research for this book, I found there are 10,082 abbreviations in health care! If you see one and forget to ask what it or the letters mean, you can type in your web browser link "healthcare abbreviations and acronyms," and this will bring up a directory you can use.
- If you do not speak English, the hospital and any of the professionals they employ are required by federal law to provide translation services. As tempting as it may be to use another family member or friend to translate, this is not always wise, as they can easily miss the full intent of what

is said. Always make every attempt to use the professional services the hospital or health entity must use.

- In your binder or notebook, you may find it is helpful to jot down key information on any of your loved one's tests or imaging results or procedures they might have done. These notes can then help you remember to ask more questions if needed.

A New Mommy, but Now with Other Responsibilities

As a new mother, we are all often scared to death of our new role. Having an infant born with birth defects and now assuming a possible lifetime role as a caregiver can be even more scary. As in all situations when you will assume the caregiver role, pay attention as the nurses and the other health care team members perform their daily tasks. Discharge, whether it is for an adult or an infant or child, will not occur until the primary attending physician says your loved one is medically stable for discharge. Because hospitals and neonatal units may vary in what they do and what you can expect, most will follow the best practice for their area and will have a list of things that must occur or be in place before a discharge is allowed. As a result, keep that notebook handy so you can jot down stuff you need either to research yourself or for asking questions.

Readiness for care at home of a neonatal intensive care or specialized unit for an infant is probably one of the most complex of discharges. The complexities of such infant discharges often pose more considerations when it comes to the availability and adequacy of community resources and support services than that used for a young child or adult. The final decision for discharge, which is the responsibility of the attending physician, must be tailored to the unique medical needs posed by each baby's unique needs. Also, each hospital may have their own criteria or goals they want to see before a baby is discharged. At a minimum, most hospitals will have the following listed, and goals for each have been accomplished:

- You have identified a second person to help you with their care; and their ability, availability, and commitment have been confirmed. Equally as important, they have been trained like you in all aspects of care for your baby, which can include but is not limited to activities such as you have been trained to do.
- An assessment of your baby's clinical status has been done, and you can recognize early signs and symptoms of an illness, as well as the signs and symptoms specific to your baby's medical condition.
- Provide care if your baby has an artificial airway (tracheostomy) or requires a specific safety precaution for the artificial airway or operation of the equipment he may be using.
- Learn how to apply any feeding tube—intestinal stoma or an infusion pump—or any mechanical and prosthetic device that requires application.
- Administer any medications, as well as learn proper storage, dosage, timing, administration, and recognition of potential signs of toxicity.
- Your baby has a sustained weight gain of sufficient duration.
- Your baby can maintain a normal body temperature fully clothed in an open bed with normal ambient temperature (20–25°C or 68–77°F).
- Your baby has established competent feeding by breast or bottle without cardiorespiratory (choking) compromise. If your baby is unable to be bottle-fed or breastfed, a nutritional risk assessment has been completed, and dietary modification for tube feedings has been instituted and tolerated, and you have been taught how to do them.
- Your baby has had a hearing test, and if they failed, follow-up care is arranged.
- All other blood work and screening have been done, and appropriate therapy has been started or set up.
- The home and all the equipment ordered are in place or ready for delivery, and if delivered, it is all set up to provide

the care required, and you and your secondary helper have been trained.

- If your infant is on life-sustaining equipment, you and your secondary helper have been trained to know not only how to perform any day-to-day task but also what to do in the event of an emergency.
- You and your secondary helper have been trained in CPR (cardiopulmonary resuscitation). CPR is the process you must follow if your loved one is to be on life-sustaining equipment at discharge, and your infant is at high risk of an emergent medical condition, and they stop breathing or their heart stops.
- You and your secondary helper have been trained on safe car seat use and how to position your baby in the car seat or even a bed. Equally as important, you have purchased a car seat that is appropriate for your infant.

A great resource to explore and do any research you may wish to do on newborn screening will be the Centers for Disease Control and Prevention website and then its Newborn Portal. This portal will give you a wealth of information on a variety of topics you may find useful.

Another resource you may want to use when you purchase or have questions about car or booster seats will be the US Department of Transportation's National Highway Traffic Safety Administration website at NHTSA.gov, and its link to "equipment" will give you information on car seats and booster seats.

Observe, Observe, and Observe

If you will be undertaking the caregiver role, regardless of your loved one's age, they will require ongoing care after discharge. You—this will include any foster parents, grandparents, or adoptive parents—will not only watch and observe what the various health care professionals do as they perform the care or services your loved one needs, but you must also be taught how to do the care. This is especially true if you are going to be caring for a medically fragile newborn or a loved one who is on life-sustaining equipment. Consequently, your actions will include asking key questions either then or making notes so you can ask later.

What happens if you are repulsed by what you see, smell, or must do; and you gag and vomit easily? It is okay to say, "I cannot do it." Any nurse will fully understand. This does not mean you are weak; it means you are honest. To say no is okay, especially if the plan is to have a discharge directly home. You must speak up, as an immediate home plan should not be considered. If you do, disaster is waiting, where charges of neglect could be filed or a readmission or death can occur.

By all means, listen to the advice of the health care team, as it will depend on your loved one's disease or injury and their prognosis before you make the move to home. The best plan they may suggest may be for a short stay in an inpatient acute rehabilitation (IAR) facility, a long-term acute care hospital (LTACH), or a subacute or even possibly a stay in a local skilled nursing facility. This allows your loved one more time possibly in therapy, where they can add strength and endurance. Or if skilled care (wound care, ventilator weaning, or completion of a course of medication) is needed, this will help make home care possibly easier. The key to home care is to ensure your loved one is medically stable for the move.

As you visit or stay with your loved one, the first things to watch for will be their facial expressions, responses, or movements. If you are seeing things you know are not normal for them, by all means, speak up and discuss your concerns with the team. Many times, such responses are due to pain or discomfort. The remedy might be a simple fix, such as an order for premedication with a narcotic before the treatment is started.

Observations such as this allow you to again ask critical questions so you fully understand what is meant or what is happening. It can also lead you to request a second opinion or evaluation by another specialist. A good example that happened to me was when my oldest daughter required brain aneurysm surgery, and shortly after her surgery, she had a stroke. During her stay in ICU, her speech was garbled, and she had uncontrolled, spastic movements of her arms and legs and a whole variety of other signs and symptoms. The worst was, she had constant tachycardia (rapid heartbeat).

As they feared a possible seizure, on admission, she was started on a new drug, Depakote, just off the experimental list and approved by the FDA. As I watched her, none of her behavior was even close to normal, so I started my own research, including review of her drugs, including the new one, Depakote. I read everything I could find on the drug, and using the list of all the signs and symptoms I observed, I compared them against the adverse list I found. Not only were many of her symptoms on the common list, but also many were on the less common list!

I took my findings to the pharmacist I worked with, and she agreed that my daughter was in danger. I then presented this information to her neurologist, and his response was that under no circumstances was this true, and he went on to call me a hysterical mother! I then demanded a second opinion from a cardiologist. He was furious I was doubting him, but he ordered it. Lo and behold, the cardiologist ordered a stop to Depakote immediately, as she was having adverse reactions and was at risk of death!

If it appears care will be required upon discharge, it is critical you watch and ask questions and request training.

- Observe any care techniques as the nurses and other team members perform their duties.
- Remember to make notes and ask questions as you observe the care.
- If it appears this same care will be needed after discharge, have them start teaching you immediately on how it is done. Do not let them merely demonstrate or, worse yet, demonstrate as you are leaving. Your teaching must be done by use of what is called the teach-back method. This means they will demonstrate the care, and in return, you must then do the care as they watch you demonstrate back what was taught. By all means, continue this type of teaching until you feel you have mastered the techniques required.

In many cases, your loved one will have a home health agency (visiting nurse) assigned to assist you with the skilled care your loved one requires. Despite this, it is critical you learn not only the actual care but also how to operate any and all equipment they may need. This will include how to troubleshoot issues as they arise and the emergency steps to take if they prove unable to be resolved.

Training—the Teach-Back Method

For your training, insist they teach you how to do whatever is needed through use of what is called the teach-back method. Teach-back training is necessary so you know what to do in an event something happens. It is also helpful when you need to assume any care required or even troubleshoot what has happened to any equipment you may be using. Teach-back training often occurs over several days or weeks. Do not let you trainer give you a onetime session if you do not feel you have learned it and have all down pat.

Teach-back training may be necessary, especially when your loved one, regardless of age, requires nursing care, such as

- maybe brushing a bedbound patient's teeth;
- giving a bedbound patient a bath or washing their hair;
- getting any patient who uses crutches or a wheelchair into a shower or onto and off a toilet;
- tube feedings or even feeding a bedbound person who cannot sit up or one who can sit but must be positioned correctly;
- medication administration (by mouth, injection, feeding tube, or infusion);
- respiratory care (oxygen or application of other respiratory devices, such as a ventilator), tracheostomy care, and application and use of a continuous positive airway pressure (CPAP) or bi-level positive airway pressure (BiPAP) or a nebulizer, which may also include chest tubes if prolonged use of such tubes will be included in the post-acute discharge plan);

- oral or possibly tracheal suctioning;
- wound care;
- bladder and catheter care;
- ostomy (bowel or bladder) care;
- getting in and out of bed or a chair or on and off the toilet;
- walking with a mobility device (cane, crutches, or walker);
- application of a brace or prosthetic or orthotic; and
- repositioning them in bed or a chair;

Depending on your loved one's medical diagnosis (regardless of age) and if he or she is considered high risk for respiratory or cardiac failure and there is not a do not resuscitate (DNR) order on file, you and any backup caregivers must be trained in cardiopulmonary resuscitation (CPR).

Remember, keep your notebook or cell phone handy so you can make notes so you can have a reminder if you must ask questions.

Rehabilitation Therapy

Observe the rehabilitation team (physical, occupational, or speech therapists) as they perform any therapy sessions. If you are taking your loved one home and mobility will be an issue, you must actively participate in any training. Key if you will be assisting your loved one to move from bed to chair or back to bed or to a commode or toilet or even repositioning them in bed or a chair is, you must have the physical therapist teach you what is called body mechanics and how to do them properly. This is critical. If you injure yourself, this means all you have done to date might be for naught, as your loved one may then require admission to a skilled nursing or assisted living facility during your recovery time.

Remember, ask questions as you watch the care, and ask the team as to what the plan at discharge might be. Will it be directly home, or will a facility be needed to help your loved one continue to build strength and endurance or continue any complex care they might need? Dependent upon your loved one's injury or illness, home may not be in the immediate future. For example, the plan may be for your loved one to be discharged to a long-term acute care hospital (LTACH) or an inpatient acute rehabilitation (IAR) or even a skilled nursing facility (SNF) or possibly even a subacute hospital. If not, will there be follow-up home health therapy or outpatient therapy ordered?

Equally as important, query the team as to what may be the equipment your loved one will not only need but what might also help you make care a little easier for you while also helping to prevent unnecessary injury as you provide the care needed. A word to the wise, while the equipment your loved one will need will, in most instances, be covered by his health plan (if it is on the listing of what is considered medically necessary), any equipment that may help make your job easier will not be. This means you may need to pay privately for such or explore community agencies that might have a loan closet.

As you watch the rehabilitation team, examples of things you will need for planning the discharge will be the following:

- You will have to alert the team on your loved one's prior level of functioning (PLOF). This is critical, as they will use this information as they set both short- and long-term goals they will be striving to reach.
- As you watch the physical therapy team work with your loved one, ensure they allow you to move your loved one about. Ensure they also teach you proper body mechanics (the movements and positions we must use as we move someone around). Learning body mechanics will assist in helping you avoid your own unnecessary back or muscle injuries. The Centers for Disease Control and Prevention and the National Institute for Occupational Safety and Health (NIOSH) website offer some great tips on the safe handling and moving of patients.
- If your loved one has tubes coming out of any part of their body, watch the team as they move him and how they place the tube or tubes. This is critical to ensure they do not come out when a change in position is made.

- As the rehabilitation team works with your loved one, equipment will be needed at discharge. Start making a list of all you will need and if they advise rental or purchase. Ask what equipment and supplies will be needed. This list will include any extra pillows, foam rolls, or blankets you may need to help keep your loved one of proper body alignment, help keep pressure sores from developing or getting worse, and help keep them as comfortable as possible.

- It is absolutely critical if your loved one will be what is termed wheelchair bound that you have the absolute right wheelchair and any seating system to help keep your loved one's body in proper alignment, and equally as important is that pressure areas are prevented whenever possible. This means the equipment will be individually custom-made for your loved one. As such, this will not be a rental but must be purchased. All this takes time. You will need authorization from the health plan, and it will take time to custom-build whatever is needed.

- Alert the team as to where the main bedroom, bathroom, and care area will be. Will it be in a bedroom or a central living area? Will the bedroom be located on the ground floor or second level? Is there a full bathroom nearby or only a toilet area? What does the bathroom look like, and will it pose problems for your loved one to access the toilet or bathtub or shower?

- If upon discharge you will need to rearrange the living space to accommodate any medical supplies and equipment you may need, make a drawing of the area so you can have the therapist make any recommendations. Best yet will be to have someone physically evaluate the bedroom, living space, and bathroom. This is critical if your loved one will be wheelchair bound. There must be enough room for the wheelchair to have the space it needs to make turns and that they can do so, and any carpet will not prevent the turns the wheelchair may do. Also, all throw rugs have been removed.

- Let the physical and occupational therapist(s) know what the entry looks like. Are there stairs to navigate to get into the house or apartment? If so, how many, and are there any turns that will be needed to navigate the stairs? Also, are there other barriers that must be cleared?

- If there are stairs and your loved one will have their main care in a second-story bedroom, how will he be able to enter and exit the room? If you are in the income group that can afford an elevator, that is great. Unfortunately, most of us do not fall in that income bracket. Thus, other considerations must be considered as to how to get him up and down the stairs.

- As you watch the occupational therapist, observe the techniques they use as they bathe, perform, or teach your loved one personal care. Ask them about possible adaptive equipment and clothing you can use to make personal caregiving either easier on yourself or your loved one. Adaptive clothing will also allow your loved one to be up and dressed in clothes other than pajamas. Also, ask about where such can be purchased. Per my research of the web, it appears such clothing can be purchased and delivered directly to your home from Amazon, Target, or JCPenney. But the occupational therapist may know of other stores to order such from, so validate with him what he recommends. Purchases such as this are considered by health plans to not be medically necessary, so this will be an out-of-pocket cost to you. Adaptive equipment can be for feeding adaptive handles, plate guards, dressing, bathing, toileting, and communication and reading devices—examples of only a few of the adaptive equipment devices you may wish to explore. The goal of using adaptive equipment is to allow your loved one to be as independent as possible.

- If your loved one has swallowing difficulties, the speech therapist will be the one to possibly perform any swallow evaluations and then make recommendations to the physicians and dietary team if food can be allowed and, if your loved one can eat, the type of food and the consistency and texture that will be the best. Also, depending on the ability to swallow, he may also recommend a substance termed thick-it. This is a substance added to liquids that basically makes the liquid almost of a custard consistency but allows your loved one to consume liquids and stay hydrated.

As you watch speech therapy and if communication will be an issue, ask them the best communication device for your loved one's diagnosis and cognitive (the ability to think) abilities. Per the American Speech-Language-Hearing Association (ASHA), communication devices may be referred to as augmentative and alternative communication (AAC). For more information on speech therapy devices, you can visit the American Speech-Language-Hearing Association (ASHA) website, and here you can conduct your own research on the Alternative-Communication or Augmentative and Alternative Communication device that best works for your loved one.

An AAC may be either augmentative when it is used to supplement existing speech or alternative when it is used in place of speech that is absent or not functional. AAC means all the ways that someone communicates besides talking. People of all ages can use AAC if they have trouble with speech or language skills. Augmentative means to add to someone's speech. Alternative means to be used instead of speech.

Some people use AAC throughout their lifetime. Others may use AAC only for a short time, like when they have surgery and cannot talk (for example, after having a new tracheostomy). The goal of using an AAC device is to help those, both children and adults, with communication or speech disorders to interact more effectively with others and help improve their language and social skills through means other than the use of gestures and facial expressions.

AAC falls under the broader umbrella of assistive technology—or the use of any equipment, tool, or strategy to improve functional daily living in individuals with disabilities or limitations. The terms *assistive device* or *assistive technology* can refer to any device that helps a person with hearing loss or a voice, speech, or language disorder to communicate. These terms often refer to devices that help a person hear and understand what is being said more clearly or to express thoughts more easily. With the development of digital and wireless technologies, more and more devices are becoming available to help people with hearing, voice, speech, and language disorders communicate more meaningfully and participate more fully in their daily lives.

To find information on assistive devices for people with hearing voice, speech, or language disorders, "Assistive Devices for People with Hearing or Speech Disorders," a great web resource you may want to explore will be the National Institute on Deafness and Communication Disorders website.

If an AAC is determined to be needed, there is a large variety of devices on the market. As a rule, they are classified into two (2) categories: no-tech and low-tech options. No-tech includes such actions as the use of gestures and facial expressions; writing; drawing; spelling words by pointing to letters or spelling words by use of finger spelling or a letter board; and pointing to photos, pictures, or written words or a picture communication board. In contrast, high-tech options include things like using an app on an iPad or tablet to communicate and using a computer with a voice, sometimes called a speech-generating device.

If your loved one's diagnosis falls into any one of the following—but this list is not all-inclusive of diagnoses, so check with your loved one's speech therapist—an AAC device may be needed.

- autism spectrum disorder (ASD)
- cerebral palsy (CP)
- if after a stroke they have aphasia
- amyotrophic lateral sclerosis (ALS)
- Down syndrome or other intellectual disorder
- traumatic brain injury (TBI)

If your loved one is a child or young adult and attending school via the school district's special education program, your child's individual education plan (IEP) must include sessions with the speech therapist. All children with a developmental or intellectual disability—from birth through age twenty-one—under the federal law called Individuals with Disabilities Education Act (IDEA), are entitled to free public education. Once enrolled and an initial IEP is developed, it must be updated annually. This is a process completed in which you should be present, and if not, have another family member or friend attend the IEP development session to ensure the IEP contains the services your child or young adult requires. You can find more information on IDEA by merely typing in "Individuals with Disabilities Education Act" in your web browser.

If your loved one is an infant or has a medical diagnosis that has affected their hearing and they are deaf, you will possibly want to investigate what is offered in your area to train you and your loved one communication skills. Again, as above, if an IEP is developed, ensure it covers what your child or young adult may need to communicate even though they may be deaf. You may also want to see what is available in your area. To see what is available in your area, visit the National Association of Deaf (NAD) website, and here you will find a variety of topics you can click on and a wealth of information will be available at your fingertips.

If your child is blind and you want to see what is available in your area, visit the American Foundation for the Blind (AFB) website and here you will find a wealth of information you can explore. Other resources may be the following:

1. Find Society for the Blind in your own location. You can call 2-1-1.
2. If your infant or child is newly diagnosed, you may visit the American Foundation for the Blind (AFB) website and here you can explore resources that may fit your child's needs if they are blind or visually impaired. You can also ascertain from them the closest schools for the blind and visually impaired. This information will be critical as you enroll your child in school, and an IEP identifies the special education classes they may require.

I know that when my own mother lost her eyesight to macular degeneration, our local Society for the Blind was a lifesaver. Not only did our chapter offer classes on cooking and how to remain independent as possible, but she also received training on walking with a white cane. She was able to purchase a wide variety of items to help her remain independent enough so she could live in an assisted living facility. Thus, she was able to purchase talking clocks and watches and a computer with voice-activated commands.

The one thing she despised and the one thing her physician did not do was alert the Department of Motor Vehicles of her blindness and the fact that she continued to drive, so my brother and I had to have that difficult conversation with her about taking her car away. (We sold it and gave her the money for taxi fare, which she never did use.) Oh my, that difficult conversation and taking her car away resulted in World War III! Despite the fact that my brother was with me, she slapped me; and after we left, she wanted nothing to do with me for at least the next six months. If she heard my voice when I tried to call her, she immediately hung up on me. So be prepared and be patient.

Dependent upon your loved one's diagnosis, another website you may wish to explore for not only for blindness but also for any illness or injury and if independent living is the goal will be the Administration for Community Living (ACL) website. Once in this website you will find an A to Z browse area. If you double-click here, you can explore a wide variety of resources that might be available in your loved one's area in which they will receive their care.

Preparing for Discharge

As you watch the health care team work with your loved one, take notes so you can ask questions either then or at the next session or, better yet, at a patient-family-team case conference. This will also help you and the health care team decide the direction the discharge plan may take.

You may feel pressure from the team to take your loved one home, or your loved one may also put pressure on you to do so as soon as possible. Despite the fact that you and your loved one may prefer home to be the plan at discharge, this may not be the best plan, especially if he requires more rehabilitation or any combination of overly complex medical care that must be done several times per day.

I cannot stress enough that if this occurs and you know you are not ready, hold your ground! Make sure the discharge plan makes good sense to do so, and it is the best for everyone involved. This also means that the home to which your loved one will be cared for will allow a safe discharge not only for you and your loved one but also for any health care worker who may be coming and going at all hours of the day or night. Equally as important, it must have

- a refrigerator for storing any medications that must be kept cool,
- a telephone,
- an emergency phone or alert system (such as Lifeline) in place,
- an emergency preparedness plan done,
- a way to heat and cool it,
- running water,
- an easy to access entry and exit,
- a plan or way to get up and down stairs, and
- any repairs or modifications that must be done to accommodate your loved one's care and mobility needs.

Critical will be that if your loved one has any lifesaving devices (primarily ventilator, any respiratory devices, or suction machines) and the equipment requires electricity and you live in a high-power outage area, ensure you have a power generator that can last several days. If not, you will need an agreement in place with the nearest hospital for them to admit your loved one and render the care required during the outage. They can do this, as laws require hospitals to have an emergency plan in place in the event of a power outage or when related or other disasters occur.

Case Conferences

Ideally, it is wise to request a case conference with all the major health care team present at least every week or so. This is especially critical if the team is hinting that discharge may be approaching. Such conferences are ideal, as they allow you to keep on top of all that is happening—is your loved one progressing or, worse yet, regressing? Plans may need to change. Team conferences also allow you to ask more questions, which can be directed to the right health care team member to be answered. If a case conference is held, this should include, at a minimum, the following:

- Hospitalist and any specialty physicians.
- Lead nurse or main attending nurse.
- Any specialty care nurses.
- At least one rehab team member. But if all three (3) are working with your loved one, ideally, it should be all three (3).
- The dietitian.
- The discharge planner.
- The social worker.
- The health plan case manager. He is critical, as he can be the health plan spokesperson to start the process for any prior authorizations of services or supplies that will be needed after discharge.

Case conferences are a great way to keep on top of all that is occurring and what the team may have in mind for the next steps for your loved one's ongoing post-acute care. As issues are discussed, this may trigger other actions you must take to be ready. Be honest with the team. Tell them if you are not ready. More importantly, if you know you will not be able to provide the care after discharge, let the team know. Be honest, and as hard as it is, try not to let guilt take hold. When guilt takes hold, the discharge to home is the wrong plan. It often ends in a readmission within a few hours or days, as care is beyond what the family or caregiver could render.

A word to the wise: as I worked with families, particularly when ongoing care was complex and would be needed, I never let them settle only on discharge plan A. I had them also think about what and where we could plan for discharge plan B. If care was extremely complex, I even helped others think about discharge plan C. Naturally, the goal should be for plan A. However, recovery from the illness or injury may not progress enough to allow plan A to occur as originally felt it will. Also, despite the fact that home may be the best place, that is not always true when dealing with a patient and what we in the medical field classify as having a catastrophic illness or injury and requiring complex ongoing care.

Like the hospital with its many levels of care—emergency room; intensive care; medical, neurological, cardiac, and telemetry units; step down units; medical and surgical units; oncology units; etc.— the same you will soon find is also in the post-acute arena. To help you find a facility or provider that may be available to continue with the care needs at discharge, hospitals are required by CMS to give the patient/family a patient choice letter. This letter allows you to choose which provider you feel may be best. Not only does this letter outline the facilities the family can chose from, but the letter will also tell you if there are any quality issues found during the facility's annual site survey/inspection.

However, you can do your own quality research if the discharge plan is to include a move to another facility or to home, and you will be using a home health agency or other outpatient provider. Before CMS came out with its provider five-star rating system, I always suggested to the families I worked with to take the administrative facility tour during normal business hours but then return unannounced during dinner or the early evening hours when administration had left for the day. This allows one to get the feel and smell of the facility when administration is not on duty. I also encouraged my families to read the state survey reports and review them for any outstanding quality issues that might be found.

When educating families on how to make an informed choice, there is a great online tool you can use to help narrow your selection. This is the Medicare compare website called Find and Compare

Providers Near You. Under the welcome tab, you can then research a variety of provider types. Here you merely click on the provider type you wish to review, and it will bring up another screen where you can type in your zip code or address, and if you have the Patient Choice letter handy, you can type in any facility names you wish to explore or consider for your loved one's post-acute care.

This site will alert you to any quality-of-care issues. Plus, it also gives you the star rating (1–5 stars) assigned after the CMS site survey is completed. Again, despite the fact that this tool is now available, I still highly recommend you do your own site visit, and ask other family members you meet as to their opinion of the place. Techniques such as this then allow your eyes, ears, and nose to help you make your own informed decision.

As any team conferences are held, be prepared to ask questions and jot down areas you may wish to further explore. You will want to know at a minimum the following:

- What are some of the various levels of care your loved one may require? Will it be a long-term acute care hospital (LTACH), an inpatient acute rehabilitation (IAR) unit, a subacute hospital or rehabilitation (SAR), or a skilled nursing facility (SNF). Or can care be rendered in an outpatient setting or at home?

- If placement is required for an infant or child, your primary option for placement will be in one of your state's subacute hospitals, designed specifically to provide care for your child. Unfortunately, each state calls their subacute hospitals by differing names; and as the demand is so small for such, facilities are limited in a state, often found only in a large metropolitan area. So this will be a major question you will ask the discharge planner / case manager or social worker about. Can the facility manage the complexity of care, and where is it located?

- If an SNF or SAR is needed, finding a facility that can accommodate a person younger than age fifty-five can be difficult. The reason is, many SNFs/SARs and the programs they offer are designed to meet the needs of fifty-five-year-olds and older.

- If a facility and at times even an outpatient clinic can be a distance from your home, does the facility have contracts in place with hotels or discounted rates or possible housing onsite for those who are not from the immediate area? Or if your loved one is a child or infant and is in tertiary hospital, does the hospital have on its property possible housing, such as Ronald McDonald House Charities, available?
- Is the facility or provider contracted with your loved one's health plan? If not, will that provider and your health plan be prepared to develop a letter of agreement (LOA) for the admission? If not, what will be your options for ongoing care?
- What is the CMS star rating for that provider?
- What will be covered by your loved one's health plan?
- What will be your out-of-pocket expenses?
- What is the average length of stay? For example, under Medicare, your loved one can have one hundred days in an SNF. But believe me, only a small percentage of patients have their skilled stay go beyond twenty days, as a utilization review of the patient progress to date shows they have plateaued, and care is now classified as custodial or maintenance. This means your loved one is to be discharged or will stay if there is money to pay the bill.

Whenever possible, you want to strive for those providers with a five-star rating. However, if a five-star is out of the question due to a long commute for you, tour local ones. If a facility is needed, there are checklists online that you can access. So as you tour various facilities, you can make notes.

To help you in your research and as you develop your own list of questions for use as you tour any post-acute facility, you may want to use a checklist like what is available either on the Medicare or on the National Institute on Aging and National Institute on Health (nia. nih.gov) websites.

Checklist for Discharge Planning

If it now appears discharge will be approaching and you are at the stage in your planning where you are doing some serious to-do lists, you may also want to start working on a list of questions you may want to ask. The list I developed below gives you some ideas of what services and agencies may be coming to your home, and it should cover all ages for discharge. However, if your loved one has violent, aggressive, or behavioral issues or is at end of life, we will discuss some additional things you may want to have in place in another chapter in this book.

Below are questions to ask the discharge planner. Keep in mind, this is only a sample. My goals were to give you an idea of some of the questions you may wish to ask, and you can jot down what is told.

Home Health Agency
Home health agency name:
Home health agency phone number: Fax number:
Main home health agency contact name: Extension:
When will services start:
Has approval been gotten from health plan?:
He/she has more than one health plan or alternate funding to help. Have they also approved it?:
What will be his/her out-of-pocket expenses for the home care?:

What services will I get?
  ➤ Nursing: _____
What type of nursing care will be provided?:
When will it start?:
How often will I have a nurse?:
  ➤ Nurse aid for help with personal care: _____
It will start when, and then how often and how many hours per day?:

Rehabilitation services will include what?
> Physical therapy (PT): _______
It will start when, and they will come how often?:
> Occupational therapy (OT): _______
It will start when, and they will come how often?:
> Speech therapy (ST): _______
It will start when, and they will come how often?:
> Respiratory therapy: _______
It will start when, and they will come how often?:
> Social worker: _______
It will start when?:
> Dietitian: _______
It will start when?:
> Ostomy nurse: _______
It will start when, and they will come how often?:
> Wound care nurse: _______
It will start when, and they will come how often?:
> IV or infusion or parenteral nutrition nurse: _______
It will start when, and they will come how often?:

Hospice
Hospice agency name:
Hospice agency phone number: Fax number:
Hospice agency main contact name: Extension:
When will services start?:
Was approval gotten from the health plan?:
He/she has more than one health plan or alternate funding to help. Have they also approved it?:
What might be his/her out-of-pocket costs?:
What care and services can I expect?:
How often will I have help?:

Home IV Infusion or Parenteral Nutrition
IV infusion agency name:
IV infusion phone number: Fax number:
IV infusion main contact name: Extension:
When will services start?:
When will all the supplies be delivered?:
Was approval gotten from the health plan?:
He/she has more than one health plan or alternate funding to help. Have they also approved it?:
What might be his/her out-of-pocket costs?:
I am learning some at the hospital. Will they help me once we are home?:
How often will they be available to help me?:
Is help available after 5:00 p.m. and weekends?:

Enteral Nutrition
Enteral nutrition agency name:
Enteral nutrition phone number: Fax number:
Enteral nutrition main contact name: Extension:
When will all the supplies be delivered?:
Was approval gotten from the health plan?:
He/she has more than one health plan or alternate funding to help. Have they also approved it?:
What might be his/her out-of-pocket costs?:
I am learning some at the hospital. Will they help me once we are home?:
How often will they be available to help me?:
Is help available after 5:00 p.m. and weekends?

Wound Care
Wound care agency name:
Wound care phone number: Fax number:
Wound care main contact name: Extension:
When will all the supplies be delivered?:
Was approval gotten from the health plan?:
He/she has more than one health plan or alternate funding to help. Have they also approved it?:
What might be his/her out-of-pocket costs?:
I am learning some at the hospital. Will they help me once we are home?:
How often will they be available to help me?:
Is help available after 5:00 p.m. and weekends?:

Durable Medical Equipment
Name of durable equipment supplier:
Durable equipment supplier main contact phone number: Fax number:
Is it ready? If not, when?:
Has it been approved by the health plan?:
He/she has more than one health plan or alternate funding to help. Have they also approved what he/she needs?:
What will be his/her out-of-pocket costs?:
Will it take training on how to operate?:
Will I get more training on how to use it?:

Equipment ordered	Purchased (P) or rental (R)	If rented, what do I need to do each month, and how will that be handled?	Anticipated delivery date	Any other info needed

Prosthetics
Name of prosthetic supplier:
Prosthetic supplier main contact phone number: Fax number:
Is it ready? If not, when?:
Has it been approved by the health plan?:
He/she has more than one health plan or alternate funding to help. Have they also approved it?:
What will be his/her out-of-pocket costs?:
Will it take training on how to apply it?:
Will I need to worry about ordering any monthly items to ensure it is used and applied correctly?: If so, what and how will I know what is needed and how many to order?:

Orthotics
Name of orthotics supplier:
Orthotic supplier main contact phone number: Fax number:
Is it ready? If not, when?:
Has it been approved by the health plan?:
He/she has more than one health plan or alternate funding to help. Have they also approved it?:
What will be my out-of-pocket costs?:
Will it take training on how to apply it?:
Will I need to worry about ordering any monthly items to ensure it is used and applied correctly?:
If so, what and how many will I need to order?:

Medical Supplies
Name of supplier for medical supplies:
Medical supplier main contact phone number: Fax number:
Have all been approved by the health plan?:
He/she has more than one health plan or alternate funding to help. Have they also approved it?:
What will be my out-of-pocket costs?:
Will I need to pick up any from a local pharmacy, as they are considered over-the-counter?:
Will I need to worry about ordering any monthly items, or will they come automatically to our home?
Other notes:

Illnesses and Injuries and Potential Recourses to Investigate

Because of the thousands of illnesses or diseases or medical conditions, this book will not begin to even cover what each diagnosis might mean. Equally as important, I cannot begin to give you all the information, tools, agencies, services, or equipment you may need or use as you care for your loved one. That will be up to you to possibly explore more on your own. If I do mention a reference you may wish to explore, I have tried to include only those federal or state agencies, as my book is by no means supporting any agencies merely advertising their product. I can just caution you to be careful. Many of the agencies do advertise placement services, and while they may be no cost to you, as they are paid by the living facilities they advertise, be careful; and again, do your research.

Many of the websites listed in this chapter and others may also be websites you may wish to explore. While duplicate, they may also be found in the Help section of this book.

Discharge Plans

During your loved one's hospital stay, your assigned discharge planner / case manager and the team should be preparing you for the discharge of your loved one. Also, at discharge, all services your loved one receives will be dependent upon their diagnosis and prognosis. A word to the wise: some patients at discharge may seem to need tons of durable medical equipment and supplies with a wide variety of health care workers coming and going to attend to their needs, but others go home with merely a mobility device, such as a walker or a wheelchair and maybe a bedside commode. Thus, all discharges are developed specifically for a patient's unique needs. As a result, a one-size-fits-all does not apply.

To give you an example of what can be done at discharge, the following may help you see that a basically mini intensive care unit (ICU) at home can be set up. It also shows you that maybe you and the discharge planner / case manager will need to think outside the box as you and the team plan your loved one's discharge plan. The following are some of the many difficult discharges I have worked on:

The mom of this baby had a normal pregnancy and delivery. However, it was found right after birth that the baby could not breathe and needed a ventilator and would be cared for in the neonatal ICU. I was the director of medical management for the health plan that was covering the baby's ongoing hospital stay, and I received a call from Member Services that the parents were filing a complaint against the hospital. It seemed the hospital was now trying to make arrangements to move the baby to a subacute hospital in Southern California.

In speaking with the parents, I found the baby was now nine months old; and despite all, the parents hoped to take the baby home. Worse yet, they were dealing with two (2) poorly trained health care professionals: the discharge planner / case manager and the social worker. The parents had never been asked about their wishes, and as my medical director and I found out on our first meeting with all, the baby had not been referred to California's then called Crippled Children's Services (CCS) program or to the area's Department of Developmental Services (DDS) and not even to Medi-Cal. The plan was to let the private health plan pay for the ongoing care.

One of our first tasks was to get the parents to apply for long-term Medi-Cal and get referrals into CCS and DDS, educating the parents on why it was necessary to complete any application. As the family lived in an older house and we knew the volume of durable medical equipment and medical supplies needed, we asked the parents to have both a county structural and electrical evaluation of the home and its ability to handle all that would be needed. It also had steps for entry into the front and backyard.

Good thing we requested both assessments, as both the flooring in the bedroom would require reinforcement, and a new electrical panel was needed, and ramps had to be built into the front and back entries. The floor could not accommodate the weight of all the medical equipment, nor would the present electrical panel handle the load of electricity needed to run the equipment. As the health plan did not cover such, as it was not considered a medical necessity, the next task we assigned to the family was to see if they could find a fraternal organization in the area that might want to take on a community service project. Luckily, we did, and both were corrected within weeks of the county inspector's report.

During this time frame, we did the following:

- We had the hospital health care professionals teach the parents how to assume the care that would be needed, and this plan included a forty-eight-hour rooming in training program for the parents.
- We had the hospital rehabilitation team work with a specialized wheelchair vendor from a durable medical equipment (DME) company to make the baby a custom wheelchair/car seat and other devices, as well as the seating systems the child needed to ensure proper body alignment. As it turned out, the vendor was a provider for the area's CCS unit but unfortunately did not have a contract with our health plan. This meant we had to do an extra contractual agreement with the company, as this allowed the parents to have the baby dually covered and without any extra out-of-pocket costs, with our health plan being the primary insurer.
- The hospital discharge planner / case manager was to order all needed durable medical equipment—hospital crib bed, ventilator, suction machine, feeding machine, wheelchair, stroller, car seat, and any seating system. This also included all the many medical supplies the parents would need for any of the DME or other services the baby's care required.
- We at the health plan went to work, working with CCS and DDS on development of a schedule for the 24-7 hired help the family would have in place for the first month. Again, with we found the agency our health plan was contracted with was not one paneled by CCS nor a provider for DDS, so this meant another contractual agreement.

Many, many meetings were held between us from the health plan, one of the nurse managers from CCS and a manager from

DDS, the attending physician, the hospital's director of discharge planning, and the DME and their respiratory therapist and the parents. It took us several months to get to the day of discharge. The best news? The baby was home for its first birthday.

In the second case, this involved a young woman who had a brain bleed (called an aneurysm) and was in a coma and on a ventilator after her surgery. As her prognosis was extremely poor for recovery, the family decided it was best to move her to a hospital in their area. (This young lady had ventured away from her home state, Eastern US, and had taken a job at our California's capital.) Unfortunately, a move such as this was not a covered benefit of a health plan, as the move was at the family's request and out of area, and she could have been moved to any one of our local inpatient rehabilitation centers. Because she was on a ventilator, this ruled out any travel by a commercial airline or land ambulance.

As it turned out, her boyfriend knew someone from work who owned a private jet. Lo and behold, the pilot volunteered his time to fly to and from the family's home area. Thankfully, only the cost of the fuel would be any out-of-pocket costs for the family. This was a godsend, as an air ambulance—or any ambulance—was not a covered benefit of health plan coverage if the move was merely for family convenience.

In this case, we had four health care professionals who volunteered their time for the flights: two (2) respiratory therapists and two (2) ICU nurses. These professionals were needed, as she would require what is called bagging—the use of an Ambu bag—as a ventilator would have been too heavy for the plane to accommodate. Thus, bagging would be required during the entire four-hour flight. Weeks and many case conferences were held as the planning continued. This was necessary, as the team had to determine when and if an attending physician and hospital could be found to accept the patient and manage her care. The team also had to measure and weigh every person and piece of equipment to ensure the plane could accommodate the weight of all persons for the flight, as well as any equipment that might be sent.

I will never forget the day she left our hospital. We all stood around with tears flowing like a river as we said, "Goodbye, honey.

You are going home." With those words, for the first time since her surgery, she opened her eyes and smiled. About a year or more after her discharge, who should come using a cane and limping down the hall on the arm of her boyfriend? The honey we had said goodbye to!

In the third case, again, the hospital discharge planning team was only focusing on one discharge plan, and that was to move this young patient to a subacute hospital in our state, which was in Southern California. Like the young infant I described above, there was little, if any, interactions between the parents and the discharge planner. Plans were being made without parenteral input, and they had called the health plan to see what options they had. In this case, the child was an eight-year-old, hospitalized with his seventh stroke in the three months before this admission, and he was now deemed stable for discharge after a five-month hospital stay. Again, no one had asked the parents what they wanted.

This child had a vast array of disabilities, including a deep decubitus (bedsore) on his buttocks that exposed bone. He was on wound care that consisted of a negative pressure wound vac, he was on a specialized bed and mattress, he was tube-fed, and he had a Foley catheter to drain his urine, which before discharge was changed to a suprapubic catheter. Additionally, he had a very stringent rehabilitation therapy plan. This was needed to help him regain any physical movement, as he had bilateral (both his arm and leg on his left side) contractures, meaning the joints of that arm and leg were in a bent and fixed position.

Like the infant described earlier, this child had not been referred to either our county's CCS (California Children's Services) or DDS (California Department of Developmental Services) programs, for which the parents completed both applications and for which he clearly did qualify for. This discharge did not require the time it took to set up, as in this case, the primary equipment would be the specialized bed and wound vac he required. Teaching of the family was started immediately, and we were able to get the child discharged to home. It was all done in less than a couple of weeks.

The fourth case involved a woman who had just turned sixty-five. In this case, she had just retired after thirty or more years of teaching and was washing her windows when the ladder she was on fell, causing her to fall as well. The bad part was, as she fell, she hit a brick planter at the base of her skull, and she became a quadriplegic in seconds. Thankfully, her friend was there, and he started CPR immediately. After a long and complicated hospital course, we found a large tertiary care hospital in the Bay Area that specialized in spinal cord injuries, and she was accepted there for the intense spinal cord injury (SCI) rehabilitation program they offered. The caveat for acceptance was, our hospital was required to accept her back once she was stabilized and was ready for discharge. As our hospital had agreed to accept her back and work on the discharge, just that happened.

She returned to our hospital still on the ventilator, as her spinal injury was so high it had compromised her respiratory system, and she would remain ventilator dependent for the remainder of her life. For her discharge plan, her gentleman friend said he would take her home and hire the help she would need. (Thankfully, they could afford to do so.) Our first duty as the receiving hospital would be getting her measured and fitted for a specialized wheelchair and seating system that would allow her to sit properly in the wheelchair. Even though she would have 24-7, round-the-clock nurses at home, we set up a training program for her male friend, especially for suctioning her and troubleshooting any equipment failure.

The house did require some modifications, such as building a ramp for entry and a wider entry door and the removal of a wall, as that would allow for better wheelchair maneuvers. The physician also changed her from a Foley catheter to what is called a suprapubic, meaning an incision was made in her lower tummy and a tube inserted into her bladder, and a tiny balloon held it in place. All in all, she remained with us for a month before her discharge. Her discharge included at a minimum the following:

- Her ventilator and a backup one for when she went outside, as well as all the supplies needed to operate a ventilator
- A suction machine, as well as a backup one, and all the supplies needed for suctioning
- Tracheal care sets to clean her trach and replace it if needed

- A medical lift with a sling seat and a split in the seat so she could be placed on a toilet
- A medical lift mounted onto her bathtub that would allow her staff to bathe her
- Adaptive equipment she could use to feed herself
- A semi-electric bed with full rails
- Wheelchair
- The wheelchair seating system
- Specialty seating cushion to help prevent pressure sores
- Suprapubic catheter supplies

About fifteen years after discharge, I ran into her gentleman friend, and he reported she had remained home all those many years and had died only a few months earlier.

The fifth case involved an elderly gentleman who did not only have severe dementia and behavior issues—outbursts of yelling and screaming and trying to harm staff—but also a large open wound on his tailbone, called a decubitus, or bedsore. This bedsore was large and deep; it went to the bone. Prior to coming to our hospital, he resided in an assisted living facility (ALF) for the memory impaired, and he was overly attached to one of the employees. Nothing worked in helping to calm him, so we contacted the facility to see what tips they could give us on how to control his behavior. Luckily, we found we could use that employee to come in and soothe him during his wound care.

To do this meant we had to change the wound care hours so the CNA could be with him during the wound care. This action alone helped us as we worked on the plan to move him to an SNF with the goal being that he would return to his assisted living facility if and when the wound healed. As we worked on the discharge, the SNF went to work in developing a contract with this CNA and establishing his hours to be there during the wound care. In this case, as without such a contract in place, the patient would have remained in our hospital. (We are required to not use any restraints for forty-eight hours before an SNF agrees to accept such a patient.) As a last resort, our hospital developed an agreement with the SNF to pay for the CNA using the charity program funds they offered.

As you can see by the foregoing, home care and odd discharge plans can be set up. Sometimes, the discharge planner and family must think about solutions outside the box. Fortunately, most of what is listed above will be a covered benefit as care for all or what is termed skilled care or medically necessary.

Items Frequently Exempt from Health Care Coverage

There are a wide variety of items or services that are considered an exclusion by most health plans, as they are considered not medically necessary. As you prepare the home for your loved one's home care, work closely with the health plan's case manager, as dependent upon your loved one's diagnosis, items that may be excluded, if there is medical literature that can support the request, the health plan may approve such using the extra contractual process.

Always check with your loved one's health plan as to what is covered versus not and also what vendor(s) they usually use. The worst thing may be if the discharge planner orders the equipment but uses the wrong vendor. If that vendor is not contracted with your loved one's insurance, a denial will be issued, and all must be reordered.

The typical health plan exclusions one may encounter as the DC plan is finalized may include but not limited to the following (if in doubt, double-check your loved one's EOC):

- Private duty nursing.
- Hourly or live-in hired caregivers.
- Enteral or tube feedings, if they are not the sole source of nutrition.
- Paying for any over-the-counter drugs or orphan drugs.
- Paying a family member to be the caregiver.
- Any home modification (building ramps, enlarging door space, removal of walls, remodeling of bathrooms, or fire and smoke alarms).

- Duplicate DME or backup equipment.
- Rental contracts for specific DME items, as many pieces of equipment, like ventilators, that run 24-7 can only run so many weeks before they require a tune-up. In the interim of the tune-up, a backup ventilator must then be rented.
- Fully electric hospital beds.
- Elevators or stair lifts.
- Over-the-bed tables and shower benches.
- Bedpans and urinals.
- Sheets and pillowcases and pillows.
- Elevated toilet seats or any elevated toilets.
- Grab bars in the bathroom or down the hall.
- Educational devices, such as braille textbooks and computers or other electronic equipment or communication boards. These may be included if your loved one is in school and an IEP is developed. The items will be covered for use in the school but must stay there. This means you may then have to purchase similar devices for use outside the school.
- Personal emergency response (PER) devices or systems.
- Environmental equipment, such as air conditioners, devices to turn lights on and off, and air cleaners and filters for such.
- Exercise equipment, weights, or treadmills.
- Nontherapeutic items or services, such as a barber or beautician for hair or nail care.
- Hand controls for an automobile or a van lift.
- Home spas or water mattresses or whirlpool or hydro bath devices.
- Handheld showerheads.

For more information on what is not covered under Medicare and often then for other health insurance plans, you can type in your web browser "Items and services not covered under Medicare," and this should bring up a web link and a booklet where you can continue your research.

Many of the foregoing items, even though they are excluded, may make your job easier. Consequently, you may need to pay for such out of pocket or make use of items you may be able to obtain using any disease or specific agency that serves culturally diverse individuals or those items you find advertised in any local want ads.

CMS defines DME thus:

- Equipment must be durable, which means it can withstand repeated use.
- It will generally last at least three years.
- It is used for a medical reason.
- It is not typically useful to someone who is not sick or injured.
- It is used in the home.

For more information on DME, if you go to your web browser, type in "Medicare coverage of durable medical equipment," and this will bring up a listing of durable medical equipment that is covered. You can also download a booklet on what is covered by using the Medicare publications web link. This will take you to a search link that will allow you to view all of the publications produced by Medicare, any one of which might be of value to you.

To help ensure the items ordered will be approved, the ordering physician is required to write the following as part of the order. Some DME items or prosthetics and orthotics devices require the physician to only write the prescription. However, there are some items and services that also require that the ordering provider show in their documentation that the order was written during a face-to-face (F2F) encounter with the patient.

The prescription for each item ordered must include the following elements and for some equipment, prosthetics, and orthotics:

1.	Patient name and ID no.:
2.	Equipment description:
3.	Quantity, if applicable:

4. Diagnosis and ICD-10 code:
5. Anticipated length of need (estimated in months, but enter 99 if indefinite):
6. Most recent height and most recent weight (may be required and are needed if the patient is obese):
7. MD signature:
8. National Provider Identifier (NPI):
9. Date of the order:

The Affordable Care Act established a face-to-face encounter requirement for certain items of DME. The law requires that a physician must document that a physician, nurse practitioner, physician assistant, or clinical nurse specialist has had a face-to-face encounter with the patient. In your web browser, you can type in "Medicare face-to-face visits," and you can then find a variety of topics that describes the Medicare process for face-to-face visits, whether it be home health care, hospice, or durable medical equipment.

If your loved one is obese and his weight or girth (measurement of waist or hips) cannot be accommodated by regular DME, your loved one's physician will need to order what is called bariatric DME. This type of equipment may not be available locally and thus must be special-ordered. Typically, this equipment will be sent directly to your home, and a local representative will come and set it up and, if necessary, teach you how to use it. If this is ordered, ensure it will be a covered benefit, as not all states and insurers in those states follow the Affordable Care Act (ACA) and the requirements for coverage of bariatric surgery. So double-check with your loved one's primary health plan to ensure it will be covered. If it is not, then unfortunately, you will be responsible for the costs of such.

Bariatric DME is used when a patient's weight is between four hundred and one thousand pounds. However, if your loved one is maybe not at that weight limit but has a wide girth (at his or her waist or hips), the physician must not only order such but also medically describe why this is required and why normal DME (designed for an average-sized person) is not appropriate. I personally had this issue arise with my husband. His weight during one of his episodes of illness was around 350, but his hips were so wide he could not fit into a standard-size commode. Just as I described, it was covered, as the physician included a statement of why such was medically necessary.

Medicare and most health plans cover at a minimum a semi-electric bed, but to be sure, double-check your loved one's EOC or call their customer services line. For information on coverage of bariatric hospital beds, you can type in your web browser "Medicare guidelines for bariatric beds," and you will find the qualifying criteria.

If your loved one may need oxygen at home, again, this is a covered benefit by CMS and health plans and can be approved for both chronic and acute medical conditions and whether it is needed short- or long-term. If your loved one will be on oxygen at home, he will also require at a minimum a semi-electric hospital bed. This will allow them to be positioned in a semi sitting position for better breathing. To qualify for coverage of oxygen, the patient will have specific respiratory markers that indicate the need for the oxygen. For more information on oxygen therapy, you can view the requirements for home oxygen by typing in your web browser "CMS National Coverage Determination (NCD) and oxygen."

Another requirement if the discharge plan will be to go home and a home health agency (HHA) or hospice agency will be providing the services is, the physician ordering such must also document that he ordered such after a recent F2F visit.

When the physician orders home health care, he must document the following if your loved one is to be eligible to use their health plan's home health benefit, certifying that your loved one meets them:

1. The patient is confined to the home (and cannot go out without taxing effort).
2. The patient is under the care of a physician or an allowed practitioner.
3. A plan of care has been established and is periodically reviewed by a physician or allowed practitioner.
4. The services are or were furnished while the patient is or was under the care of a physician or allowed practitioner.

As a rule, most home health agency visits start within forty-eight hours of discharge. However, that can be moved up if it is critical that a nurse sees your loved one sooner. Home care by a home health agency or hospice provider will be discovered in greater detail later in this book.

Discharge Barriers

Not all discharges go smoothly, and delays can be encountered. Possibly the number one reason for the delay, especially for discharge to an SNF, will be your loved one's diagnosis and prognosis and subsequent level and intensity of care needs required, as many may be too complex for the post-acute providers to manage. In other cases, the complexity of care or possibly the medication to be given is not approved for home use, or a state's nurse practice act does not allow nurses to administer the drug outside the hospital setting.

In most delays in discharge, these occur as the result of how a state has developed their code of regulations to how they will enforce any CMS rules. For example, in California, the regulations for SNFs and other health care facilities are termed the California Code of Regulations, Title 22. Under Title 22, the staffing for an RN in an SNF reads, "For every 99 patients there must be a Registered Nurse (RN) on duty and awake for 8 hours during the day hours." Believe me, many SNFs use this as a guide and do not deviate. So they meet this requirement. However, this frequently means this RN is also the director of nursing. This then means all care on the three shifts—days, evenings, and nights—is then provided by licensed vocational nurses (LVNs) and nurses' aides.

As a result, it is important during case conferences, especially if it appears the discharge is looming, that your loved one's level of care needs and hours and frequency for care serve as the driver for placement and for what post-acute level of care will be needed. Thus, your loved one could possibly go to any or all of the following (with the exception of the DD facilities) before they are able to be discharged to home:

- Inpatient acute rehabilitation (IAR) unit
- Long-term acute care hospital (LTACH)
- Subacute
- SNF, or in some states referred to as a subacute rehabilitation unit (SAR)

If your loved one has a development delay (DD) or intellectual delay (ID) and he is eligible for DDS services, he may be discharged to an SNF. But in most cases, it is to hopefully discharge them back to the previous LOC where they live (either at home or in what is called a residential care facility or res care facility or an intermediate care facility, or ICF). However, due to advances in technology and medical practices, the DD and ID populations and their caregiver are living longer and are now requiring a higher LOC than they lived in prior to their current illness or injury, and they often now will require placement in an SNF.

This is true even though all states offer a LOC termed intermediate care facility-DD. Whether it is the ICF-DD-H (habitation) or ICF-DD-N(nursing) or ICF-DD-CN (critical nursing), their new LOC need is above what the ICF is licensed to provide.

In California, the Department of Developmental Services (DDS) also provides a LOC statewide that provides basically an ICU level of care for DD or ID individuals who are medically stable and do not require daily physician visits or the specialized imaging or laboratory services offered by an acute hospital. The facilities are staffed 24-7 with RNs and LVNs and provide care for ventilator or patients with overly complex medical care needs. These homes are referred to as ARFPSHN (Adult Residential Facility for Persons with Special Health Care Needs).

Because criteria for admission to an IAR, LTACH, or subacute is stringent, many patients only have one choice for placement, and that is to find the right LOC. The discharge planner / case manager often must do a statewide search of facilities that can possibly meet the LOC needed after discharge, this means you may not have a choice, and your loved one must then be placed out of area.

The following are other common barriers:

- The weight of the patient, if over 250–300 pounds, poses a problem, as most SNFs do not have bariatric equipment. This means that out of the reimbursement they receive from health plans and Medicare or Medicaid, they have to rent any and all equipment required.
- There are no beds available. Either the facility is full, or the beds are empty, as they do not have the staff to work all shifts.
- The patient is combative or abusive to staff.
- The patient has an infectious disease, and the SNF does not have a private room. Or they have an old ventilation system, and the infectious disease can then be airborne in the facility and affect others.
- Patient has a history of alcohol or drug abuse.
- Patient has a dual diagnosis for both a mental health condition and for a physical illness or injury.
- The facility does not have a dedicated wound care or an infusion nurse when more-than-once daily treatments are needed, and the SNF only has an RN on the day shift.
- The patient has end-stage renal disease (ESRD) and requires dialysis and also has specific dietary needs.
- The patient has a trach and must be suctioned more than three times per shift.
- Patient has a bedsore, and it is at a stage IV.
- Patient is under the age of fifty-five or a child or youth meeting and is classified as a child or youth with special care needs.
- The staff is untrained in complex care.
- The patient has a developmental or intellectual disability, and they have behavior issues and complex medical care needs.

- Patient has limited financial resources and has not yet applied for the state's Medicaid program, as assets remain too high.

Barriers to a home plan may include the following:

- Landlord or fire marshal restrictions or laws may be a consideration if your loved one previously resided in a rented house or apartment.
- There is no elevator in the building.
- There is no running water.
- There is no way to control the temperature of the living area.
- There is a delay in getting all the services and supplies into the home.
- The HHA or hospice agency is short-staffed, or a weekend or holiday weekend is approaching. If I knew a weekend or holiday was approaching, I always made every attempt to have the doctor order the discharge for no later than Wednesday. Why? Because often, the physician who will be assuming the case may also be taking off early for a long weekend; and while he may have someone on call, that physician will not know the patient. When such occurs, you can pretty much count on an unnecessary readmission.

Summary

This chapter may have been a little scary, but this book is to educate you on all that is going to be needed as you start in your role as the caregiver for your loved one. I strongly encourage you to purchase a spiral notebook for note taking. This will assist tremendously, as you need to and should ask questions to the team. Keep in mind, you may now also be the eyes, ears, and voice for your loved one.

All discharges are totally different, and there is not a one-plan-fits-all. Thus, every discharge plan must be individualized for each patient. That is why I am giving you so many websites. This will allow you to do your own research—and if you are not trained on how to use a computer or even your phone to its fullest capacity, one of your team members may be one of your own (children or a grandchild or a neighbor or a friend)—and you can be informed as you work with the team on the discharge plan. One of the main purposes of this book is to help you be an informed consumer.

Again, do not be afraid to say no if this means you will have some help and take a break. It is critical in your new role that you learn to take care of yourself mentally, physically, and emotionally. You are no good otherwise.

CHAPTER 2

Getting the Home Organized and Prepared for Caregiving

THE HEALTH CARE team is saying your loved one will soon be discharged, or the doctor is saying you need to get a caregiver to help you. This means if your loved one is at the point where they need total care, have severe dementia and may wander, or have a tendency for violence, your big worry will be what you are to do to accommodate such needs. The goal of this chapter will be outlining some key information and tips to help you as you evaluate your loved one's home and make it ready for you to assume his care. If in the hospital, hopefully, in one of the case conferences, you are able to ask the many questions, such as the following:

- When is discharge planned?
- Who can you expect to help you?
- What durable medical equipment (DME) and supplies will be needed?
- From what agency will be used for home care?
- What company will be delivering the equipment, and when can you expect all to arrive?
- How will your loved one be transported home?

- If care must continue upon discharge and you will maybe be responsible to provide some, when and how will you be trained?

If there will be a wide variety of medical supplies and equipment, keep that list handy, as it will help you as you evaluate the space that will be used for the bedroom and the bath area and hallways, at a minimum.

As indicated earlier, one of your best resources will be to discuss your home's interior and exterior with the physical and occupational therapist and see what they recommend. Or better yet, query them if they can make a home visit to help you assess the space needed. The interior areas that will need the most attention will be the bathroom, bedroom, hallways, positioning of the doors, and width of the door opening. This will include the layouts and dimensions of each area. Additionally, you must not forget the exterior—both front and back doors and any steps both inside and outside—and good lighting. If modifications are needed, these can take time. So this may mean, if your loved one is ready soon for discharge, placement in a skilled nursing facility (SNF) or assisted living facility (ALF) may be needed in the interim.

Note: Medicare is the only health plan your loved one has. Medicare never covers home modifications, such as ramps, widening of doorways, or improving wheelchair access. Thus, if modifications will be needed and funds are limited, you will have to do your own research as to who can do it for you.

Research shows that if your loved one has a managed care plan, there is a chance modification may be covered if medical necessity for such can support the need. But you must do your homework as to where the money will come from if home modifications are needed. One resource may be your loved one's state Medicaid program, but it is rare they cover such. While Medicaid benefits vary by state, they all have some form of long-term care program available that may help. Also, if most modifications are covered, coverage will include the cost of the materials, but not the labor.

Some resources to assist with covering the costs for home modifications, especially if labor is not covered, will require research on your part as you explore what is available in your loved one's community. You may also want to explore the following to see if it can offer to pay or perform the services:

- A volunteer fraternal organization will take on the actual labor needed for the home modifications as one of their service projects. Research shows that Wikipedia has a full listing of fraternal organizations you may want to explore.

There are a variety of resources that might be able to assist with any needed home modifications. To find information on home modifications, this will require research on your part, but the following companies or organizations offer such services if you meet their requirements. The companies and organizations are as follows:

- The Home Depot and their foundation and national partnerships.
- Veterans Administration Program and one of its grants, such as the Home Improvements and Structural Alterations (HISA).
- Wounded Warrior Housing and Home Modifications and their Operation We Are Here Program.
- The National Rehabilitation Information Center (naric. com) and their I Have a Disability Program.
- Rebuilding Together—this organization uses a wide variety of corporate companies to offer their program.
- The American Red Cross has a program to assist military families.
- Gary Sinise Foundation and its many sponsors and the RISE ("Restoring Independence and Supporting Empowerment") project (Reference: RISE | Gary Sinise).
- Habitat for Humanity and home modifications, and they have two weblinks you may wish to explore—the Critical

Home Repair site or their Aging in Place with Habitat for Humanit (Habitat for Humanity site).

- If your loved one has a developmental or intellectual disability and they are deemed eligible for their state's developmentally disabled services program, under their individual program plan (IPP), which is a plan developed for all clients and home modifications are needed, DDS will cover all materials and labor.

Evaluating the Home

The following are many tips and suggestions I have given to the families I worked with over the many years. Thus, as you review your home and the area where your loved one will receive his care, some of the key areas to consider will be the following:

a) Where will your loved one's bedroom be located, and does it have a full bath nearby?
b) Is it upstairs or down?
c) How easily can one get to the bedroom and bath area, and are the doorways wide enough and without barriers, such as moving around a wall or a corner?
d) How about the doors for the entry and exit to the house?
e) Are there stairs anywhere, and if so, are they straight up or curved?
f) Is there one or two handrails?
g) Is there a threshold to enter the house, or is it zero clearance?

General Safety Tips

Many of the following tips I have learned over the years of working with the rehabilitation team, so your best source will be to ask questions to them, especially since newer products, including much newer technology, are now readily available.

Make sure all throw rugs and any loose or bunched up carpet or loose tiles and any clutter or any type of cords lying around are removed. Any one of these issues can be the cause of a fall or of the wheelchair tipping over, causing any variety of injuries. As a rule, carpet, if it can be replaced with tile or laminate flooring, do it, especially if your loved one is in a wheelchair or has frequent bouts of diarrhea or incontinence. This is necessary, as carpet is hard to navigate in a wheelchair when it is on the floor. And if incontinent, cleanup and odor elimination are easier if the area is not carpeted.

Critical as you evaluate the bedroom or any room your loved one may use, especially if in a wheelchair, will be to ensure the doorway width is at least thirty-six inches. This width is then wide enough to accommodate a standard wheelchair or walker. Better yet, if it can be forty-two inches, this helps, as it will allow your loved one's hands to not be scraped as they enter or exit. Two (2) more tips: (a) make sure that the door has swing clear hinges, as these will allow the door to swing totally open and that (b) there is a lever-style handle and not a doorknob, allowing them easier access to opening the door, if they are able.

If our loved one tends to wander, the only time you may not wish to consider the lever-style doorknob is for the front or back entry doors. In any case, you will want to investigate and install the right locks or doorknob covers. If you do install locks, install them out of sight, either above or below eye level. And to ensure your loved one does not lock themselves or even you in a room, keep an extra set of keys handy or possibly hidden on top of the doorframe. Better yet, you may want to install keyless locks, which can be opened by a code, a remote device, a fab, or even your cell phone.

Another device you may want to consider is a simple door alarm that can help alert you if your loved one has dementia and attempts to leave the home. Technology is here, so investigate what may work in your situation, should it be programmable door locks, sensors that can alert you of movement, or audio or video monitors. By all means, if your loved one is total care with or without a variety of equipment and you will be sleeping in another room, you may want to invest in a baby monitor, one with both a camera and also audio features.

Below are some other general safety tips.

- If you have glass doors, place stickers on the glass to help your loved one see them and not walk into the glass, possibly breaking it and causing serious injuries.
- If you have a swimming pool and your loved one has dementia or is a child, fence in the pool area and add locks to the gate.
- If your barbecue grill is a concern, lock the cover and access to gas tanks and remove all fire starters.
- Check the garage and back or side yards for safety hazards, like gasoline, tools, or ladders, and block access if they pose a danger to your loved one. If you have a golf cart or riding lawn mower and your loved one has dementia or another brain disorder that makes him an unsafe driver, place the keys in a safe place; otherwise, they may try to use this as a means of transportation.
- Ensure you keep cleaning and laundry supplies in a central area, and it has a lock on the door where such is stored.
- Install locks on all fence gates to help prevent wandering.
- If your loved one is one who has a brain disorder of any sort and tends to wander, take the time to sew in and label all clothing with tags where you can write in washable ink their name and address, at a minimum. Also, make every attempt to write identifying information on glass cases or their wallet and shoes. If they will wear it, have them wear a medical alert bracelet or necklace; or better yet, if they will wear a watch, invest in one of the GPS watches now on the market.
- As you prepare the home, ensure smoke and carbon monoxide detectors are working, and the batteries are fresh. They should be replaced twice yearly. A good habit to follow will be to replace them every January 1 and June 1. If you do this, make sure you add the information to a calendar you keep for all your reminders. You will also want to

ensure you have a fire extinguisher, you know how to use it, and it is working properly.

- If there are guns in the home, consider removing them or other weapons; and if not, store them in a locked cabinet.
- Make sure all medications, even yours and any over-the-counter medications, such as aspirin, are in a locked drawer or cabinet.
- As you ready the house, ensure all razors, safety pins, and other sharp objects are locked up.
- Possibly eliminate extra electrical outlets, and cover those not considered necessary with a solid plate covering.

The Bedroom

The important thing to consider if your loved one is total care and to make care easier on you, if possible, attempt to have your loved one's bedroom on the first floor. But it must be near running hot and cold water and have a tub or shower. If it is upstairs and your loved one is total care, you then will need to consider the installation of an elevator if you have the funds and if the home has the space to accommodate such. If not, consider a chair lift system designed for stairs. Key will be to ensure it can accommodate the weight of your loved one. As a rule, this may be an uncovered item under your loved one's health plan. But check it out, as some managed care plans may possibly cover it.

If your loved one will have a large amount of durable medical equipment, such as a bed, ventilator, suction machine, oxygen, or wound vac, or even if you are doing home peritoneal dialysis, not only will you have all the equipment to tend with, but each will also have a variety of medical supplies as well. Thus, you must take into consideration not only the weight of all the equipment but also how and where all can be stored. Keep in mind, you want as much as you can for the care your loved one requires handy, and not in an area where you must lug all to the caregiving area.

For storage of items, I would suggest a portable shelving unit or, better yet, plastic storage drawer units. If at all possible, store such in the closet or under the bed, as this will help keep the area clutter free; and equally as important, it allows the room to not look like a hospital room. If you do store the items under the bed, ensure the space you use is one where when the bed is in its lowest position items will fit.

If the house is older, you must consider the type of flooring. If wood, you may need to have a building inspection to ensure the floor can accommodate the weight of the equipment, all the supplies needed, and your and your loved one's weight and any volunteer's weight. In addition to the flooring, if your loved one will have a large amount of equipment that must be powered by electricity, you must ensure the home can accommodate the electrical output required. Again, this may involve having a county inspection of both. If either one or both fail, this means home modifications are in store, as the home will not be safe. This also means they must be done before you can safely bring your loved one home. Consequently, if your loved one's medical condition is starting to stabilize and they soon will be declared medically stable for discharge, placement may be required in the interim.

If your loved one will require a hospital bed, there are several things to consider.

1. Bed linens and pillows or extra pillows and any bed rolls or positioning pillows are not a covered benefit for health plans, including Medicare and Medicaid. If you do purchase sheets, for the bottom sheet, purchase the type with deep pockets and ones with bands on all four corners to help secure the sheet and prevent it from bunching up in the middle of the bed with movement. If your loved one is bedbound, you may want to also consider a transfer sheet, which will help you turn and reposition him. A transfer sheet helps reposition a patient's body. These sheets consist of two sheets, one on top of the other. Once you get both sheets under your loved one, the sheets easily slide against each other, making it easy to reposition your loved one in his bed.

2. You will want extra flat sheets you can fold in quarters so you can fashion what is called a pull or turn sheet. Better yet, for a sheet that can serve as a pull or turn sheet, as well as to protect the mattress (if your loved one is incontinent), purchase what is termed hospital sheeting from a local yardage store. This is made of rubberized material covered with a soft cotton covering. The best feature is, this is a washable product and can be cut into widths to fit the bed. For this, I would suggest you purchase five yards, as you can cut them into a yard each, and you will then have five sheets you can have handy. Sheeting such as this helps cut the costs of using the disposable underpads, commonly referred to as chux.

3. If your loved one is incontinent, to help keep the urine or stool smell to a minimum, one of your best resources for cleaning will be plain old white vinegar. You may also want to make in advance any cleaning solution made of bleach and water. For this, the Centers for Disease Control and Prevention (CDC) recommends the following:

    a) Follow the label directions on the bleach product. Check to see if you need to wear any protective equipment, such as gloves or eye protection.

    b) Never mix household bleach (or any disinfectants) with any other cleaners or disinfectants. This can release vapors that may be very dangerous to breathe in.

    c) Make sure you have good ventilation while using bleach products indoors (for example, open windows and doors to allow fresh air to enter).

    d) Use regular, unscented household bleach. Most household bleach contains 5 percent–9 percent sodium hypochlorite. Do not use a bleach product if the percentage is not in this range or is not specified. This includes some types of laundry bleach or splashless bleach, which are not appropriate for disinfection.

e) Follow the directions on the bleach bottle for preparing a diluted bleach solution. If your bottle does not have directions, you can make a bleach solution by mixing five tablespoons (one-third cup) of bleach per gallon of room temperature water or four teaspoons of bleach per quart of room temperature water. In your web browser type in "CDC disinfecting with bleach" and you can then find the information you may need.

There is another tip I learned many years ago, when my mother took care of my dad after his back surgery and paralysis in the late forties, which at that time meant a full-body cast and bed confinement for over a year. The staff at the hospital taught my mom a tip to help prevent friction burns on his elbows, heels, and butt. This tip was to sprinkle small amounts of dry cornstarch on the sheets. It worked, as while bed-confined for over a year, my dad never had one friction burn. However, before you do make use of such tip, double-check with your health care team if this is safe to use. The only exception may be if there is any broken or open skin areas.

As you ready the home and at this point your loved one is free of any open pressure sores, and you want to ensure you keep it that way, you can type in your web browser "preventing pressure ulcers." Here you will find a wide variety of articles you download and read and use to help you reach and maintain this goal.

Another tip to help you in your caregiving role will be possibly the use of the new voice-activated devices, which can be set to remind you of events. These devices let you record times for medication and caregiving activities, such as turning or other tasks you must perform, reminders for the refilling of meds or ordering medical supplies and medical appointments, or maybe even reminders for birthdays or anniversaries.

The Bed

Generally, a room size of ten by twelve is a sufficient amount of space for a standard hospital bed. But if your loved one requires a bariatric bed, this may be too small for both the bed and any items he may need, which includes not only other DME but also any medical supplies. Keep in mind, you want to conserve your strength, so make every attempt to create a centralized area for his care. This includes space not only for the bed but possibly also the patient lift system, any mobility devices used, such as a wheelchair or walker, and then space for a cabinet or shelving to hold all the ancillary supplies that may be needed.

In the past, working with a therapy team, they always had me advise patients and families that typically, the space needed for use of wheelchairs and such is as follows: You should allow for at least three feet of clearance around the bed, but as much as a five-foot clearance may be necessary, as this ensures the bedroom is wheelchair accessible. So allow a five-by-five floor space for turning. This floor space for turning must also be taken into consideration in other parts of the house as well.

For the bed, the health care team will help decide if your loved one can use a regular hospital bed or if a bariatric bed or possibly another type of specialty bed is medically necessary. This will include any special bed. For most health plans, coverage for a hospital is limited to only a semi-electric bed. It is rare that a fully electric bed is medically necessary for patient care. However, for the most part, a semi-electric bed is the one most often recommended. The big drawback will be, while this type of bed will let you adjust the head and foot of the bed, to move the height does require that you crank it by hand. If your loved one requires a special bed, this will require more documentation from the physician that supports the medical necessity of the bed. Unfortunately, this process can take extra time for approval, so if a special bed is identified, ensure the health plan has been notified and any delays in discharge are avoided.

For the bed, you must also ensure side rails are ordered. If your loved one can help in turning himself, then as a rule, one-half rails are all that are needed. However, if they are total care and you must move them side to side as you change their positions or if they tend to try to get out of bed, full rails are the ones you will want to have.

To keep covers from applying pressure to your loved one's feet and toes, you should also consider a bed cradle.

If your loved one can assist in moving up and down in bed and has the arm strength to help with moving, then you will also want to consider either a bed trapeze that fits onto the bed or, if not, one that is called a free-standing trapeze. The nice thing about a free-standing one is, it can be moved from room to room should you be able to use it to help him or her get in or out of a chair.

If your loved one is a child or youth or even an adult with a developmental disability and has behavior issues, discuss with the team what type of bed will be best. Often, this includes a bed with some type of net closure that surrounds the bed. Enclosed cribs or enclosed beds may be medically necessary for recipients with diagnosis of a developmental disability when the nature and severity of their illness, injury, or disease meets all the following medical criteria.

- The behavioral necessity for an enclosed bed is documented and described in the medical record.
- There is clinical documentation that underlying behavioral issues have been proactively addressed with appropriate behavioral interventions and modification without success.
- Other less restrictive forms of bed restraint/accommodations have been employed without adequate success, such as increased caregiver monitoring, alarm systems, padding bed rails, or placing mattress on the floor.
- An ordinary bed cannot be modified or adapted by commercially available items to meet your loved one's needs.
- There is no other appropriate and reasonably feasible alternative method for providing safe bed/sleep care.
- The request for the enclosed bed is not for caregiver convenience or due to lack of caregiver monitoring for your loved one's safety.

If your loved one is one who rolls around in bed or is a safety risk in a chair or has a behavior issue, investigate with your loved one's doctor what restraint(s) may be the best one(s) to use. Restraints are used for a variety of purposes, such as to immobilize a person or extremity, to control behavior, or to prevent your loved one from pulling out tubes, rolling out of bed, or falling out of a wheelchair. Also, there are both restraints for use in a bed and for a wheelchair, and they can be either a belt or vest type. As you investigate such, also explore what will be one you can use in a car, if your loved one can sit in a car.

If your loved one is basically bed confined or has a pressure sore, you will want to discuss with the health care team and doctor what mattress type will be best. Will it be a gel or gel-like pressure mattress pad? Do they need an alternating air mattress or low air loss mattress system or water pressure pad for a standard mattress? Or might they need another type of bed called an air-fluidized bed? If your loved one is one who is confused and will attempt to get out of bed unattended, you will want to consider a bed alarm or, as mentioned above, the use of a restraint.

To help you as you perform any tasks, while not considered medically necessary and an item that will not be a covered benefit, you may want to consider having a table by your loved one's bed. This will allow you to have any supplies handy as you perform a task.

The Bathroom

A key area to evaluate will be the bathroom. If your loved one can walk but can only walk short distances, you will need to know that within the distance, he can safely walk to get to and from the bathroom. If it is not, you may want to ask the physical therapist if a bedside commode may be a piece of equipment he may need. This item is a covered benefit of insurances, and this also may make it easier for you as you assist them when a toilet is needed.

If a commode is needed, you will also want to ask the therapist if this should be a regular commode with the arms attached or if a drop arm device would be better. Another device you may want to consider if they do recommend a drop arm one will be the possible use of a slide board or a patient lift system. If either is recommended by the therapy team, ensure they teach you how to use them.

If your loved one can use the toilet, a necessity will be the following:

- You will need the installation of grab bars on both sides of the toilet, if space allows.
- If not, you can purchase a raised toilet seat with arms; or if a raised seat is not needed, you or someone you hire can install armrests that are secured in place by a normal toilet seat.
- If you must move your loved one to the commode or toilet and to do so you must use a patient lift system, ensure that when the sling seat is ordered, it has a slit in it so you can easily undress them, and the opening can let them pee or poop without any hassle.

As you evaluate the bathroom, you must consider how you will or how your loved one will be able to take a shower or take a bath; and as you evaluate either one, be careful with the use of bathmats. They can often get waded up and cause a fall. Your best bet will be to use some type of nonslip stickers or strips you can stick on the flooring or just outside the shower or tub.

By all means, a walk-in shower will make it easier for you, but there are things to consider as you evaluate the shower.

- Is there zero clearance to enter (no threshold to step over).
- Install a grab bar, as this will stabilize your loved one if they can stand.
- Another device will be a shower seat. While a shower seat is not a covered benefit of most health plans, as it is not considered medically necessary, it will be an item you will have to purchase. However, it will help you as you help your loved one shower. An alternative is, if your loved one has a bedside commode, use that as a shower seat.
- Another device frequently recommended by the therapy to purchase will be a hand-held showerhead.

- If the bathroom has room, you may want to consider a walk-in shower, as this will eliminate any threshold to step over.

If your only choice for bathing is a bathtub, then you must evaluate how you will get your loved one in and out of such, and you must carefully consider yourself for this task. Evaluation of yourself is critical, as the biggest number of back injuries for caregivers comes from helping your loved one get in or out of a tub. If this is so, then you must consider how you will be able to use it. Two options will be the following:

1. Consider a transfer bench. If able to assist you, this will allow your loved one to move from their wheelchair onto the bench. These benches often extend beyond the actual tub with two of the legs on the floor and the other two in the tub. The benches most often will have a back rest as well and side bars to help move onto the bench. Despite the side bars, it is wise to also consider grab bars in the tub area in the event your loved one can stand, and this will make bathing their private area easier.

2. To help avoid injury for yourself, you may want to consider using the patient lift system you may already be using in the other areas of the house. However, the bathroom must be big enough to accommodate it. If not, you may want to consider the purchase of a hydraulic lift and seating system, whether it is electric or hand operated. There are many devices on the market, so let the therapy team help you make the right choice. Another choice for a lift system, if the bathroom is big enough, will be to install a ceiling lift.

As indicated earlier in this book, regular DME items are designed to accommodate weights of about 250 and some even 300 pounds. If weight is greater than this, you must then consider bariatric equipment for your loved one. As you consider any equipment, ask our rehabilitation team what they recommend and what the weight limit is for any and all items used.

The Kitchen

Another area to evaluate will be the kitchen, and as you do so, ensure the refrigerator is working properly. This is key, as many medications, formulas for feedings, and nutritional items will require refrigeration. You do not want a refrigerator that often will unexpectedly freeze food or solutions for no reason. You also will want to ensure you have a lock on it if your loved one wanders and is on a special diet and can get to food other that at mealtime or snack time.

In addition to installing locks possibly on the refrigerator, you may need to do the same for a pantry or cupboards where food is stored. If your loved one has any sort of brain disorder and he may have a tendency for violence or other aggressive or wild behavior, while for some homes the installation of childproof locks on drawers may work where sharp or glass items are kept, this may not be the need if your loved one has a tendency for rage if the situation is one that bothers him. In this case, a lock with a key or cell phone control may be the best to use. For the stove, install childproof knobs, and keep any matches or other lighters in a secure place. Another consideration if they are violent and will throw things is replacing any dishes and glasses with melamine or plastic ones.

Play Area for Your Child or Developmentally or Intellectually Disabled Loved One

If your loved one has a developmental or intellectual disability, you must consider space for a play area, where you can have it equipped with any number of fun and the right sensory-specific toys or games or fidget toys or other equipment their therapist recommends. This will allow your loved one, regardless of age, to play or have the education and therapy recommended.

Space for Key Documents

As you ready the home for your loved one and their needs and while you may have such in your cell phone, set aside an area where you can keep a notebook with key phone numbers and addresses, as well as your appointment or reminder calendar. For the phone numbers (make sure you include the phone number for the poison control center in your area, as you never know when your loved one, especially if with a challenging behavior, may accidently ingest something poisonous) and other addresses and reminders, I always recommend a three-ring binder with plastic page protectors. This then allows you to update pages with information as it changes (for example, your volunteer list and their names and phone numbers or as new health care team members are added or replaced). By having this handy, if you should become ill yourself, others can easily find the information they may need.

Another key thing to consider will be to have in a central location—and you have alerted family members of where it is—will be any key medical information on your loved one and yourself. If your loved one has an advance directive, it is wise to have that posted. So if emergency personnel enter the home, they can see it immediately and know your loved one's wishes. Again, dependent upon your situation, if there is a possibility they can be destroyed by your loved one, find a place to lock them up, but also tell the family where the key is.

To assist you or any volunteers you may use, consider the use of a white board to write down specific dates/days and times for care and appointments.

Below are more tips.

1. It is wise to put a lockbox on your front door with an entry key to the house. This will allow emergency personnel to enter the home should your loved one have an emergent event, and you are the only one home and attending to him. If you do have a lockbox, make sure you notify the fire department of the code to use for entry.

2. As you prepare the home, it is wise if you take the time to either set up an app on your phone or work directly with the local grocery store to set up an account. Many stores will also accept your Supplemental Nutrition Assistance Program (SNAP) or state's EBT card (Electronic Benefits Transfer), where you can order groceries ahead of time and either have them delivered or available for pickup by you or your volunteer.

3. You will also want to discuss with your loved one's health plan or his assigned case manager what mail-order pharmacy has a contract with the health plan. By using the mail-order option, you will get a three-month supply of meds. This will not only save you time for the pickup, but you will also only pay for two months' worth instead of three.

4. If your loved one is on life-sustaining devices or if your loved one has challenging behaviors, alert—not only with your loved one's name but also with a brief description of potential needs or issues you want them to be aware of—the fire department of the fact that he will be coming home. This will allow them to be prepared should an emergency arise, and they are aware of your loved one's special needs or issues.

5. Take the time to call utility companies and alert them of your loved one's medical condition, and at the same time, ask if there are discount programs for which you may qualify. They also need to be aware of your loved one's medical condition, especially if they are on life-sustaining equipment. This will allow, in the event of a power outage, your home to be on the list for immediate services for reconnection.

Pets

Pets are a wonderful addition to any home, and they can be of great comfort to your loved one. However, they can also pose issues with tripping and then possible falling. If this could be an issue, you will then want to consider having a secure area where you can keep your pets. Also, as you prepare for any weather-related emergency, don't forget to pack an emergency to-go kit for your pet.

Other Considerations

The following information is just tips on what to expect if your loved one requires any of the following devices, many of which may also have a battery backup unit. If the device does have a battery backup, it is key to ensure you follow the manufacturer's instructions on how and how often to charge the system. This means you need to schedule when the device should be charged. At the same time, if you have extra medications, you set up a schedule of when to review them for expiration dates and the ordering of new ones.

Note: If the discharge date is known and set, Medicare and the health plans will not pay for early delivery of DME items. Thus, the DME will be delivered, as a rule, the day before discharge. The only exception will be if your loved one is on life-sustaining equipment, and you must be trained on them. These often can be delivered to the hospital a week or so in advance of the discharge. However, discuss all with the hospital discharge coordinator / case manager.

Oxygen and Other Respiratory Devices

Medicare and insurances cover the rental of oxygen equipment and its accessories, as well as other respiratory devices, such as ventilators, CPAPs or BiPAPs, humidifiers, nebulizers, and other such devices, under the durable medical equipment (DME) benefit when your loved one's doctor prescribes it for use in the home. Health plans follow the guidelines established by CMS for Medicare. These guidelines include the following:

1. For oxygen and its supplies, Medicare or your loved one's health plan will help pay for oxygen, contents, and supplies

for the delivery of oxygen when all these conditions are met:

- Your loved one's doctor says your loved one is not getting enough oxygen.
- His health may improve with oxygen therapy.
- His arterial blood gas level falls within a certain range.

2. If your loved one meets the conditions above, Medicare helps pay for

- systems that provide oxygen,
- containers that store oxygen, and
- tubing and related supplies for the delivery of oxygen and oxygen contents.

3. Medicare may also pay for a humidifier when it is used with your loved one's oxygen machine. If your loved one has Medicare and uses oxygen, the equipment can be rented from a supplier for thirty-six months. After thirty-six months, the supplier must continue to provide oxygen equipment and related supplies for an additional twenty-four months. Basically, the supplier must provide equipment and supplies for up to a total of five years if your loved one has a medical need for oxygen and meets the criterion.

4. The monthly rental payments to the supplier cover not only the oxygen equipment but also any oxygen accessories and services.

- Tubing or a mouthpiece
- Oxygen contents
- Oxygen machine maintenance
- Oxygen machine servicing
- Oxygen machine repairs

What happens after thirty-six months of oxygen rental?

- The supplier must continue to maintain the oxygen equipment (in good working order) and furnish the equipment and any necessary supplies and accessories as long as your loved one needs it until the five-year period ends. If this remains the case and your loved one meets the criterion, the supplier can't charge you for performing these services.
- If your loved one uses oxygen tanks or cylinders that need delivery of gaseous or liquid oxygen contents, Medicare will continue to pay each month for the delivery of contents after the thirty-six-month rental period, which means that your loved one will pay the 20 percent co-payment of the Medicare-approved amount for these deliveries.
- The supplier that delivers this equipment to your loved one—if your loved one medically needs them for up to five years—owns the equipment during the entire five-year period.
- If your loved one's medical need continues past the five-year period, their supplier no longer must continue providing the oxygen and oxygen equipment, and your loved one may then choose to get replacement equipment from any supplier.
- A new thirty-six-month payment period and five-year supplier obligation period starts once the old five-year period ends for the new oxygen and oxygen equipment. Your best source to review and educate yourself on oxygen and equipment coverage will be the Medicare government site. In your web browser type in "Medicare and oxygen," and this will bring up the information you may need.

If your loved one will be on oxygen 24-7 and is up and about, discuss with the DME provider the feasibility of having an oxygen concentrator in place of any tanks. This is by far safer. Equally as important, it will have a small unit that can be carried like a backpack that is fillable and with the little unit lasting up to six or so hours. The best part? Such units allow your loved one some freedom to move about and even leave the home for short periods of time.

In your web browser, you can find information on what Medicare covers as stated earlier by typing in Medicare site or if your loved one has private insurance by typing in your web browser the insurance company's name and then the type of oxygen or respiratory equipment you want more information on.

Suction Equipment and Supplies

Suction equipment is a medical device that is considered medically necessary, and as such, it and any supplies are considered medically necessary. Because the machine will require you to rinse the tubing as you suction your loved one, this means once out of the hospital, health plans do not cover a new tube for each time you suction. However, when you have your loved one home, the home health agency nurse will teach you that sterile technique, like what you saw in the hospital, will not be needed in most cases, as you are not spreading germs like what may occur in a hospital. This means you can switch to what is termed clean technique.

The home health nurse will teach you how to care for the suction tubing between uses and how to keep it clean between uses. He will also teach you how to make the saline water you may need as you suction your loved one. Saline water is basically made with boiled water and salt, and once the salt dissolves, it is kept in a sterile jar with a lid you either wash in a dishwasher or boiled. For sterile water, it will be made fresh every twenty-four hours.

What is clean technique the home health agency nurse will teach you? It is basically good and thorough handwashing and maintaining a clean work area as you perform the caregiving task needed.

Patient Lift System

Another item to consider if you do have to assist your loved one and they are total care will be moving and getting up and down with the use of a lift system. While there are now more than the old hand-cranked Hoyer lifts, you may want to consider an electric lift versus one that fits on the ceiling. However, if that is the one selected, this will be only for the bedroom—unless the bathroom/toilet area is large enough or can be modified to accommodate a ceiling lift there as well. As mentioned earlier, as a lift system and the sling are considered, it will be wise to find one with a slit in the seating area to allow ease of going to the bathroom.

Lift Chairs

As you prepare the home for your loved one, you may want to consider a lift chair. This is a recliner that can make into a bed or can allow a person to rise from a sitting position to standing. This type of chair may, in many instances, be covered by Medicare and many health plans, if your loved one's physician will order such and supply the medical necessity need.

Home Dialysis Equipment and Supplies

If you and your loved one decide that doing home dialysis is the option you would like, your loved one's dialysis coordinator can talk you through the requirements you must consider and then have available. This will include not only consideration of where the dialysis will occur (bed or chair) but also—and equally as important—the space required for the dialysis equipment and all the supplies. As a rule, the dialysis provider often recommends storage of a six weeks' worth of supplies.

To do home dialysis, you as the caregiver will be required to have four to six weeks of training before you can assume such care.

Infusion Equipment and Supplies

Diseases commonly requiring home and specialty infusion therapy include infections, gastrointestinal diseases and disorders, dehydration, congestive heart failure, multiple sclerosis, rheumatoid arthritis, hemophilia, immune deficiencies, neurological disorders, and more.

Infusion therapy can either be for the administration of drugs or possibly the administration of nutrition—when your loved one cannot consume or digest food and must have what is termed parenteral nutrition.

For administration of either, your main requirement will be possibly a refrigerator to store the solutions in. Other equipment will be an IV (intravenous) pole to hang the bag from and then storage for any related dressings or tubing that will be needed. To assume any such infusions, your loved one must have a central line inserted before discharge, and you must be trained before you can do them. For any dressing changes, these will often be done by the home health nurse.

Wound Care Equipment and Supplies

The wound care supplies your loved one requires will depend on the type of wound. Supplies can consist of merely gauze and tape and the solutions to clean the area to actual negative pressure wound therapy (NPWT) devices and all the supplies you will need to use the device and make the necessary dressing changes. While the vac is applied and stays on twenty-four hours per day, it will require dressing changes two to three times per week.

NPWT uses a machine called a wound vac, wound vacuum, or pump to help with wound healing. Suction from the machine removes excess drainage from the wound and pulls wound edges closer together. NPWT promotes healthy tissue growth by increasing blood flow to your loved one's wound. NPWT also reduces bacteria that cause infections.

While many of your loved one's dressing changes will be performed by a nurse who specializes in wound care, it is important you have been taught at least some basics of the care prior to discharge. In your training, you should have also been taught how to troubleshoot equipment malfunction, and you may also have been taught what to do if there is excess drainage between scheduled dressing changes.

Diapers and Incontinent Supplies and Catheters

As a rule, diapers and any incontinent supplies are not covered by Medicare, and coverage varies among other health plans. If your loved one has a health plan, check with their customer services department or your loved one's assigned case manager. Medicaid varies from state to state, and in some, incontinence supplies are only covered for elderly, disabled, or children with complex health care needs. Incontinence supplies benefits under Medicaid typically start for children with complex health care needs at the ages of three to four, because that is the age where children usually develop self-toileting skills. To receive incontinence supplies through Medicaid, the recipient must obtain at least one of the following:

1. Physician's prescription with qualifying diagnosis
2. Prior authorization (PA)
3. Letter/certificate of medical necessity (LMN)

One example of a state that covers incontinent products is California, and you can find more information on incontinence supplies at their website and the policy on incontinence supplies.

California's Medi-Cal program provides incontinence products to eligible individuals but has a monthly cap on the amount it allows for such supplies. Medi-Cal covers incontinence supplies when prescribed by a physician for use in chronic pathologic conditions that cause incontinence to the insured individual. These medically necessary items include protective underwear, disposable underpads, bladder control pads, and reusable underwear. For coverage, the individual must be actively enrolled in a California Medicaid plan. Medi-Cal does not reimburse for incontinence supplies for recipients younger than five years old unless incontinence is due to a chronic physical or mental condition, such as cerebral palsy or developmental delay. To receive incontinence supplies from Medi-Cal or a state's Medicaid plan, your loved one must have the following:

- A medical condition that requires incontinence supplies (i.e., autism, diabetes, Down syndrome, Parkinson's disease, etc.).

- Prior authorization (if necessary) and documented proof within the last six months from a physician stating the medically necessary items.
- The estimated amount of incontinence supplies needed per day.

Coverage for diapers and other incontinent supplies is a benefit allowed by a state's DDS services for a developmentally or intellectually disabled person, and dependent upon the state, coverage may be allowed under the state's Children and Youth with Special Health Care Needs program.

Coverage for Urinary Catheters, Tracheostomy, and Other Ostomy Supplies

For all urinary catheters, tracheostomy, and other ostomy supplies, all will be a covered benefit of health plans and Medicare and Medicaid, but each will have specific limits per month on how many can be obtained. Most health plans follow Medicare criteria in what is allowed per month. Since coverage varies by health plan and Medicaid, if you have questions regarding what and how many as well as what other supplies might be covered, it is best to either do a web search or call your loved one's health insurance's member services department as you seek answers.

Note: If the equipment or supplies arrive and they do not fit your loved one correctly or they are not what was ordered, do not sign off on delivery of such. You do not want to accept them if not right. If this occurs, this may delay the discharge, so keep the team aware of any issues.

Another note: As you decide on the equipment needed, especially if it is life-sustaining, make every effort to only rent the items. This will allow the rental contract to cover the costs for the routine servicing such devices require since they run 24-7. This means the items must be basically overhauled every so often, and as part of what is needed, a replacement device will be needed in the interim. If you purchase the devices, this means you are responsible not only for the servicing of the device but also for the rental of the replacement device in the interim.

Violence and Aggression

By all means, discuss your loved one's diagnosis and tendency for violence with his mental provider on treatment options that may be tried. You may also wish to discuss what actions you can take if they have a tendency for violence and punch holes in walls and doors or break windows in their rage. A solution you may want to discuss will be to possibly install plywood or plastic sheeting on the walls and high enough to prevent wall destruction. For windows, you may want to install plexiglass or tempered glass windows; and for doors, consider installing possibly fiberglass or steel doors. For items in the room, consider pillows or soft objects they can throw. Key to whatever you do is to discuss all with the treating provider, as the addition of such could result in your loved one taking their rage out in other destructive ways.

Summary

As you can see, getting the home ready for your caregiving role can take some time to do, and there is a wide variety of things that will need attention. There is so much to consider not only for the care of your loved one but also how to make the care as easy as possible for you. You also will want to get as much as you can done before your loved one comes home, as home caregiving will take over and may be time-consuming.

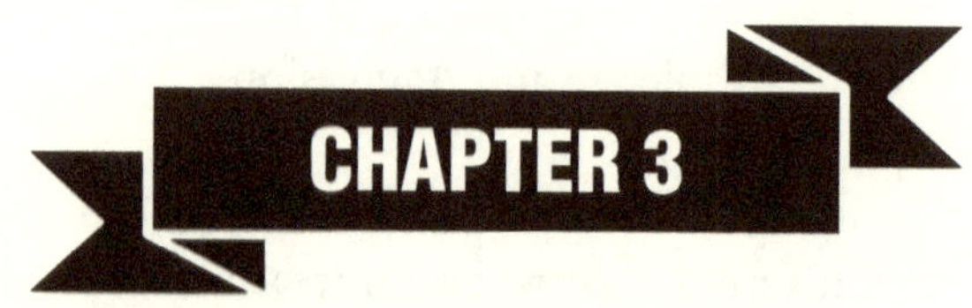

Emergency Preparedness

MOST CAREGIVERS ARE trying to balance their caregiving with other responsibilities at work, at home, and in other areas of their life. This means that while you may already be busy working or being a housewife or a husband doing regular chores, you now have bigger, newer, and more challenging ones added to your plate. So be prepared!

A key as you start this preparation is to, again, keep that notebook or cell phone handy. This will not only allow you to continue to make notes for your ongoing research on various topics, but it will also serve as a helpful reminder of all that needs to be done. Your reminders can then be used as you develop your to-do list.

As with the hospital, you will now be building your posthospital team. This team will include some from your hospital team, but in most cases, your team will change. An example of who to include in your post-acute hospital team may be the following:

1. There are two (2) to three (3) who will continue from your hospital team.

   a. First is the private health plan—if military insurance, TRICARE—case manager. Or if your loved one's illness or injury is work related, your primary contact will be his workers' compensation (WC) assigned caseworker. WC is only available if your loved one's illness or injury is work related, and there is an active claim. If WC is involved, his private health plan will not be involved at all. Private health insurance is only applicable if the WC claim is denied or if a settlement has already taken place.

b. The pharmacists from the main pharmacy that supplies the medications.

c. If English is not your primary language or you have difficulty understanding what is said or if you, like many of us, lack the technology skills needed to use your phone or computer, you will want to have a person who can assist you as part of your team. This is necessary so you can continue your research on topics while allowing you to build your skills so you are an informed consumer or, better yet, your loved one's case manager.

2. Your loved one's primary care or any or all specialty doctor(s) offices or clinics, including any mental health counselors who may have treated him and have indicated they will continue to see him after discharge. While this team member—many times, it's the office manager—may not be the doctor, he will be your link to the doctor if more medical information is needed.

3. If you have enrolled your loved one in any of his state's Medicaid waiver program, such as the HCBS (Home- and Community-Based Services), you will want that case manager as one of your team members.

4. If you have applied for your state's Supplemental Security Income (SSI), your assigned caseworker will be one to add to your team. This person will be your main link to assist you in maintaining or getting the hours and services you may need under any program your state may offer that allows for in-home support services (IHSS) or a personal care attendant (PCA).

5. If you have applied and been approved for any services provided by your state's agency that provides developmental services or any program designed to assist children with special health care needs, you will want to include one or both case managers who will be assigned to your loved one's case.

6. Dependent on the posthospital discharge plan and if the plan is for placement before going home, this may include the discharge planner / case manager or social worker at any or all facilities used. Post-acute facilities are useful when your loved one progresses and has reached a point in their care where they no longer require the care and services provided by the acute care hospital, but they are not at a point where home care may be a safe plan.

Sadly, this list can change if your loved one does not progress or reaches a stage where they no longer meet the guidelines for that level of care. He must then be discharged to possibly a facility designed for long-term care or even home.

So be prepared to keep your team list updated, as it may change, as your loved one may be one of those patients who, as we who work in health care call, must bridge the continuum of care as they move from one facility to the next.

The continuum of care post-acute facilities may be any one of the following:

a. *Inpatient rehabilitation facility (IRF).* This is usually after a major spinal cord or brain injury of other major neurological or muscular disorder.

b. *Long-term acute care hospital (LTACH).* This is often used when a person fails ventilator weaning, and attempts are made to totally wean. Or it may be used for very complex wound care or other complex care beyond what a skilled nursing facility (SNF) or a subacute rehabilitation (SAR) can manage.

c. *Subacute facility.* These are facilities that offer a level of care that is designed to provide comprehensive care to someone who has an acute illness, injury, or exacerbation of a disease process; and they no longer need the diagnostic equipment provided by the acute hospital. While there are more adult subacute facilities available nationwide, there are also pediatric subacute care facilities. These facilities provide a level of care that is needed by a person who is less than twenty or twenty-one (depending on the state) years of age and who requires the uses of a medical technology that compensates for the loss of a vital bodily function. Pediatric subacute facilities vary by state and name (not all are referred to as subacute), and if your discharge planner / case manager or social worker has not given you a list to choose from, you want to do your own investigation and comparison if more than one is in your state. This means, you may be required to call your state's Division of Licensing and Certification (DLC). Or in some states, it may be the Department of Health and Human Services or the Department of Insurance to find out more about such in your state.

d. *Skilled nursing facility (SNF).* In some states, this is referred to as a subacute rehabilitation (SAR).

Others to include in your team might be:

- If the plan is to home directly, this will include at a minimum the home health agency (HHA) or hospice nurse and possibly the nurse attendant and social worker. If linked to hospice and you are religious, this can include the chaplain. It may also include your own religious leader.
- If your loved one's care plan includes durable medical equipment (DME), prosthetics, orthotics, enteral or parenteral feedings, or medical supplies, this will include your point person at the agency from which the items and equipment are ordered.

- While this may seem strange and is a professional used only annually, you need to include a dentist or dental hygienist as part of your team. This professional is critical, especially if your loved one hates it when someone or something touches their mouth or teeth (called sensory defensiveness). Thus, daily brushing and mouth hygiene will be a huge chore, if not impossible. For such dental care, this type of care is termed adjunctive dental care, and it is considered medically necessary. It is then a benefit available under your loved one's health plan. However, this type of procedure does require a prior authorization, as this often requires the procedure to be done in a hospital or outpatient surgery center, where your loved one can be sedated.
- Do not forget your local or online support system buddies. They are and can only be a wealth of information but also, equally as important, a point of contact just to be able to take a short break and talk.

Appointing a Lead Case Manager

One thing to keep in mind as you think of all those who may be on your team is, once home, you will have so many team members, many of whom will be from various agencies, and each will be called a case manager. You must have one of those difficult conversations with all and insist on one of them becoming the lead case manager. This, in many cases, will be the home health agency or hospice nurse. Once it is decided who will serve in that role, they can then be the link for information need on topics, as well as the point person to ensure the right case managers have what they may need to do.

Assigning one case manager as the primary point person will not only help you, but equally as important, it will also help your loved one's doctors and the health plan's case manager so they are not be overloaded with multiple calls for the same purpose. So once your loved one is home and the many case managers are there, you must make this a priority request.

Your To-Do List

Once you have started to develop your team, do not forget to add those family and friends who have volunteered to help. Far too often, we often say, "No, I can manage." This is not the time to be brave and think this way.

If a friend or a family member asks "How can I help?" stop and think and let them know if they can and what task you may need help with. If you have some ideas ahead of time, take time to list the tasks you may need or would like help with, and try to give an approximate time. Let them choose. Then write down who, when, and what they may do.

As you do your list, include all the things that you regularly do (or want to do) in a week and separate out those you will need to do. Your list may include help with caring/playing with your children or transporting them to school or after-school events, maybe even some simple caregiving tasks, preparing a meal, help with tidying up the house, or doing simple yard work. The list will be designed to help you.

Write all these tasks and who has volunteered to help on a separate list. Make sure you keep your list in a visible place, where people who want to help will see what needs to be done. Be sure to include any relevant details that may assist them as they assist you. I have also suggested to families that they then keep a calendar handy so they know if anyone is coming that day or not.

While you can find forms for such online, you can make your own, and it may look like this.

Task	Time of day, week, or month to do it	Name of volunteer	Days and hours they can come	Phone number

Planning and Getting Prepared for Any
Personal Emergency or Crisis

While it may not seem important now, it may be at some point. I have always suggested to families to take time to plan for any unexpected, emergent event and to do it ahead of time. Unlike while hospitalized where staff is available immediately, when home, this is not the case. Preparing ahead of time for a crisis or emergent situation will help ease the stress knowing that you will both be safe and supported.

Think about the situations below and whether you have a plan in place should any of them occur.

- There is a sudden deterioration in your loved one's medical condition.
- Your loved one is on lifesaving equipment, and it fails, and your attempts at troubleshooting are not working.
- There is a prolonged power outage (more than twenty-four hours).
- You are suddenly unable to provide care, whether it is from a temporary or possibly permanent illness or injury.
- Your loved one falls, and you are unable to lift him.
- Your loved one wanders away or gets lost.
- There is a disaster, and you must evacuate the home due to an unexpected event, such as a fire, flood, or fallen tree.

Be Prepared Just in Case There Is a Health Crisis

Included in your plan, you will want to stop and think of all you may need in the event of an emergency. So as was your work on your to-do list, you need to think about emergency planning. As you work on this, one key element will be to make copies of any documents that pertain to health care or financial decision-making. This includes the following:

- Advance directive for health care or your state's Physician Orders for Life Sustaining Treatment (POLST) or Medical Orders for Life-sustaining Treatment (MOLST).
- Financial power of attorney form.
- Copies of any Medicare or health plan identification cards and Evidence of Coverage (EOC) handbooks.
- Make a list of names, addresses, and phone numbers (not only in your cell phone but also on a separate written list) for you and possibly for any key family members or friends or other advocate you feel is needed. If your loved one has a guardian or conservator, include the appointed agent's name and any phone numbers.
- Add other names and phone numbers: your loved one's primary physician, health plan case manager, and home health agency or hospice nurse.

This will help ensure future health care and financial decisions are carried out according to your or your loved one's wishes. It is also useful if questions arise about care; the hospital staff has access to someone who may be able to assist in the situation.

How Do I Prepare for an Emergency?

If there is a disaster in your area that will affect transportation, power, or other essentials, as you prepare for any possible crisis, a great point of contact will be to see what your local American Red Cross may suggest. For more information on how to prepare for emergencies, you can type in your web browser "American Red Cross how to prepare for an emergencies," and the information you need will be there. Their plan is called 1-2-3, and as you will see once in their website, it contains a wealth of information to help you plan.

Another website you may want to use as you prepare your home and loved one(s) for a potential disaster or an unexpected emergency will be the information you may find on the Ready.gov website. With natural disasters occurring as they do, you may also wish to download the FEMA (Federal Emergency Management Agency) weather app on your cell phone. This can help alert you of any bad weather that may be approaching while also allowing you to activate your emergency plan(s).

Plain Old Telephones versus Cell Phones and Emergency Response Systems (PERS) or Medical Alert Response Systems (MARS)

In this day of telephone and computer technology, many of us have discontinued our landline phones (the plain old telephones that sat on a table or nightstand), and we have moved strictly to using handheld cell phones. However, this may not be a wise decision for a caregiver who now is taking care of a loved one whose medical condition can change in the blink of an eye. Or if one occurs during a major storm or disaster and there is a power outage, you will need help immediately. The American Association of Retired Persons (AARP) has a website you may wish to explore to help you make the decision as to what is the correct action for you to take and help decide if keeping a land line phone should be included in your emergency plan.

Thus, as you develop your emergency preparedness plan, you need to consider not only what telephone is best but also what is called a personal emergency response system (PERS) or medical alert response system (MARS). Again, AARP has another educational website you may wish to visit that can help you make the right decision on selection of a medic-alert device. This website covers options and the various types of devices available. To access information, type in your web browser "AARP medic alert devices." Information here should assist you as you make an informed choice.

Alerting the Local Fire and Emergency Response Team

If your loved one will be returning home on lifesaving equipment, even if you elect for lifeline or a medical alert system, one resource you should consider as you set up your emergency preparedness plan will be to contact your local fire and emergency response department. If you place a lockbox on your door, remember to give them the code to open the box should you be alone in the house, attending to your loved one's emergency. By alerting them ahead of time, if a disaster hits, you may need them to respond as quickly as possible.

Dependent upon where you and your loved one lives, you may want to discuss with your local fire department what and how it is going to be best to set up an evacuation plan, especially if you live in a high-rise building. Remember, elevators will not be working, and stairwells can pose the largest obstruction for evacuation. So plan on how to get out.

To help you as you plan for an evacuation event, you may wish to conduct your own research on the topic by searching various websites on the topic. However, two of the best ones will be the Safety. info.com website as well as the National Fire Protection Association (nfpa.org). Both websites contain a wealth of information on a wide variety of disabilities, giving you tips on what to do and consider.

Help During an Emergency

As you create your emergency plan, it is essential you contact and enlist the help of neighbors, relatives, and friends so you have someone who can possibly be available to assist should an emergent event occur. Again, make a list of who may be available to help, including their phone numbers, and have it not only in your phone but also posted in a visible place.

Alerting the Power Company

Regardless of the fact that your loved one may or may not be on life-sustaining equipment, notify your local power company of the fact your loved one is home and disabled. This call can be twofold.

- Ascertain if you and your situation is eligible for any financial discounts.

- Discuss any programs they may have in place for an emergent event.

Do not forget, power is also critical to help keep the temperature in the home right, so see if they have any recommendations you may wish to consider. Remember, in an emergency or disaster, regulating the temperature in the home may not be possible, and there may not be any warning of approaching danger, so make what plans you can ahead of time.

Also, many utility companies keep a priority reconnection service list and map of the locations of power-dependent customers for use in an emergency. Ask the customer service department of your utility companies if this service is available. Note that even if you are on the priority reconnection service list, your power could still be out for many days following a disaster. Thus, it is vital that you have power backup options for your equipment. If none is available, make arrangements for admission to the nearest hospital.

Power for Lifesaving Equipment

Wherever you live, if your loved one will be returning home on lifesaving equipment—this is not limited to breathing machines but can include home dialysis, suction devices, nebulizer, and even the refrigerator if medications must be kept cold—it will be necessary that you see if an alternative source for power may be needed. Again, do your research and make an informed decision on what is best for your situation and area. Absolutely, do not rely on merely the words of a salesperson. Your situation is not to run your refrigerator or other electric devices as a power generator may do.

Your need is to find the right one, one that, if needed, can run for several days. If you cannot afford a power generator or it is not one allowed by your landlord, the only alternative will be to have your loved one taken to the nearest hospital (all hospitals are required by law to have such a plan in place specifically for this purpose). Here your loved one will remain until it is safe to return home. For information on how to plan for emergency power when your loved one is dependent upon electric or battery-operated assistive devices, your best resource will be information you will find on the ADA website at adata.org. Here you can download a checklist of issues you must consider.

Backup Breathing Device

If your loved one will be coming home on life-sustaining equipment for breathing, double-check with his doctor if you should possibly also have a self-inflating resuscitator, a mask attached to a bag to use if the ventilator is not working. An example brand is Ambu. If this is felt wise, ensure you have the hospital train you on how to use it.

If your loved one is an infant, there are three types of devices being used to ventilate this age group: a self-inflating bag (bag valve mask, or BVM), a flow-inflating or hyper-inflating bag (commonly called an anesthesia bag), and an infant T-piece resuscitator. If your loved one's physician agrees this may be needed, ensure the hospital respiratory staff will train you on its use before discharge.

Batteries, Flashlights, and a Plain, Old-Fashioned Battery-Operated Radio

As you are preparing your emergency plan, remember to have an adequate supply of batteries available. Batteries will not only be for such devices as flashlights but also possibly a battery-operated radio. This will allow you to keep on top of any critical information you may need in a disaster for putting your evacuation plan in motion. Unfortunately, batteries, flashlights, and such radios are uncovered benefits of a health plan.

If your loved one has any power equipment (for example, a scooter, wheelchair, or portable suction device), the equipment will come with an extra battery. However, make sure you set up a reminder to ensure it is charged as recommended by the maker.

Monitors, Alarms, or Detectors

As you work on your emergency plan, do not forget to install or, if already installed, adding fresh batteries to any smoke, carbon dioxide (CO_2) or fire alarms, or detectors. If your loved one will be or already is one who wanders, consider the following:

- Install motion detector or bed, window, and door alarm(s).
- Install dead bolts for exit doors.
- A personal GPS (termed a global positioning system) might help.
- In your yard, ensure there is a fence, and any and all gates are locked.
- For windows, there are many types of locks for windows. For example, there are locks that will allow the window to open, but the opening will not be large enough for an escape.
- For doorknobs, look into the possible installation of a doorknob that fits loosely over a regular doorknob. This will allow the knob to turn, but it will not allow the door to open.
- You may also want to post Stop or Do Not Enter signs on doors.
- Some of your best sources for such information will more than likely be from
- The physical therapist working with your loved one.
- To assist you as you plan for how to manage your loved ones if they have dementia and a tendency to wander, you will find a wealth of information on either the Alzheimer's or National Institute on Aging-Dementia websites.
- If you have found a support group, see what they may recommend.

As part of your planning for a wandering loved one, you may wish to consider the following as well:

- Ensure your loved one carries some kind of identification or wears a medical bracelet.
- Alert your neighbors should they see them wandering about.
- Label all clothing, including shoes and any mobility devices (canes, walkers, or wheelchair), with their name and address.
- Keep a recent picture of your loved one in case police or other search groups are to be used.
- Keep an article of clothing your loved one has worn and that has not been washed. This can be used if police or other search and rescue animals are used.
- If you or your loved one is deaf, a resource you may wish to explore or purchase will be a smoke alarm that is designed for the hearing impaired. You can find information on both the National Fire Protection Association (nfpa.org) and the National Association of the Deaf (NAD.org) websites on what might be the best smoke alarm to obtain for the disabled or hearing impaired.

If your loved one has been diagnosed with a developmental or intellectual disability, in their daily life, any change in their routine can trigger an outburst of violence or agitation. If so, this must be taken into consideration as you develop your emergency plan. If an emergency arises, keep as calm as possible, and use any techniques you may have learned in the past for helping to keep him or her calm.

Ready-to-Go Kit

As you prepare your emergency plan, one key thing to include will be a ready-to-go kit for both your loved one and you. This will allow you to grab it when an emergent event occurs, and everything is hurry-scurry.

Your loved one's kit should contain, at a minimum, such documents as the following:

- Picture of them
- Copies of the key legal documents described earlier
- Listing of all his medications, including doses and frequency taken
- Listing of most recent immunizations
- Listing of all allergies, food or others, and typical reactions

As you prepare your kit(s), do not forget to ask your loved one's physician and health plan about ordering and having on hand an extra supply of all medications and medical supplies for your loved one's to-go kit. If this is allowed, then a critical factor to include will be a plan on how you will rotate them, especially if there is an expiration date.

The kit may also contain, of course, possibly slippers and any hygiene items and maybe even an extra change of clothes. If your loved one wears glasses, maybe an extra pair; and for hearing aids, include more batteries or a battery charger. Remember, we all have varying needs, so make attempts to include what they may use on a routine basis. If your loved one has a service animal, do not forget their kit as well.

If your loved one has a developmental or intellectual disability or has dementia and likes a specific item or task to help keep them busy, be sure to include such items (for example, that may be a color book and crayons, stuff to fold, or a specific blanket or toy).

If your loved one has a specific developmental or intellectual disability or mental illness that affects their behavior, you may want to develop something like the following. Remember, this is your loved one, so list the information that you want the hospital to know about him. You can also make it on a bright-colored paper and have it laminated so it can follow him and can then be stored for future use. Your list will describe your loved one, but it may include such as below.

You may want to add a
picture of your loved one.

My name is ____________.
My nickname is ____________.
My birth date is ____________, so I am ____________.years old.
My main diagnosis is ____________.
I speak and understand ____________.
(If deaf or blind, you may add this.)
I am deaf.
I am blind.
(If possible, list how they communicate.)
I can communicate through ____________.
I am allergic to ____________.
I am sensitive to ____________.
(This may be certain smells, certain touches, certain tastes, certain
    sounds, or certain lights.)
I hate it when ____________.
I love it when ____________.
My behavior if I do not like something may be ____________.
(Describe what most often happens—hitting, screaming, hair pulling,
    biting self, having a drop attack, or falling down.)
If you have questions, you can call the following ____________.
(If a conservator or guardian is appointed, include their name and phone
    number.)

Your Own Ready-to-Go Kit

Your kit will carry those items you may use daily either for hygiene and an extra set of underwear and clothing. Make sure you include any medications you may be on. Also, do not forget such items as an extra cell phone charger.

Remember, the kits are specific to you and your loved one's needs. Once assembled, keep them in a designated place and have them ready in case you must leave your home quickly. Make sure all family members and any volunteers know where the kits are kept. Once back home, replenish the kit so it is ready again.

Emergency and Evacuation Plan

As you work on your emergency plan, do not forget to include a plan for a safe emergency evacuation of your home, especially if your loved one is bed confined or has mobility issues. This plan will also be critical if stairs must be used. Thus, your plan must include the following:

- What device or devices are appropriate for your loved one's mobility issues? (Can they walk or not? Are they bedbound due to being in a coma or unresponsive? Do they have multiple neurological or muscular issues that prevent mobility?)
- Who will be your helper?
- How will you exit if a stairway is an issue?
- How will you exit if you live in an apartment or high-rise building?
- If your loved one is exceptionally large or fat, investigate what may be the device—this will be termed a bariatric device—you may need to help move him. If your loved one is exceptionally large or fat, you will need to enlist the help of more than one volunteer. So remember to include their names and contact information on any list you make for the volunteers who may be available to assist you.

For your emergency and evacuation plan, you will want to research what device may be the best to use. In addition to any patient lift or hoist devices you may have to help with the day-to-day caring of your loved one, you will also need to investigate what may be the right device to assist in any emergency evacuation plan. For example, on the market today, you will find such devices:

- An evacuation or escape chair is a device designed for persons who have mobility challenges.

- A transfer or slide sheeting is incredibly useful and incredibly easy to use, as it is designed to be used to aid with the movement and transfer of a patient and to eliminate the need for lifting a patient. Use of this type of device helps ensure the transfer is easier, safer, and more comfortable for both you and your loved one.

- If your loved one is or will be on an alternating air mattress, you may want to consider what is called an evacuation or escape sheet. These sheets are designed to be used with an alternating air mattress. If used, it is permanently fitted under the alternating air mattress. Thus, it is there whenever an emergency may arise.

- If your loved one is not on an alternating air mattress, then research and consider an evacuation mattress. This is a mattress that is designed for persons who would not be able to comfortably get into an evacuation chair or where evacuation chairs may struggle (for example, when evacuating an individual down a spiral staircase). An evacuation mattress will be essential for moving a bedbound or a person who is unconscious or in a coma. Evacuation mattresses are suitable for all types of stairs, including spiral staircases. An evacuation with an evacuation mattress must always be done by two operators. To use this device, your loved one will be strapped onto the mattress using webbed strapping. The feet are placed into the attached foot sack and head secured into the safety headrest, ready for evacuation. The mattress is then easily pulled across the floor and downstairs to a place of safety.

For your research on how and what you may need as you develop your emergency and evacuation plan and what will work in your situation, you may want to visit the following websites:

a. the Centers for Disease Control (CDC) website on emergency preparedness for disability and health as well as the hyperlink to the state-by-state guide to resources for evacuation planning,

b. the Escape Mobility website and information they offer on an evacuation mattresses for a bed confined or disabled person,

c. and any one of the many websites that offer an evacuation or escape chair you may wish to consider.

Summary

Because we never know when a natural disaster will come or when one may become ill and require hospitalization or shelter, it is critical, if your loved one is bed confined or has special needs due to an illness or injury or has a developmental or intellectual disability, to have a to-go kit ready should they be required to leave the home.

CHAPTER 4

Start of Care

AS EXCITING AS it may be, this day and even some immediately following can be stressful and frustrating, not to mention scary. The good news is, depending on your loved one's medical condition, if he, especially if an infant or child, is on very complex treatments or on life-sustaining treatments, the hospital will have made every attempt to ensure either shortly after your loved one's arrival home or at the time of arrival that there will either be a home health or hospice nurse. As a rule, your loved one's medical needs will dictate what type of nurse will be there. So if your loved one will be receiving ongoing skilled care, then the nurse who will meet you will be from the home health agency. In contrast, if it is decided hospice would be the plan, the hospice nurse will be there.

Because this is going to be a busy day, remember to keep your notebook handy so you can write down questions. Or if you are using your cell phone for voice reminders, make sure it is charged. Hopefully, as part of your preplanning and getting the home ready, a neighbor or family member has volunteered to bring in meals. This will allow you to not have to worry about a meal and cleanup. If you find there is a time you can rest, take the time to do that. The whole day and probably many days following can be emotional and, in fact, at times overwhelming. So take the time to express your feelings, and take some deep breaths. And yes, it is okay to cry if you need to.

Remember, it is just as important to take care of yourself as it is to take care of your loved one.

The Important Message from Medicare

As your loved one's discharge approaches, if he has Medicare Part A—this will be the original Medicare plan, a Medicare managed care plan, or TRICARE for Life or if the Medicare plan is the second payer), the hospital is mandated to give you or your loved one if they have decision-making capacity a letter termed the Important Message from Medicare, referred to as the IM letter. This same letter should have been issued within two days of admission and, again, given just prior to the discharge. This letter outlines how to file an appeal if you or they are not in agreement with the discharge and plans. In the body of the letter, it will explain appeal rights and what Quality Improvement Organization (QIO) has the Medicare contract for your loved one's state to handle such appeals.

There are two QIO agencies that serve Medicare and perform the appeals (both for the original Medicare plan and any Medicare Advantage plan your loved one is enrolled in). These two QIOs handle not only any expedited appeals and the processes required, but they also help beneficiaries with complaints or quality of care concerns. The two agencies are KEPRO and Livanta.

If you are unfamiliar with which QIO serves the region in which your loved one lives, you can type in your web browser, keproqio. com or livantaqio.com. Here, you will find not only the information you may need but also the correct phone number.

Not only will the letter tell you who to contact, but the letter will also give you the phone number to call. If you file such an appeal, this type of appeal is termed an expedited appeal, as it is issued during the receipt of care. This means once the QIO is notified of the desire for an appeal, they have seventy-two hours to issue their decision, whether they agree with the hospital and the discharge plan or whether they agree with you that the discharge is not safe.

All sample letters that might be issued to a Medicare beneficiary (original Medicare or a Medicare Advantage) can be found on the Centers for Medicare and Medicaid Services (CMS) website or CMS.gov/BNI website.

If you file an appeal, the hospital is also mandated to send a copy of all your loved one's medical records and also issue another letter. This one is called the Detailed Notice of Discharge (DND). This letter explains in detail the plans for discharge.

During the time the QIO reviews the medical records, your loved one can continue to remain hospitalized without any financial responsibility. However, once the QIO renders its decision, if they agree with the hospital, your loved one's financial liability starts at noon of the day following receipt of the QIO's decision. If they agree with you, your loved one can remain hospitalized until a safe discharge can be set up and you agree.

If you continue to feel the discharge plan the hospital has arranged is not safe, you can file another appeal. However, at this point, if you do file another appeal, you may receive not only another Detailed Notice of Discharge (DND) but also a hospital-issued notice of non-coverage (HINN). If so, the HINN will inform you of any financial liabilities, which is generally a summary of the total hospital daily charges, you or your loved one can financially be responsible for if you continue to oppose the discharge and denial.

Transportation Home

By the time of your loved one's discharged, the hospital discharge planner / case manager will be working with you for setting up the type and mode of transportation. As you work with them, advise them of any steps (how many and where) or hazards or possible obstructions the transportation provider may encounter as they bring your loved one home and into the house.

Depending on your loved one's medical condition, in most cases, he will more than likely be sent home by either gurney or wheelchair van or, in some cases, even by a nonemergent ambulance. Payment for such will depend on your loved one's health plan. For example, if he only has the original Medicare plan and no second health plan, since Medicare does not pay for gurney or wheelchair transportation, this will be a cost he must assume in full. However, Medicaid does cover such for eligible individuals. If it is a nonemergent ambulance and your loved one has the original Medicare, then your loved one will be responsible for 20 percent of the costs.

This initial transportation will be set up by the hospital. Future trips to medical appointments will require you to set them up, and what is set up will depend on your loved one's medical condition. To qualify and have your loved one's health plan pay for the services, your loved one's physician must complete the form termed Physician's Certification Statement of Medical Necessity. This form requires the physician to attest to the fact that your loved one meets the requirements listed on the form.

Other than coming home from the hospital, each time nonemergency transportation is required, you must arrange for the transportation in advance, as the provider must ensure that not only is the physician statement on file but also that a prior authorization from your loved one's health plan is on file for each trip.

The good news is, once an initial Physician Certification Statement of Medical Necessity for NEMT is filled out, the physician can request up to sixty days in advance the need for such when it is known nonemergent transportation will be needed for follow-up medical appointments. An example of requirements for NEMT can be seen from a Medicare Part B administrative contractor, Novitas Solutions, and these requirements can be seen on their website.

Like so many states and its criterion for their Medicaid plan, gurney or wheelchair services require that a prior authorization must be on file. The same will be true for other health plans. The only exception to having a prior authorization on file is the original Medicare plan; no prior authorizations are required. But the claim is subject for retrospective review. This means the claim will be reviewed to ensure the need is medically necessary. If not, the claim will be denied, and the cost of the trip will be your loved one's financial responsibility.

For Medicare coverage and other health plans, when a nonemergent ambulance is needed, your loved one must meet specific criterion to qualify. If he is insured only under the original Medicare plan, coverage for this type of transportation will be paid under Part

B. However, remember, Part B is for outpatient services only. And for such services, your loved one's co-pay will be 20 percent of the costs.

For a full explanation of Medicare and emergency and nonemergency transportation, you can type in your web browser "Medicare.gov/publications," and in the search box type in "Ambulance Transportation," and here you will find a booklet that fully describes Medicare and transportation. If your loved one's insurance is from a private health care insurance company, you can also search the internet for the insurer's policy on transportation.

To assist with transports, most diagnosis-based nonprofit groups can assist with this. Some examples are American Cancer Society, American Heart Association, and American Lung Association. There are many more groups that can be found local to your area by searching online.

Who Might Be at the House

As indicated, your loved one's medical condition and the types of equipment and services he requires will help determine who may be at the home upon his arrival. His medical condition will also help decide how soon the providers and agencies will be there. For example, if your loved one is on life-sustaining equipment or they are deemed terminal and death is near, in most cases, they can meet at arrival or shortly thereafter by either the home health nurse or the hospice agency nurse, at a minimum. If not, services may not start for at least forty-eight hours; and if a long weekend, possibly longer.

In all cases, when a home health agency or placement will be needed for post-acute care, the hospital is required by law to give you a patient choice letter. This letter outlines the providers you have a choice to choose from, all of whom are Medicare-participating providers in the local geographic area.

However, be advised, if your loved one's health plan is a managed care organization (MCO), your choices will be limited to the providers the MCO contracts with. The same will be true if your loved one is under the age of twenty-one and is eligible for your state's Children and Youth with Special Health Care Needs (CYSHCN).

The agency requires providers to be paneled, which means the provider is required to meet specific criterion for treatment of children and young persons. For a listing of programs offered, see the Health Resources and Services Administration, Maternal and Child Health Bureau website.

It is thus important to do your homework and that you know which list you can choose from. If you choose one outside the MCO's provider network or one who is not paneled, care will be denied. This means there may be some very frantic days between discharge and switching of your loved one's care from one agency to opening and start of care by another.

The only exception to this rule will be if the contracted provider is unable to provide the level of care or services your loved one requires, and a noncontracted provider is found that can. In such cases, the MCO and provider, if both agree, can work together, and a letter of agreement (LOA) can be developed for the provisions and payment for the services.

If a home health or hospice nurse is present when your loved one arrives home, do not be surprised if you have a wide variety of health care professionals in the home. These can include, as mentioned, the home health nurse, but it also can include the following:

- The home infusion agency nurse may be there to ensure all equipment and supplies are in place and possibly to ensure any infusion lines are working properly. If it is time for the first dose of home medications, the nurse may administer the medication(s) or solution(s) or watch you as you perform the task.
- The DME company's respiratory therapist will help set up any equipment and ensure it is working correctly or possibly work with you on any additional training.
- If your loved one has a wound vac, the nurse from the wound vac provider may perform the initial home care plan for the wound care or continue training you.
- The case manager from your loved one's health plan or if the illness or injury is work related and your loved one is

eligible for workers' compensation, a case manager may be there as well.

- The case manager if your loved one was deemed eligible for his state's Department of Developmental Services (DDS) or the case manager from your loved one's state Children and Youth with Special Health Care Needs (CYSHCN) program may also be present.
- If your loved one is one who is diagnosed with a serious mental health condition, you may even have a case manager from the division of his health plan that provides the utilization reviews and case management services needed for your loved one's mental health coverage.

Key is, if you have a wide variety of case managers either initially or coming to your home while all for differing reasons, it often helps to have them decide who may serve as the primary case manager for general issues that arise. In most cases, as the home health agency nurse will be in the home the most, it may be wise to have him serve in this role. This helps to have one point of contact for you and your loved one's physician as well. However, every case is different, as well as the situation requiring attention or possible change in orders.

I can recall many years ago during the height of AIDS (acquired immunodeficiency syndrome) epidemic a young lady who was in the end stages. In this case, she had seven case managers, all from different agencies with none of them coordinating any care between one another. The poor husband was so confused, and he frantically called us, the health plan, to see what he could do. He was confused, as with any changes in her condition, he had been instructed to call all seven! We quickly arranged a case conference, and the end result was, one case manager (the home health agency nurse since she would be there daily) was deemed the primary contact for all questions and answers to flow through. Not only was the husband relieved, but so was the attending physician. In the future, when we had a big case such as this one, we always suggested one to assume the lead case manager when possible.

Developing the Care Plan

At a minimum, if the case managers from your loved one's insurer or mental health department and possibly DDS or CYSHCN are present, each will be responsible for developing their own organization's requirements for a care plan. As they do so, make sure they seek your input as a minimum as the plan is developed. Equally as important, it is wise if they collaborate on the development of the plan with any others who may be developing a care plan. This will ensure items or services are not duplicated or gaps are not present and that goals match, and you are not struggling to meet far too many goals. More importantly, any care plan without input from you is worthless. If it is, it is doomed to failure, as it is not your loved one's plan but the organization's!

While each care plan will be developed following the case manager's organization requirements, care plans will include basically four key components.

1. A thorough intake and initial assessment of your loved one's medical condition, as well as the needs for any of the medical conditions listed and what your loved one's physician ordered. As the case manager works with you and your loved one, they will also gather information on a variety of topics, such as past and current health conditions and what health services your loved one used, socioeconomic and financial status, prior living situation and work history, what you do for fun or socialization, your and your loved one's religious or cultural beliefs, and prior cognitive functioning. Another critical element to be collected will be your and your loved one's understanding of the disease and current condition, as well as, if your loved one is cognitively able, their perceived seriousness of their illness or injury and their commitment to compliance to the plan and ability to manage some of the ongoing symptoms or changes, if such are needed.

2. Identification of all services that may be needed to assist with the care and when and how such will be implemented.

3. Identification, by working with you and your loved one, on setting both short-term and long-term goals and the actions that may be needed to accomplish them. As goals are discussed and decided upon, they must be what we in the health care industry describe as SMART. This means they must be specific, measurable, achievable, realistic, and time-bound. As a rule, it is wise to only set no more than three at a time, and as the goals are set, the case manager will also include what actions may be needed to accomplish them. If more than three goals are set at a time or if actions are not listed, you and your loved one can be overwhelmed and disappointed. When you and your loved one have clear goals with realistic actions and time frames for achievement, you will be more often involved and willing to work on achieving them; and if your loved one is involved, they will also be more involved in their own treatment and recovery.

4. Identification of how often your loved one's situation and care plan require monitoring and evaluation to ensure it is progressing as planned. Your loved one's progression or regressing will determine the frequency of the monitoring plan. It is crucial to ensure your loved one is getting his care at the right time and that changes are made as required.

In all cases, a copy of the plan(s) must be given to both you and your loved one's physician(s).

The primary goal of the care plan is to decrease any unplanned hospital admissions, decrease emergency department use, identification of any health services that may be needed, and help limit any out-of-pocket expenses while improving your and your loved one's experience, quality of life, and satisfaction with care.

OASIS

While any one of the case managers will be working on the development of a care plan, once the home health agency nurse has completed any treatments ordered by the physician, the next duty they will perform will be to complete the CMS-mandated form called an OASIS form.

OASIS is the acronym for home health's Outcome and Assessment Information Set, and it is a patient-specific, standardized assessment form to plan care for patients receiving home health services. The instrument is also used to determine reimbursement and measure quality. The Outcome and Assessment Information Set (OASIS) is a comprehensive assessment designed to collect information on nearly one hundred items related to your loved one's demographic information, clinical status, functional status, and service needs.

CMS requires the form to be completed by either the home health nurse or the therapist, and it is done upon admission, discharge, transfer, and change in condition for all Medicare and Medicaid, nonmaternity, and nonpediatric beneficiaries. The data collected is done via direct observation and possible interviews of your loved one or you, as the caregiver. This form is used to calculate each patient's reimbursement rate under the Prospective Payment System (PPS), the payment methodology CMS uses to pay the provider.

Eligibility for Home Health Agency Care

To be eligible for home health agency services, CMS and all other insurers have stringent guidelines that must be followed if payment is to occur. If your loved one has only the original Medicare, coverage for the home health services will be allowed either under Part A or Part B.

To be eligible, your loved one must meet two criteria.

1. Be in need of skilled services as long as the need is part-time or intermittent (part-time or intermittent means a few

hours per day to do the care or a few hours per week). This means care is generally given for about an hour each visit. Do not let the word *intermittent* confuse you and make you feel you will have part-time help. Unfortunately, this is not true. Be prepared that if a home health agency is coming to the home, this means care will be given approximately an hour each visit or the length of time it takes to either perform the actual skilled care services or teach the care to the caregiver. As a rule, most patients are seen approximately three (3) or less times per week.

2. The other criterion is, your loved one must be homebound, which does not mean they are bed confined or bedbound. Homebound means the following:

- Your loved one will have trouble leaving the home without help (like using a cane, wheelchair, walker, or crutches or special transportation or help from another person) because of his illness or injury; and leaving may cause further injury.
- Leaving the home isn't recommended because of their medical condition, and leaving the home may harm or exacerbate your loved one's current medical condition.
- Your loved one is unable to leave the home because it would cause major effort.
- It is important to note that not having transportation, such as owning a car, does not qualify for homebound status.

Examples of patients who may qualify to be considered homebound can include but are not limited to the following:

- A patient on a ventilator or other life-sustaining devices
- A patient who is paralyzed from a stroke and confined to a wheelchair or requires the aid of crutches in order to walk

- A patient who is blind and senile and requires the assistance of another person in leaving their place of residence
- A person in the late stages of amyotrophic lateral sclerosis (ALS) or another neurological disorder and is unable to leave the home
- A patient who has just been discharged after surgery and is suffering from resultant weakness and activities
- A patient with a psychiatric illness that is manifested in part by refusal to leave the home

What Is Skilled Care

Skilled care is defined as care, such as nursing or rehabilitation therapy services, that can only be safely and effectively performed by or under the supervision of licensed professionals or technical personnel, and it is given under the direction of a physician. Basically, it is health care given when skilled nursing or skilled rehabilitation therapy is needed to treat, manage, and observe a medical condition and evaluate the progress. It is only given by written and signed orders from the ordering physician. The primary skilled care can include any one of the following:

1. Intravenous or intramuscular injections and intravenous feeding.
2. Enteral feeding (i.e., tube feedings) and if the feedings are a new treatment.
3. Management of nasopharyngeal and tracheostomy secretions requiring suctioning.
4. Insertion and sterile irrigation and replacement of suprapubic catheters.
5. Application of dressings involving prescription medications and aseptic (sterile) techniques.
6. Treatment of extensive decubitus ulcers (bed sores) or other widespread skin disorder.

7. Heat treatments that have been specifically ordered by a physician as part of active treatment and that require observation by nurses to adequately evaluate the patient's progress.
8. Initial phases of a regimen involving administration of medical gases (oxygen).
9. Rehabilitation nursing procedures, including the related teaching and adaptive aspects of nursing, that are part of active treatment, such as the start of a bowel and bladder training program.

Rehabilitation therapy may not be as intense as it is during hospitalization, but physical therapy will focus on continuing to restore functional mobility so your loved one, if possible, can do some of their own activities of daily living (transfer, bathing, dressing, and grooming) without any falls or injuries. Rehabilitation services are covered only when the services are specific and safe and an effective treatment for your loved one's condition. The amount, frequency, and time period of the services need to be reasonable; and they need to be complex, and only a qualified therapist(s) can do them safely and effectively. Exercises may consist of restoring range of motion (ROM) and possibly techniques to improve mobility and ambulation so that your loved one is no longer homebound and can transition to outpatient therapy.

If an occupational therapist is available, they will continue to work on teaching personal care techniques while a speech therapist will continue with any swallowing or speech techniques started while hospitalized. For therapy services, the services of a physical therapist (PT), speech-language pathologist (SLP), or occupational therapist (OT) are a skilled therapy when the inherent complexity of the service is such that it can be performed safely and effectively by or under the general supervision of a qualified and licensed therapist. To be covered, the skilled services must be reasonable and necessary for the treatment or for the restoration or maintenance of function affected by the patient's illness or injury with the plan of care developed by a qualified therapist, not an assistant. With therapy, reassessments must occur every thirty (30) days. If the treatment is performed by an assistant, a qualified licensed therapist must reassess the patient every fourteenth and twentieth therapy visit.

If teaching you to serve as the caregiver is the primary reason for the home health care, teaching (from the nurse or therapy team) may be for but is not limited to the following:

- Teaching of self-administered injectable medications or a complex range of medications.
- Teaching a newly diagnosed diabetic or caregiver all aspects of diabetes management, including how to prepare and to administer insulin injections, to prepare and to follow a diabetic diet, to observe foot care precautions, and to observe and understand signs of hyperglycemia and hypoglycemia.
- Teaching of self-administered medical gases or other respiratory treatments (oxygen or nebulizer treatments). If your loved one is on a ventilator, teaching will be for all care and techniques to ensure the ventilator is functioning correctly and so you know how to troubleshoot if issues arise.
- Teaching of wound care where the complexity of the wound, the overall condition of the patient, or the ability of the caregiver makes teaching necessary.
- Teaching care of a recent or new ostomy or where reinforcement of ostomy care is needed.
- Teaching of new self-catheterization techniques.
- Teaching of Foley or suprapubic catheter care. If the catheter must be changed, this will be a task traditionally performed by the nurse or, in some cases, the attending physician.
- Teaching of new self-administered gastrostomy or enteral feedings via a percutaneous endoscopic gastrostomy (PEG) tube.
- Teaching of care and maintenance of peripherally inserted central catheter (PICC) or central venous lines and administration of intravenous (IV) medications through such lines.

- Teaching bowel and bladder training when bowel or bladder dysfunction exists.
- Teaching how to perform the activities of daily living (ADLs)when the patient or caregiver must use special techniques or adaptive devices due to loss of function.
- Teaching transfer techniques from bed to chair to ensure a safe transfer and using proper body mechanics if help is needed.
- Teaching proper body alignment and positioning and timing techniques of a bedbound patient and using proper body mechanics.
- Teaching ambulation with prescribed assistive devices (AD) that are needed due to a recent functional loss, and if you are needed to assist, use proper body mechanics.
- Teaching prosthesis applications and care of the device and any gait training.
- Teaching the use and care of braces, splints, and orthotics associated with skin care.
- Teaching the preparation and maintenance of therapeutic diet and possibly hydration limitations.
- Teaching of proper administration of oral medications, including signs of side effects and avoidance of interactions with other medications and food.

Note: If the care and services provided can safely and effectively be given by a nonmedical person, like yourself, and done so without the supervision of a nurse, this care is not skilled nursing care; it is termed custodial or maintenance care.

One key post-acute care need may be laboratory blood draws. If this is the only medical need from the home health agency, this will not be a covered benefit. This means you must make arrangements to have your loved one transported to a nearby laboratory that can perform the services and one in your loved one's health plan provider network.

In addition to the nurse or therapist for skilled care, other home health services can include: a medical social worker and a home health aide to help with any bathing and personal care. In all cases, any care given must be tailored to meet your and your loved one's needs, which includes taking into account your and your loved one's diverse values, beliefs, and social and cultural needs. It also must be given to you in a language you can understand. This means, the provider must use a language interpreter services line when communicating with you if your primary language is not English.

Payment for Care

If your loved one's insurance is from the original Medicare, any home health agency services will be paid by Medicare, and your loved one will not be required to pay any out-of-pocket costs. The only exception will be if the home health agency orders any durable medical equipment (DME) or medical supplies. In this case, if your loved one does not have a second health plan, there will be a 20 percent co-payment for such. If your loved one has a managed care plan or another type of health care coverage, there may be a charge or co-payment for each visit when a health care professional that provides care sees or treats your loved one.

Unlike home health care, if your loved one has the original Medicare, where there are no limits to the number of times and the physician can recertify home care services health plans, this is not true for Medicaid or other health plans. Each will vary with the recertification timeline, as well as the costs per visit. Key is to check with the health plan or read the health plan's Evidence of Coverage (EOC) for recertification and co-payment details.

There are services that are not paid for by Medicare and a health plan. (The main exceptions will be if your loved one has a long-term care policy or their illness or injury is work related.)

- Twenty-four-hour-a-day care at your home.
- Meals delivered to your home. Many communities have a food delivery service, such as Meals on Wheels, that provides meals to shut-ins and the elderly.

- Homemaker services, like shopping and cleaning, that aren't related to your care plan.
- Custodial or personal care that helps you with daily living activities, like bathing, dressing, or using the bathroom, when this is the only care your loved one requires.

Requirements for the Home Health Agency

For your loved one to receive home health agency care, the agency must be one that is Medicare certified, and the services must be ordered by his physician. To have the home health agency's care covered by your loved one's health plan, all of the following conditions must be met:

- Your loved one must be under the care of a doctor, and your loved one must be getting services under a plan of care created and reviewed regularly by a doctor, who has determined that the care your loved one needs requires the specialized judgment, knowledge, and skills of a nurse or therapist. To need this care, your doctor must decide that your loved one's condition will improve or be maintained by the services provided by the home health agency, and the care ordered is reasonable and medically necessary.
- To certify the care, your loved one's doctor must do a face-to-face (F2F) visit either in person or via a video or telehealth with your loved one. The F2F helps determine the type of care required, which may be one or more of the following:

  - Intermittent skilled nursing care (other than drawing blood). Medicare defines *intermittent* as skilled nursing care that's needed for fewer than seven days each week or daily for less than eight hours each day for up to twenty-one days. When skilled care is needed, the services must be performed by a registered nurse or a licensed practical nurse. If care is from a licensed practical or vocational nurse, a registered nurse must supervise the care.

- o The care given will be done by the nurse, or if you have been taught the care, the nurse will observe you to ensure it is being done correctly. Do not be confused if the nurse teaches you differently from what you were taught in the hospital. This means the hospital, to help prevent the spread of germs, will teach care using what is called sterile technique. However, once your loved one is home, in most cases, the technique to use when changing dressings or even suctioning will be called clean technique. This means washing your hands, keeping a clean area to work, and maybe reusing some supplies more than once.

- As mentioned earlier, the doctor ordering the home health services must certify your loved one is homebound.
- If your loved one's care is skilled, then he will qualify for two additional home health agency services. These will be a home health aide to help with bathing and personal care and a medial social worker to help with social or emotional concerns that may interfere with your ability to perform the tasks needed. Both services can be allowed, but as with other care, the doctor must order such. Note: Neither of these nor occupational therapy considered a stand-alone service. Your loved one must have other qualifying skilled needs from a nurse or physical or speech therapist.

Before your loved one starts getting any home health care, the home health agency must inform you if any items or services they provide will not be covered by Medicare and also how much each will cost. This should be explained both by talking with you about it and also in writing. The written notice is called an Advance Beneficiary Notice (ABN). If services will not be covered, the ABN must be given before any services and supplies are given to your loved one.

For more information on home health care, you can visit the Medicare.gov/publication site and in the search bar type in "Home Health," and you will find a booklet that describes what Medicare covers. This site has a vast array of booklets that you may want to download, and it is well worth your time to review this site and choose the documents you find you may need in your caregiver role.

Pediatric Care

If your loved one is an infant or small child and they require very medically complex care for a medical condition, prior to any discharge, your teaching and preparation for the discharge will, in most cases, be far more intensive than that provided for an adult. As a rule, a medically complex pediatric patient may be one who has the following:

1. At least one or more chronic conditions that cumulatively affect three or more organ systems and severely reduce cognitive or physical functioning, such as the ability to eat, drink, or breathe independently, and that also require the use of medication, durable medical equipment, therapy, surgery, or other treatments
2. A life-limiting illness or rare pediatric disease
3. A chronic condition or a serious, long-term physical, mental, or developmental disability or disease, including any of the following: cerebral palsy, cystic fibrosis, HIV/AIDS, blood diseases (such as anemia or sickle cell disease), muscular dystrophy, spina bifida, epilepsy, severe autism spectrum disorder (ASD), or serious emotional disturbance or serious mental health illness

Making Use of a Day Care Center

A resource you may want to explore to help take care of yourself whether your loved one is a child or an adult will be a day care center or, depending on your loved one's medical care needs, possibly a day health care program. Note: There is a vast difference between a day care center and one that is licensed as a day health care center.

1. A day care center is designed to provide care and companionship to persons who need assistance or supervision during the day. This type of center is often referred to as a social program. The main benefit is that it offers relief to you or the family. If nothing else, it will allow you to relax possibly during the time your loved one is at the center or, if you are one who is also still working, to continue working.

2. In contrast will be a day health care center. These centers offer a more intense program and offer health and therapeutic care for persons with a serious medical condition and will provide not only skilled care but also care that may include physical and occupational therapy and administering medication. The intent of the program is to offer some care for your loved one so as to avoid nursing home placement.

As with all health care, states vary as to what is provided at a day care center since not all states license and regulate adult day care centers. Thus, do your homework, as it will be important to learn about the care and types of services provided by the center in your loved one's area. In all cases, it is strongly recommended you visit the center and ask questions. And do not only talk to the staff. If other families are there, ask them key questions too so you will feel comfortable if you use it for your loved one.

While an adult day care center is not covered by Medicare or the Veterans Administration, it may be part of your loved one's Medicare Advantage plan, and it may also be covered by your loved one's state Medicaid plan. Definitely, this will be a benefit allowed by your loved one's Department of Developmental Disabilities. Again, it is dependent upon your loved one's health plan coverage or other coverage for benefits you may have homework to do.

If the day center is for adult day health, this is covered by most health plans, including a managed care plan, the Veterans Administration, TRICARE, and programs that serve Children and Youth with Special Health Care Needs. This is also a level of care that is often a benefit if your loved one has a long-term care insurance plan. However, a word to the wise, to use the long-term plan, many require a waiting period of sixty to ninety days in advance of getting or paying for any services.

States vary with the coverage they allow for a child under the age of twenty-one who needs a pediatric day health care center. To find such in your loved one's community will be to call 2-1-1, or if your loved one is eligible for developmental disability services or the state's CYSHCN, the case manager assigned to his case can help you locate and get your child enrolled.

Hospice and Palliative Care

Starting hospice is one of the hardest decisions we have to make, as the reality that death is possibly near is now a fact. Thankfully, in today's health care arena, we have many choices about the health care services we receive. Over the years, we have had some end-of-life choices, including the support needed, with hospice and palliative care being two. Both have a purpose, with palliative care focusing on providing relief of pain and symptom management for a wide variety of illness and is not limited to helping during the last six months of life, when curative treatments are no longer an option.

The goal of hospice care is to improve the quality of your loved one's last months, weeks, days, and hours by working with a team of professionals to provide comfort and dignity during the end stages of life. Hospice addresses all distressing physical symptoms, with a special emphasis on controlling your loved one's pain. Equally as important, it provides the emotional, social, and spiritual impact of the disease not only for your loved one but also for you and any family members or friends. Thus, the focus of hospice care will be on you and your loved one, and this will include a variety of bereavement and counseling services for you and your family members for up to a year after your loved one's death.

Like hospice, palliative care is a field of medicine that specializes in providing relief from pain and teaching how to manage the symptoms of a serious illness and how to cope with the side effects from medical treatments. The availability of palliative care does not depend on whether your condition can be cured, and it is not designed to be time-limited. In contrast, hospice is designed to help the patient and family during a minimum of the last six months of life.

Unfortunately, many elect to enter a hospice program too late and do not receive all the benefits traditionally allowed. Sadly, this fact is supported by the National Hospice and Palliative Care Organization (NHPCO) in a report they did in 2021. This report indicated that only 10 percent of Medicare beneficiaries received hospice care for two days or less in 2019. Twenty-five percent of beneficiaries received care for five days or less, and 50 percent received care for eighteen days or less.

These very short length of stay (LOS) in hospice are unfortunate, as they are definitely too short a period of time for patients and families to fully realize the benefits the program is designed to provide. Hospice is a person-centered, interdisciplinary team approach to care and offers a wide variety of services when the program is selected. So if time allows, work with the health care team and get your loved one enrolled in a program as soon as possible. Not only will they have the care and services they need to remain as comfortable and pain free as possible, but you will also have the emotional and grief support you need during the time your loved one is in hospice. Equally as important, you will have the bereavement support you need after his death.

Choice of Agencies

As with the home health agency or other providers your loved one may need at discharge, the hospital is mandated to give you choice in the selection of the agency to perform the hospice services. As mentioned above, for home health agency care, the agency selected must be a Medicare-participating provider; and if your loved one has a health plan that is not Medicare, the provider must still be a Medicare-participating provider. Equally as important, it should be one that is contracted with your loved one's health plan. If not, care will be denied, and the financial obligation will be placed onto your loved one.

If the health plan has more than one hospice agency in its network, then you can use the Medicare.gov compare website to help in your selection. Another option will be to discuss this with other health care professionals or even friends who have used such in the past as to which one they worked with and were satisfied with the care and services received. To help you choose a hospice, you can also use the questions found on the Medicare.gov hospice checklist website.

Pediatric Hospice Care

Children with special care needs who are terminal will not only possibly have a larger amount of care needs than an adult. Equally as important will be to ensure you are mindful of your emotional needs and ask for help. It is also important to ensure respite is included in your child's plan of care or as the case management plan is developed.

Key as you select the hospice provider will be, as I am advising you throughout this book, familiarizing yourself with the types of services you can expect from the provider. The hospice will be no different. Hospices that participate with Medicare will offer the same basic services, as each provider must offer services in accordance to Medicare regulations.

For more information on hospice, you can use the CMS.gov/publications website and in the search bar type in "Hospice Care." Here you will find a booklet that explains hospice care benefits. These regulations outline what a hospice must minimally provide to patients enrolled in hospice under Medicare. The Medicare rules have been adopted as an industry standard. Thus, the rules apply to all patients under hospice care regardless of insurance coverage. If for some reason the agency is not a participating provider for Medicare, do not use them, as your loved one's claim for payment of such will be denied.

If time permits, it may make sense, like much of what you are doing as you prepare for your role, to explore the hospice options available in your loved one's geographic area. Always take the time to ask questions, and by all means, if you have a choice, pick the one you feel comfortable with. I always advise the families I work with to bring someone with them so both of you can pay attention and make notes.

Also, let your instincts help you decide what will be the right agency to meet your loved one's and your own needs. If the agency marketing representative is trying too hard to sell you on their agency, all I can say is, listen to your instincts. Once you have selected the hospice agency, let your hospital discharge planner / case manager or social worker know who you wish to be the provider. Once enrolled in hospice, the hospice benefit covers all costs related to your loved one's care.

Enrollment

To get your loved one enrolled in a hospice program, only the hospice doctor and your loved one's regular doctor can certify he is terminally ill and has a life expectancy of six months or less. After six months, your loved one can continue to get hospice care as long as the hospice medical director recertifies (at a face-to-face meeting) that your loved one continues to meet the criterion for hospice services to continue.

At one point, this meant a face-to-face had to be done in a physician's office. However, many changes have occurred in health care since the COVID pandemic. One of them has been that the face-to-face (F2F) requirements to help decide on a benefit are now more relaxed for most health plans. The good news is, Medicare and most health plans now allow an F2F visit to be performed using audio or visual telehealth. The bad news? If your loved one's primary insurance is Medicaid, many states still require an on-site F2F visit with the doctor. If you are in doubt about your loved one's Medicaid requirements, your best resource on this topic will be to contact your local area's state hospice association. To find a hospice agency in your loved one's area you can find one on the National Hospice Locator website.

The Election Statement

Before a hospice care team can step in and begin to help the family, the terminally ill person must state in writing that it is their intent to seek palliative care instead of curative care. This means that all care will now focus on improving quality of life and relieving pain rather than on life-prolonging treatments. For cases when the terminally ill person is unable to communicate or make decisions regarding their own treatment, the person holding a medical power of attorney, often a close family member, can make medical decisions on their behalf and initiate the hospice request.

This written statement is known as the Hospice Election statement and it must include:

- Identification of the particular hospice that will provide care to the patient.
- The patient's or representative's, as applicable, acknowledgment that the patient has been given a full understanding of hospice care, particularly the palliative rather than curative nature of treatment.
- The patient's or representative's acknowledgment that the patient understands that certain Medicare services are waived by the election.
- The effective date of the election, which can be the first day of hospice care or a later date but cannot be a retroactive date.
- The patient's or representative's designated attending physician, if they have one. Include enough detail to clearly identify the attending physician. This may include but is not limited to the physician's full name, office address, or National Provider Identifier (NPI).

- The patient's or representative's acknowledgment that the designated attending physician was their choice.
- The signature of the patient or their representative.
- Information about the holistic, comprehensive nature of the Medicare hospice benefit.
- A statement that although it would be rare, there could be some necessary items or services that will not be covered by the hospice, because the hospice has determined that these items or services are to treat a condition that is unrelated to the terminal illness and related conditions.
- The statement would also include information about possible beneficiary cost-sharing for hospice services.
- Notification of the beneficiary's or representative's right to request an election statement addendum that includes a written list and a rationale for the conditions, items, drugs, or services that the hospice has determined to be unrelated to the terminal illness and related conditions; and that expedited advocacy is available through the Beneficiary and Family Centered Care-Quality Improvement Organizations (BFCC-QIO) review if the beneficiary or representative disagrees with the hospice's determination. If you recall, we have previously discussed the two QIOs (Kepro and Livanta) that are available to assist you on any Medicare appeals or to address quality issues. So if you have a quality concern, contact your loved one's QIO directly.

By signing this form, this means that all care will now focus on improving quality of life and relieving pain rather than on life-prolonging or curative treatments. For cases when your loved one is unable to communicate or make decisions regarding their own treatment, this means, as stated earlier in this book, an advance directive was done, and you or whoever is named to be your loved one's proxy for decision can be the one making the choice to start hospice.

Note: Even if you or your loved one elects hospice now, it can be stopped at any time. This may happen when life expectancy improves or when new treatments become available, and you wish to try some possibly curative treatments.

The Plan of Care (POC)

All hospice care and services offered to you and your loved one must follow an individualized written plan of care (POC), which will be based on the orders of your loved one's attending doctor and will meet your loved one's specific needs. Once your loved one is assessed, the hospice team working with you and your loved one and his attending physician will establish what is called the POC.

Your loved one will be eligible for hospice if they have been diagnosed with a terminal illness and given a life expectancy of six months or less should the disease run its expected course. To be eligible does not require your loved one to be bedbound. As the POC is developed, the hospice medical director must agree with your loved one's doctor and his assessment on the need for hospice.

As the case is reviewed, three things will be taken into consideration that will validate that hospice is the right choice.

1. Despite treatment, your loved one is showing no improvement.
2. Your loved one's primary goal is to be as pain free and as comfortable as possible, and seeking a cure is no longer the important issue.
3. Your loved one has had an acute health event that has resulted in possibly one or more of the following:

   - Frequent hospitalizations in the past six months.
   - They are not able to be sufficiently hydrated or nourished, or their appetite is decreasing, or they have trouble swallowing, resulting in a significant weight loss (10 percent or more) within the past three to six months.
   - They have had a change in mental, cognitive, and functional abilities.

- Inability to complete daily tasks, like eating, bathing, dressing, or walking, due to weakness or fatigue.
- Recurring infections or increasing pain.
- A desire to stop treatment or to not go to the hospital.

What Services Are Provided Under the POC?

The initial home visit usually takes about one to two hours. Prior to the visit, to help keep the time of the visit not too tiring and help the nurse as the POC is developed, he will have reviewed your loved one's medical record, as this allows the nurse case manager to concentrate their time doing the following:

- An assessment of your loved one's medical condition and asking a variety of questions, at a minimum to include information about your loved one's ability to move about, sleep, their appetite, any weight loss, recurrent infections, and reasons for recent hospitalizations.
- A review of your loved one's medications. This means they will go over with you the names, dosages, and frequency of administering your loved one's medicines. He or she will also compare that list against what was ordered at the time of discharge, and if there are issues found, the ordering physician will be notified of the differences and, if changes are needed, the meds to be delivered overnight or as soon as possible.
- A review with you of the types of hospice services available beyond medical care. This includes any social work and counseling services, assistance with advance care planning, the fact that a home health aide will be available to help with bathing and personal care, chaplain services, the possible availability of pet therapy, and as mentioned, the delivery of medical equipment, like walkers or shower chairs, that can help with the care needs.
- If for some reason the hospice nurse is unable to get out to the home within forty-eight hours and the patient and

caregiver are in need of immediate contact, sometimes, the medical social worker assigned to the team can come out first and do a preliminary case open prior to the nurse's first visit.

Hospice care generally includes the following:

- Any physician visits related to your loved one's medical care, and any orders written will focus on pain control and symptom management.
- Basic nursing care and even therapy (physical, occupational, or speech) services if the need is identified and are given following written orders from your loved one's physician and agreed upon by the hospice medical director.
- Durable medical equipment, such as a bed or other devices, to help your loved one move about or those needed for pain relief and symptom management.
- Medical supplies, like bandages or catheters.
- Drugs for pain and symptom management.
- Aide and homemaker services.
- Access to a member of the hospice team twenty-four hours a day, seven days a week.
- Counseling and social support to help you and your loved one, including any immediate family, deal with any psychological, emotional, and spiritual issues.
- Guidance with the difficult but normal issues associated with accepting that end of life is imminent.
- A break (respite care) for caregivers, family, and others so you all can take care of yourselves.
- Volunteer support. Volunteers may do things such as prepare meals or run errands or may do light housework.
- Counseling, social services, and spiritual grief and bereavement support for you and your family to help you grieve. In most hospices, this also includes therapy and support to any minors who are involved with the patient, some examples being music or art therapy.

- Dietary counseling.
- Short-term inpatient care for pain and symptom management.
- Inpatient respite care to give you a break.
- Bereavement follow-up and counseling for all friends and family involved in the patient's care for one year after the loved one's death.

What Is the Cost of Hospice?

When under a hospice program, once you and your loved one made the choice for hospice, hospice pays for all care and services other than those listed below.

- If your loved one has medications and the medications are for the terminal disease, these medications will be paid by the hospice benefit and not from a Medicare Part D plan or your loved one's health plan. If the medications will not be covered, someone from the hospice agency will tell you which ones are not covered, and they or you must contact the health plan to find out why.
- If your loved one continues with care that is not related to his terminal care, then medications taken for that condition will be paid from Medicare Part D or your loved one's health plan pharmacy benefit. For these, he remains responsible for any co-payments for these drugs.
- If your loved one is admitted to an inpatient hospital for respite and you can have a break, there will be a 5 percent co-pay of the Medicare-approved amount for the stay, with the amount needed for the stay not more than what would have been the deductible for the year.
- If for some reason an inpatient stay is needed in a skilled nursing facility and there are no skilled needs, then the financial responsibility of paying for room and board and possibly other charges will not be covered by hospice, and you or your loved one will be responsible for such charges.

Your Team

You and your loved one and any family members are the most important part of a hospice team. At this point, the team serving your loved one will include the case manager from your loved one's health plan and, if your loved one is developmentally disabled, the case manager from your loved one's agency assigned to provide DD services. The same applies if your loved one is a child or youth and is eligible for his state's Children and Youth with Special Health Care Needs program. Added to these professionals will be any one of the following from the hospice agency:

- The hospice physician
- Nurses or nurse practitioners
- Social worker
- Pharmacist
- Physical and occupational therapist
- Speech-language pathologist
- Hospice aide
- Volunteers
- Chaplain

While the hospice team will be led by the hospice doctor, you can also choose to include your loved one's regular doctor as the attending medical professional who supervises your loved one's care. The same with the chaplain. If you have your own religious leader, you can certainly use them in place of the hospice chaplain.

Hospice Benefit Periods

The hospice benefit is designed for persons with a life expectancy of six months or less, if the illness runs its normal course. If your loved one lives longer than six months, they can still remain in the hospice program as long as the hospice medical director or other hospice doctor recertifies that your loved one is terminally ill. You also will have the right to change hospice providers should you not be satisfied with the current provider.

The hospice benefit is allowed to provide care for two ninety-day benefit periods, followed by an unlimited number of sixty-day benefit periods. After the first ninety-day period, the hospice medical director or other hospice doctor must recertify that your loved one remains terminally ill, and they can continue with the hospice program.

However, if your loved one's health improves or they go into remission and hospice is no longer needed, your loved one will be discharged (or graduated) from the program.

Hospitalization Once in Hospice

If hospitalization is needed for the terminal care, it often is for the management of pain or symptoms or to give you a break. In simple terms, if it is to give you a break in your caregiving role, such is termed respite care. If respite is needed, the hospice agency will arrange for this, and it will be provided at no cost to you or the family. If respite is needed, Medicare and health plans will cover up to five days, during which your loved one will be admitted either to a hospital or skilled nursing facility.

If hospitalization is needed and it is related to your loved one's terminal illness and reason for hospice, the hospice provider must make the arrangements. The cost of the inpatient hospital care is covered by your loved one's hospice benefit, and thus, any charges will be paid to the hospital by the hospice provider via the contract the hospice provider and hospital have in place. However, be advised, if you take your loved one to the hospital and the hospice provider doesn't make the arrangements, this will be your financial responsibility. In most cases, this will mean you are financially responsible for all charges.

Care Needed When Not Related to the Terminal Condition

If your loved one has a medical condition that arises and it is not related to his terminal condition that qualified them for hospice, you can make the arrangements to take him to the emergency room for possible admission, all of which can be done without the hospice agency's involvement. Thus, after your loved one's hospice benefit starts, he can still get covered services for conditions not related to their terminal illness. For example, your loved one has a diagnosis of a brain tumor. But suddenly, he develops severe abdominal pain, and imaging reveals they have found gallstones. Any costs related to the treatment of the gallstones are definitely not part of your loved one's brain tumor or reason for hospice and terminal care. This means the care and services needed to treat the gallstones will be covered but under your loved one's health plan. In cases such as this, your loved one's out-of-pocket expenses will be whatever the deductible and co-payments would normally have been.

Stopping Hospice

As stated earlier, you always have the right to stop hospice care at any time. If you choose to stop hospice care, you'll be asked to sign a form that includes the date the care of your loved one care will end. Stopping hospice care is a choice only you can make, and you shouldn't sign or date any forms until the actual date that you want your loved one's hospice care to stop. Key pointers when you stop hospice are the following:

- If your loved one had a Medicare Advantage plan or other health plan, notify them of the fact you have decided to not continue with the hospice program for your loved one. To do so, you will need to give them the notice you signed, stopping the hospice benefit.
- If your loved one has a Medicare Part D plan, they likewise will need a copy of the notice you signed to stop hospice services. Otherwise, you may receive denials for any prescriptions filled.

Hiring Help

If you have the finances to do so, you may want to consider the possibility of hiring help to help you with the care of your loved one. This care will be in addition to the care or services being provided for your loved one from either the home health agency or hospice agency. Hiring help can definitely help you conserve your own energy and help ease the burdens of caregiving. The hours you need help and the level of the professional hired will depend upon what you plan on having them do and how many hours per day they will work.

Hired help, especially if care is to help with any custodial care (bathing, housekeeping, and meal preparation), is not a benefit of any health plan. Thus, it is only reimbursed through private pay arrangements with the caregiver or agency. Below are the other options for payment.

- If your loved one qualifies for SSI (Supplemental Security Income) and has hours allocated for in-home support services or a personal care attendant (IHSS or PCA).
- Has a long-term care (LTC) policy.
- The Veterans Administration offers a variety of programs to help pay for hired help in the home. You can find a wealth of information on the VA.gov caregiver website. This same website also has links to other resources you may want to explore, and you will find that on this weblink listed under Support Veterans Topics.
- If your loved one is eligible for his state's developmental or intellectual disability services.

If more care is needed outside what the home health agency provides and the care is skilled, you may want to explore what will be available to help cover the costs by working with the case manager from the following:

- Your loved one's workers' compensation plan.

- Your loved one's health plan, including TRICARE. Skilled care of this type is often only covered in lieu of hospitalization. Coverage for this will only be allowed under the health plan's extra contractual process, as without the extra help, your loved one will require placement in a long-term acute care hospital, a subacute hospital, or a skilled nursing facility if it can provide the level of care needed.

Under federal law, for children under the age of twenty-one, if your loved one requires skilled nursing care beyond what is provided by the home health agency, such care can be provided under the state's EPSDT (Early and Periodic Screening, Diagnostic, and Treatment) program. For information on the benefits allowed under EPSDT, you can find all on the Medicaid.gov EPSDT website.

Hiring help can relieve you of some of the tasks you are responsible for, freeing you to have some time for yourself, catch up on sleep, or socialize with family or friends. It is also helpful for long-distance caregivers or those who continue to work while also serving as the caregiver. Hiring help can provide the added care and assistance your loved one needs when you cannot be there to perform the care yourself.

Note: As you think about hiring a caregiver, you will need to take into consideration your and your loved one's needs. Some areas to assess may be the following:

- Personal care (bathing, eating, dressing, toileting, and grooming)
- Household care (cooking, cleaning, laundry, and shopping)
- Health care (medication management or taking your loved one to physician appointments or any outpatient services, such as physical therapy)
- Emotional support (companionship for you or performing meaningful activities with your loved one)

If the care needs are more custodial—bathing or personal care—or for household duties, your costs will be in the eighteen- to twenty-dollar range per hour, compared to what it will be if technical skilled nursing care by a registered or licensed vocational nurse is provided. For nursing care, the range can be much higher and will depend on the state's and the agency's rate for the nurse and other costs they must cover. If you use an agency, they often require a four-hour minimum for the help you hire.

While it may seem cheaper to hire caregiver staff on your own, there are many drawbacks to this. If you hire on your own, this means you are responsible for hiring, firing, and supervising, as any employer may be required to do. You are also responsible for payroll taxes, workers' compensation insurance, and unemployment insurance. Worse is the fact that if the caregiver is sick or doesn't show up or if they want vacation time or time off, you have no one to replace them. The same applies if they start work, and then you find they do not have the skills to perform the care. This means you must then terminate them and start the hiring process all over.

If you do hire on your own without using a placement agency, by all means, do a background check. This means that as you interview them, request references you can call, and verify if they are able to do the care needed, how satisfied they were, if they were reliable, and other critical issues you may want to explore.

As you do your homework on hiring caregivers, your best websites to search will not be those that are advertising their services and thus are a for profit agency, but center your search on such sites as:

- American Association of Retired Persons (AARP) and Caregiving
- The Caregiver Action Network
- National Institutes on Aging and Caregiving
- Area Agency on Aging and Caregiving
- Department of Health and Human Services and the Administration on Aging and Caregiving

In addition to doing a background check, you will also want to validate that your homeowners insurance had medical coverage should someone be injured on your property. A word to the wise, use your instincts as you interview, and investigate anyone you hire privately.

You can still be misled, and this brings me to my own story. I was one of the first nurses in Sacramento in the early 1970s to suspect Dorothea Puente of possible patient deaths. She was always prim and properly dressed and was so doting on her clients. We all would say, "Gosh, too bad others don't have a caregiver such as Dorothea." To help you understand what happened, her patients before she was finally arrested for murder were single people without nearby family. Later, we found out she always had them sign over their Social Security checks. As doting as she appeared, her patients were always near death when admitted.

It was during the hospitalization of a patient that I was informed by an Adult Protective Services (APS) worker of the fact that our local APS office had been monitoring Dorothea for some time. It appears they had been alerted by another state of the fact they were investigating her for possible digitalis poisoning of her husband. However, charges were never filed, as he had been cremated before charges could be filed, and Dorothea had skipped town.

In this call, I was alerted to call our patient's physician of such. Sure enough, when I notified our patient's physician, laboratory tests were drawn, and the results were positive for high levels of digitalis in her blood. Unfortunately, Dorothea slipped town before APS and the authorities could arrest her. This same scenario occurred a few years later, when another patient was admitted with digitalis poisoning. Again, we found out Dorothea had skipped town. She was finally arrested several years later when bodies were found buried in her backyard. So be careful. You never know.

Summary

Two of the most important home care services your loved one or you have an option to choose from will be home health agency or hospice care. Each has their own purpose and criterion for the services they provide. However, each can be invaluable to help you in your caregiver role. This is especially true if you are not in a position to financially afford a home health aide to help with the bath and personal care your loved one will require.

As with all health care, to be a Medicare-certified provider, the Centers for Medicare and Medicaid Services has stringent regulations designed specifically for the care and services the individual provider must follow. These are called the conditions of participation, or CoPs. To help you find the right provider that will help you in your situation, make use of the questionnaires and tools available online as you make your choice.

The costs associated with each service will vary. For home health, as this care is considered outpatient care, in most cases, you will find your or your loved one's out-of-pocket costs will be 20 percent if there is no secondary health care plan to help pay the bills. For hospice, most cares are provided either at a very low out-of-pocket cost (in some cases, it may be five dollars), or there will be no charges. However, if you elect to get care for the terminal condition outside the hospice benefit, the services will be denied and your or your loved one's financial responsibility. Again, with hospice, if your loved one has a medical condition that arises that is not related to the terminal medical condition that qualified him for hospice, your loved one's health plan or Medicare will pay for such care. Hospice will also not pay for any care they do not arrange. So work closely with the hospice agency to minimize any costs.

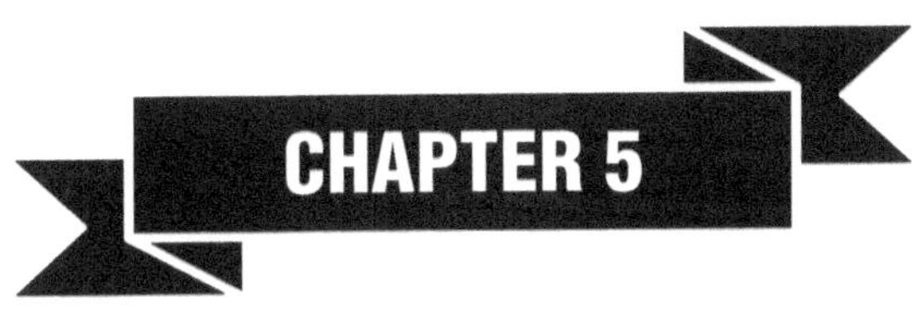

End of life—Planning and Caregiving

THE TERM *END of life* refers to the support and medical care given during the time surrounding your loved one's approaching death. While you may feel this means care only in the moments leading up to your loved one's death, when breathing ceases and their heart stops beating, it does not. Many people live with chronic or catastrophic illness or injuries often for years or months before death occurs, and while death, in most cases, is not wished, it may be in some instances, especially as you see your loved one progressively get worse and possibly have a prolonged period of suffering.

History of End-of-Life Battles

As you may recall, over the past many years, there have been some court cases that centered on end of life for several people when the family was in conflict over what to do, or they were in disagreement with the medical team's recommendations. Probably the ones that come to mind will be Karen Ann Quinlan in 1985, Nancy Cruzan in 1990, and then Terri Schiavo in 1990–2005. All three were young women whose families and medical teams did not agree on allowing their loved one to die.

In two of the cases, Karen Quinlan and Nancy Cruzan, both families wanted their loved one to have their life-sustaining care discontinued, and the medical team disagreed. Both cases ended in a court battle with both families winning their case. However, it was the Cruzan case that set the stage for what is now the right to die. For more information on a surrogate's right to terminate life-sustaining treatment you can view such on the American Medical Association's website.

In the Terri Schiavo case, she collapsed in 1990 after a cardiac arrest and suffered severe, irreversible brain damage due to lack of oxygen. Her husband argued she would not have wanted prolonged artificial life support, but in contrast, her parents said she would. The case went to court, and the battle of what to do dragged on for fifteen years with her finally dying in 2005, thirteen days after the final removal of her feeding tube.

Hospitalized as End of Life Approaches

While your loved one may be hospitalized when his end of life comes and there is no advance directive of his wishes, you may be faced with the decision of ending any life support, which refers to any combination of machines that is keeping your loved one alive as their own organs have failed or shut down. When such a discussion must take place, this conversation may include your loved one's attending doctor, as well as the unit social worker and possibly even the hospital chaplain. All will be present to give you the information and support you need as you make an informed decision about withdrawal of life support.

This decision will more than likely be one of the hardest decisions you have to make. Critical at this time will be the fact that the health care team is talking and guiding you, as testing has already proven the part of your loved one's brain that controls life has ceased functioning. Once this happens, there is no recovery. If you cannot make the decision to remove the life support, while your loved one will have their body there, medically, they are not. It is the machine that is performing and making it appear they are alive. In cases such as this, the decision is then often a prolonged one, as it is one that must be made either by the hospital ethics committee or even by a court of law.

You may ask, what are ethics, and what is an ethics committee? Ethics are, simply stated, the rules that help direct our lives and help us decide what is good or bad. An ethics committee is made up primarily of the physician leader for the hospital; other doctors from such hospital departments as medicine, surgery, or psychiatry; the medical director over the palliative care team; the hospital administrator; the social worker; the chaplain; the chief nurse; the director of quality; the hospital director of risk management; and community representatives, such as a lawyer or someone with advanced training in ethics who specializes in theology or philosophy. The goals of an ethics committee are to basically

1. promote the rights of patients,
2. help with case consultations and decision-making when there are differences in what to do, and
3. promote fair policies and procedures to help achieve good, patient-centered outcomes.

Several years ago, the physician consultant I was working with and I were asked to do a presentation on the problems facing advancing ages, including those who were classified as the developmentally and intellectually disabled. The following are some of the excerpts of what we prepared to present. Unfortunately, with the COVID pandemic, this presentation was placed on hold. But some of what we planned to discuss is appropriate to include now as I do this chapter on end of life.

In this discussion, we were going to present the fact that we are seeing so many advances in medical technology and improved care techniques. This means our population is seeing many elderly people living far longer than in the past. Included in this group are the developmentally and intellectually disabled and their aging caregivers. With this increase in longer life, we are seeing the following:

*   There are more persons with dementia, persons with multiple chronic medical conditions, and persons who are living with what is termed the frailty syndrome. Frailty is

not a disease but a combination of the natural aging process combined with a variety of chronic medical problems, causing an increased risk of declining health and bodily functions. Frail older adults are at increased risk of falls, disability, hospitalizations, and death. Frailty symptoms include generalized weakness, exhaustion, slow gait, poor balance, decreased physical activity, cognitive impairment, and weight loss. Thus, the management of frail patients must be individualized, and this category of patients is those most appropriate to benefit from palliative care and the support and symptom control offered.

- There is an increase in deaths related to heart disease, cardiovascular disease, Alzheimer's disease, chronic lung disease, diabetes, and accidents. Any one of these can cause problems with swallowing and choking, which then leads to aspiration pneumonia or, if bed or chair confined, possible sepsis from bedsores or from a urinary tract infection often due to incontinence. (Most often, this can be from improper care after your loved one pees or poops and is not cleaned properly or if they require a catheter—a little tube inserted into the bladder—to drain urine or pee. For men, this often is due to a medical condition called prostatic hypertrophy—enlarged prostate, which obstructs pee from passing.)

As end of life approaches and the medical team asks you to have that difficult conversation with your loved one or possibly to make the decision for them, as you are the proxy or your loved one's agent. Here are some questions you may wish to ask the team.

- Explain to me why this is necessary.
- Are you doing all you can?
- How uncomfortable will my loved one be?
- Will my loved one be in pain?
- What can be done for the pain?
- If you withdraw treatment, how long will it take to die?

- What might we expect to see happen in the next few hours, days, or weeks if we continue the current course of treatment?
- Will treatment provide more quality time with me or the family?
- Tell me what to expect if we go home and provide the care. Who will help us?
- What happens when my loved one stops eating or drinking? What should I do?

Home When End of Life Approaches

Most patients prefer to die at home, and when they make that request, we in the health care field make every attempt to honor that wish. To help you as the caregiver of your loved one, one of the most critical and best resources we will help you set up will be hospice. Hospice is often considered the gold standard for end-of-life care, as the goal is to improve the quality of life during your loved one's last months, weeks, or days.

Here is a brief history of hospice: The hospice program as we know it today was started in 1967 by Dr. Dame Cicely Saunders in the UK when she founded St. Christopher's Hospice. In 1969, Dr. Elizabeth Kübler-Ross then published her book *On Death and Dying*, with the book focusing on interviews of the dying patients and the benefits of dying at home and the right they should have to die with dignity. Then in 1986, the Medicare Hospice Benefit was implemented. Over the past many years, legislation has even modified it further.

When possible, working with the hospice team, there are ways to increase the likelihood your loved one will have a peaceful death. Let's hope it will be following any end-of-life and after-death wishes he requested in their advance directive. If an advance directive is not in place, it may be due to any number of reasons, such as "I don't want to think or talk about that" or "I can beat this" or "I'm too young." Whatever the reason, it was never completed, nor was it the topic allowed to be talked about.

If he is able at this point to communicate their wishes, you may once again try to have that difficult conversation with them. If he agrees, you can then download a form or possibly, the hospice agency may have such you can use. In any event, as indicated earlier in this book, a health care team member cannot witness this type of document. This means you must either hire a person who is certified to notarize such documents or find two neighbors or friends who can witness it.

Pain

As you work with the hospice team, there will be many ways they may teach you as to what you or other family members or friends can do to help keep your loved one comfortable, particularly as the final days approach. Discomfort during the dying process can often be seen by changes in how your loved one acts. Knowing how much pain someone is in can be difficult.

If your loved one is unable to communicate, this means you need to watch for clues, some of which may be increased agitation, crying, groaning, or moaning. Or they may become more restless and possibly flailing (wildly flinging or moving) their arms and legs about or having their fists gripped tight or their legs pulled up. You may also see facial expressions such as frowning, grimacing, or grinding of their teeth. Or their heart may be faster, or they perspire profusely, or their complexion may be redder or paler than normal. Possibly one of the biggest changes you may see will be how they breathe. It may be slower or more rapid. Or the most frightening will be the different sounds they make as they breathe.

The key as you observe your loved one is to pay special attention to any of these as you care for him. While techniques may have already been addressed by the health care team as to what to do and how, in all the confusion or the discharge and all you have to do, you may forget. Do not be afraid to ask if you feel there is anything you need more teaching on. Discuss all with them again, and request tips you may need to relearn how to ease and comfort your loved one.

You may even want to do some online research on managing pain to help you better understand what is happening, and this may lead to other questions you may want to ask the team or doctor. Your questions may also include having them go over any or all the techniques on how to administer the medication and what signs and symptoms to look for. Included in this discussion, another key may be to have them give you some suggestions on how to care for your own emotions and feelings. Your loved one's care team has been thoroughly trained in all this, yet here you are, the newbie, often with little or no training on what to do when or how. Yet you are expected to step in and do it. So one key is, learn to speak up when you need help or don't understand it all.

Because the dying process is so hard on us as caregivers, especially if pain is out of control, it is not uncommon that you may feel overwhelmed. This may also be combined with a variety of mixed emotions, such as feeling helpless or even guilty that you wish your loved one will pass away so they are out of pain. By all means, it is critical you discuss these feelings either with other family members, your hospice team, your support group, or your mental health professional. Again, it is okay to cry and be sad during this most stressful time.

While not everyone dying experiences pain, for those who do, pain is possibly one of the biggest causes of many of the actions listed above. Thus, one of your primary focuses must be how to help keep your loved one as comfortable as possible.

- Listen to what the health care team says, and with all the hype of addiction we are hearing is happening in our society, addiction will not be the case for your loved one.
- The doctor may prescribe the medication round the clock, so this means you will have to set your clock so you can administer the medication(s) as prescribed.
- The main thing is, do not let the pain get out of control. If it gets out of control, it is far harder to get it back under control.

End-of-life pain, chronic pain, or pain typically associated with diseases such as cancer, shingles, sickle cell, fibromyalgia, migraines, arthritis, or slipped disc or sciatica often requires pain medication that is far stronger than your typical over-the-counter pain medications, such as aspirin or Tylenol, can offer. Thus, in an effort to control pain, your loved one's doctor will often prescribe medications referred to as narcotics.

Narcotics are drugs, such as codeine, morphine, hydrocodone, oxymorphone, buprenorphine, or fentanyl. Your loved one's pain medications may then either come as a pill (and even some are combined with aspirin or Tylenol), or it may be a suppository, meaning you have to put it in your loved one's rectum, or by patch, called a transdermal patch, as it is applied to the skin. Or it may be a lozenge that dissolves under the tongue. In many cases, the medication is either given as an injection into a muscle or vein. If it is by vein, your loved one should have an intravenous line in place, which will be another care need and area you will need to watch.

If the medication is given by vein, your loved one may already have in place what is called a central portal line, as they may have been getting curative drugs in the past. This is a line that is surgically inserted directly into a major vein, usually in the neck, chest, or groin. Once inserted, it can be used for long-term infusions; and while it will require meticulous—a very thorough or a very strict process on how to do it—sterile technique, which usually the home infusion nurse will change, for dressing changes, it can remain in place for up to a year.

However, most infusions and intravenous medications, including intravenous narcotics, will be given by what is called a peripheral IV. This is a small catheter that is inserted in a vein in your loved one's arm, leg, hand, or foot. It is also the most common way your loved one will receive any IV therapy, which is short-term, usually a few days. Once the catheter is in the vein, it will be secured in place by a transparent dressing that helps prevent it from becoming dislodged. If the IV line will be needed longer than six days or so, your loved one may need to have what is called a PICC (peripherally inserted central catheter) line inserted either by the infusion nurse, if he has been trained in this technique, or at the hospital.

Struggling with pain, as most of us know, can be draining, and it does not only increase our fatigue level but also makes us irritable, angry, and short-tempered. This will be the same with your loved one. If they are still able to communicate, this can make it even harder on you as you try to provide the care you think they need or as you try to communicate with your loved one in a meaningful way. In response, they may fight you, try to or actually hit you, swear at you, or even say hurtful things to you. Do not take what they say personally.

Due to the nature of caring for someone in your private home, other visitors' behavior is not monitored as closely as it would be in the hospital setting. For this reason, it is important to be vigilant about the people who have access to your loved one's narcotic medications. There have been instances of family members or friends helping themselves to the patient's narcotics. In one instance, a drug-addicted sibling was stealing pills from the patient and melting them down and injecting them. That person overdosed on the drug and caused an issue that the family never should have had to deal with. In another case, the patient's own daughter was taking her morphine pills and had to be taken to the hospital due to an overdose.

In the final stages of dying, if your loved one's pain remains unresponsive to the pain medication regimen their doctor has prescribed, the doctor may then prescribe what is referred to as palliative or comfort sedation. This type of sedation will make your loved one unaware and unconscious (a deep sleep), eventually leading to their death. The term "comfort care" is used to describe a set of the most basic palliative care interventions that will provide immediate relief of symptoms for your loved one when they are very close to death.

As you watch your loved one die, this is possibly the most stressful of any of your caregiving duties. Often, by the time your loved one is in the final or end stages of life, you may be physically and mentally exhausted. As said multiple times in this book, ask for help and take the time to take care of yourself.

Importance of Bowel Care

The key for care if your loved one is on any pain management regimen—bowel care is very important anytime anyone is on pain management plan even if not on hospice—is a strict bowel management plan so they pass feces as normally as possible. This means, while also giving their doses of pain medications at the right time and as prescribed, you must also follow a plan for a routine, daily bowel care program.

This program will be prescribed by your loved one's doctor, and it may include, if their disease can tolerate it and it is not contraindicated, a high-fiber diet and one with increased drinking of water. In most cases, the bowel regimen will include a bowel softener, possibly a laxative or suppository or in some cases even an enema. (If you have never given an enema, this is something your loved one's home health or hospice nurse can teach you.) The bowel regimen must also include, if any one of the foregoing is administered and there is no bowel movement, the next steps you will have to take.

Thus, as with the pain medication record keeping, you must also maintain a record of your loved one's bowel movements. How often is a bowel movement occurring? What is the consistency (hard, soft, or liquid)? Was it a large or a small one? If a next step regimen is needed, what did you give, and what was the result? The goal is to keep your loved one from getting a painful fecal (poop) impaction in their lower bowel.

A fecal impaction is different from constipation. Constipation is when it is difficult to poop, but you can. However, if left untreated, the poop continues to back up and causes a buildup that becomes a hard lump that then obstructs the lower colon, and it becomes so hard that it is impossible to pass. The initial symptoms of fecal impaction include discomfort and abdominal pain. It progresses, and it may cause abdominal bloating and discomfort and even pain, nausea, vomiting, confusion, and bleeding. Sometimes, liquid stool may leak around the blockage. If this occurs, do not mistake it for diarrhea. When an impaction occurs, your loved one will require what is called manual removal. In plain terms, this means it must be dug out. This is done by using a lubricated (greased) glove. A finger is then stuck in the rectum, and stool is attempted to be broken up and removed.

Other Signs Seen at End of life

As end of life approaches, whether it is months or weeks, suddenly, you may see other changes in your loved one. These may be any one or more of the following: increased fatigue and weakness, decreased food and fluid intake, breathing changes, heart rate changes, and color changes. They may have decreased urine (pee) output, and the color may change and may not be as yellowish as in the past but browner or even at times red. They may become incontinent of both urine and bowel and have body-jerking movements, or they may even move their hands around their face as if picking at something.

Fatigue and Weakness

As your loved one becomes weaker, you may need to help them walk; and as this worsens, they will eventually become bed confined. If this happens and they were not prior to this, it means you will possibly need to take on more care needs, such as turning them frequently and also using meticulous (remember, this means thorough) care, such as making sure the areas touching the sheets are not wrinkled or wet, their bottom is kept clean and dry, and rub the skin gently if it is reddened. If the skin is starting to break down, then apply cream or balm to help keep the area from possible further breakdown.

If you have other family members or friends there and they are not embarrassed by such care, make sure the hospice nurse explains to them why such activity is critical; and if necessary, he teaches them how to perform such tasks. This will include proper movement and position to use that will help teach them the proper body mechanics they must use to prevent injury to themselves.

Decreased Food and Fluid Intake—Feed and Hydrate or Not

As end of life approaches, some common forms of digestive issues may include nausea, vomiting, swallowing difficulties, or loss of appetite. The causes, as well as the treatments, will vary, and you need to keep notes on such so you can discuss it with the doctor or health care team to see if there is a way to help ease such issues. Dependent on the cause, the treatments as well will vary. Definitely, medications may help relieve nausea and vomiting, which are often common side effects of strong medications.

Losing one's appetite is a normal part of dying, and going without food or water is generally not painful. The key to helping your loved one when they lose their appetite is to not force them to eat or drink. The team will more than likely have some recommendations, but one of the simplest ways will be to offer only small portions or sips of their favorite food or liquid. Sips can be given, but only if there are no swallowing or choking issues. If these are present, the team may suggest you use a product called thick-it. This is a product that is over the counter, so it can be purchased without a prescription. The key to its use is, the product is stirred into liquid, and the liquid will thicken, and this is a way to allow your loved one to stay hydrated, if hydration is part of the recommended treatment.

This area is possibly one of the hardest for you or any family members to understand. It is natural to think we must eat and drink to keep our strength and endurance up. After all, eating is one of the pleasures of life for most of us. For us working in health care, eating is often something we know may not be of any help and may even worsen the condition of your loved one. So even when we hear families say "If they don't eat, they will starve" or "If they don't drink, I know they will feel thirsty," we know this is not true.

Studies have shown this is not the case when a person is dying. An example of such a study can be found on the BioMed Center and its BMC Palliative Care website. In fact, food and fluids can cause stomach discomfort. Or in some, if they are not peeing, it can cause what is called fluid overload, which means the lungs fill with fluid.

When decreased food and fluid intake occurs, part of the care you will now give will include good mouth care and keeping the mouth and lips clean and moist. This may be by applying a gel (like Vaseline) to the lips to keep them soft, but this can be contraindicated if your loved one is on oxygen. Another method will be to use a washcloth dampened with water or even a mild mouth wash so you can wipe out their mouth and even run it over their teeth. Hospices often provide what is called toothettes. It is basically a small sponge on a lollipop stick that can be moistened and used to wet lips and gently clean the mouth. If these are not provided by your hospice or home health, you can purchase them at a medical supply store.

Breathing Changes

Breathing changes is often one of the first sign you may see. This may be rapid and fast breathing, such as panting, as your loved one struggles to breathe. Or it may be short, shallow breathes, and in any case, you may feel like they are suffocating. Some of the types of breathing changes you may hear may seem like funny words to you, but the medical terms are as follows:

- *Cheyne-Stokes.* In this type of breathing, your loved one may alternate between deep, heavy breaths to shallow ones or even no breaths at all, which is referred to as apnea. In this case, use of oxygen does not help or hinder the breathing. This type of breathing does not mean they are uncomfortable. This type of breathing is a normal part of the dying process and will occur as the brain area that controls our breathing slows down or stops.
- *Noisy breathing.* This is often due to secretions or fluid buildup in the upper part of your loved one's respiratory track, such as the trachea, and your loved one may make gurgling sounds. This type of breathing is referred to as the death rattle and is probably going to be the most upsetting to you and your family. While this type of breathing will

not bother your loved one, it can be alarming to you or the family.

To help treat this, you may need to frequently change your loved one's position, turning them on their side or elevating the head of the bed. If your loved one is receiving an IV and if the health care team is present, they may slow it down or discuss with you discontinuing it altogether. Often, caregivers are convinced that they can improve this condition by suctioning the patient. This is not recommended, because it really does not relieve the congestion and can be very uncomfortable to the patient.

- *Agonal breathing.* This type of breathing is very shallow breathing where shallow breaths are passed through the lips (it can resemble how a fish breathes). This type of breathing generally means death is near.

Skin Color Changes

As your loved one's body slows down, so does their circulation of blood. At this point, you may see funny bluish discolorations or splotches (called mottling) on the hands, feet, and knees. Along with the skin changes, you may feel their skin starting to get cooler. Your first reaction will be to think they are cold, and you can certainly add another blanket. However, when this happens, it is a part of the dying process.

During this time, you may also see some breakage in their skin, especially on their butt and shoulder blades or bony areas on their spine. When this occurs, keep the areas as dry as possible, and you may even want to use a gel, such as petroleum jelly. Also, you may want to purchase an over-the-counter balm called Bag Balm. This is a salve we in health care often have recommended to patients for use on dry skin. Bag Balm was actually developed in the late 1800s and was originally used to soothe dry, irritated skin on the udders of cows.

Another skin issue you may see is dryness on parts of the face and eyes. Again, these can be cared for by placing a warm washcloth over the eyes or by applying a dab of eye cream or gel around the eyes.

Changes in Levels of Consciousness, Delirium, and Confusion

As death approaches, your loved one may sleep more and possibly even sleep deeper, and they become less arousable. When they do wake up, while some may be clear, others will be very confused, and they may say things that make no sense at all to you. They may also talk about seeing a loved one who has died before them. I know as my mom was nearing her end of life, she often told me she saw my dad and would describe what he was doing; and as she was talking to me, she often had a conversation with my dad. She would even describe in vivid detail what my dad was wearing and where they were—often in our hometown and the club they loved to go to with friends, where she and my dad would cut a rug, as she would say. So let them talk. As hard as it is not to correct them, let them talk.

When your loved one becomes unresponsive, it indicates that the illness has progressed, and the patient is nearing the final stages toward end of life. This can take a great toll on you and other family members. Even when unresponsive, it is critical you continue to make every attempt to comfort them by holding their hand, speaking softly to them, or playing soft, soothing music to help keep the surrounding environment peaceful. This allows you the ability to also monitor their pain and manage it throughout the remainder of the active dying, transitioning, and imminent phases as death finally comes.

Staying close to someone who is dying is often called keeping a vigil. While it may be comforting for you and your family members to always be there, it can also be tiring and stressful. Unless your cultural or religious traditions require it, do not feel that you must stay with your loved one all the time. If there are other family members or friends around, let them take turns and sit in the room so you can take a break and address your own emotional and spiritual needs.

During this time, there may be a pet that your loved one is particularly close to, such as a dog or cat. You will find that this animal is often very insistent about being on the bed or chair with the patient. Many patients want their beloved companion to be very close to them at this time, and it should be allowed if at all possible.

Importance of Communication and Use of Comfort Measures

As indicated, the end stages of life may not happen in the blink of an eye. If your loved one remains able to communicate, it is important you let them express their feelings. It is not uncommon for them to feel depressed or anxious or have fears of the unknown or even what will happen to you and other family members after they die. If you see or hear this, let them express their feelings; and if necessary, encourage them to speak with the hospice social worker. Possibly, they will help to counsel your loved one.

Another way to get the emotional support your loved one needs will be to take advantage of the technology we have today. This means, if your loved one is already linked to a mental health counselor, they continue; and hopefully, the focus of the counseling will be on the end-of-life emotional issues your loved one is experiencing. The best part is that all can now be done via video conferencing, and your loved one is able to conserve their energy by not having to leave the house.

Thus, as with all of life, it is critical you and your loved one communicate, doing so as often as the occasion may call for it and using terms they hopefully can understand. Proper communication is even more critical when you are dealing with a child or a person with dementia or a person with a developmental or intellectual delay. In any case, it is best to have simple but direct conversations with your loved one, as using indirect words as you talk with them may cause confusion or an inability to comprehend what is said. If you have a hard time having any direct and simple conversations or even those difficult conversations, use the resources you will have from your loved one's medical team. This in many cases will be the social worker or possibly the chaplain. They may also be there to support you when such conversations are needed.

Sometimes, when having those difficult conversations or those that center on your loved one's feelings of death and your loved one is one with dementia, is a child, or has a brain injury or developmental or intellectual delay, it is often best that you not only speak simply and directly but also that you talk with them through open-ended questions to help them better understand. If your loved one asks about death, as hard as it may be on you, be honest with them and listen if they also want to talk about it.

Again, if you are not aware of how to use open-ended questions, your team social worker may be your best source to help you. One of the best resources I have found that will help you in talking to your child or your loved one who has the IQ (the official term is "intelligence quotient," and it is our ability to reason and solve problems) of a young child about death is at the Children's Hospital of Orange County (CHOC) website. This is a site I would suggest you read to find tips that may help you as you have this difficult discussion with your child.

If you are having a hard time yourself with understanding what is being said or the severity of your loved one's medical condition or even their prognosis (prediction of how long they might live), make sure you let the team know you do not understand and request they use simple ways to tell you. The best way is to have a family member or friend there to help explain things in a way you can understand. Remember, there is nothing wrong with saying you do not understand and request that whoever is speaking use simple ways, maybe even including drawing a picture or giving you an example so you can understand as best as you can what they are saying.

Communication is important if your loved one can talk and understand, but a must will be providing a comforting environment as care is given or time is spent with your loved one. Comfort measures may be merely sitting and holding hands or massaging their hands or feet, dimming the lights, playing soft and soothing music, or reading to them. Basically, just being present and near may be the main joy you convey and they feel.

As you provide care for your loved one and the team is not there, remember to write down questions as they arise. While many of them probably can be answered by a team member, there will be some that must be addressed by the doctor, and you are not sure what to say or ask. It is okay to request help from your loved one's nurse, social worker, or even health plan case manager. One of them may be available to help advocate for you or even be present when you discuss your questions with the doctor. If English is not your primary language, ensure as you meet with the doctor that a translator is available to tell you in your native language what was said.

Do Not Be Afraid to Ask or Say Yes if Help Is Offered

Family and friends may wish to provide you with some help with the care of your loved one or possibly even for you so you can take some me time. This will be the time, if not done already, that you use either the list of tasks you developed as you were getting organized and preparing all for your loved one's homecoming. If not done already, here is the sample list again. As you do your list, include all the things that you regularly do (or want to do) in a week and separate out those you will need to do.

Be sure that all basic instructions for care are clear to the person caring for your loved one if you are going to be out of the home for a while. Volunteers from the hospice program are trained in how to handle changes in your loved one's condition while they are with them and will usually remain calm. However, a friend or family member may not be sure to react to certain changes in your loved one and will sometimes panic if there is an unexpected change. They may even call 911, not knowing what else to do.

In order to prevent paramedics from taking your loved one to the hospital or taking lifesaving measures, such as life support, make sure you have a do not resuscitate order posted prominently on the refrigerator or wall above the patient's bed that has been signed and dated by their physician and renewed every ninety days. While the paramedics may understand that these are not your wishes, they are bound by law to do everything if they do not have or see that order.

Your list might include help with caring/playing with your children or transporting them to school or after-school events; if not home-delivered, possibly picking up groceries or medications; maybe even some simple caregiving tasks; preparing a meal; help with tidying up the house; or doing simple yard work. Another task might be to have someone keep your online blog possibly on Facebook or via email or a telephone tree, updated with changes in your loved one's life.

Whatever list you create will be designed specific to your needs. Include in the list who will be there to help, and make sure you keep your list in a visible place, where people who want to help will see what needs to be done. Be sure to include any relevant details that may assist the volunteers in what might be needed for whatever task. I have also suggested to families they then keep a calendar handy so they know if anyone is coming that day or not. You can purchase schedule books with room to write details on each day and time of the week, such as a day planner, or you can find forms for such online. Or you can make your own, and it may look like this.

Task	Time of day, week, or month to do it	Name of volunteer	Days and hours they can come	Phone number

Again, providing comfort and care for your loved one at any stage in caregiving can be physically, emotionally, and mentally draining and exhausting. Thus, do not be shy, and do not think you can do it alone. Ask for help, and then accept it. Also, do not hesitate to suggest a specific task for someone who might offer to help. Friends and family are usually eager to do something for you; they often just don't know what it is or what to do.

In the end, consider that there may be no perfect death, so just do the best you can for your loved one. The deep pain of losing someone close to you may be softened a little by knowing that when you were needed, you did what you could.

Summary

End of life is a natural part of the human experience. If it is properly prepared for, it can be a peaceful and easy time for all involved. One of the most important things is to remember we all desire dignity and respect not only in life but also, equally as important, as end of life approaches.

Dealing with end of life will possibly be one of the most difficult tasks we have to do. During this time, you, like so many in the same role, will more than likely be on an emotional roller coaster. So as you provide the care your loved one needs, it is just as critical you do not ignore your own or that of the immediate family and the emotional or spiritual support you all may require.

Keeping your loved one as comfortable as possible will be the primary focus of some of the care you give them. While this might include any measures needed for pain control, it also means giving them the emotional support they need, especially if they remain alert almost to the end.

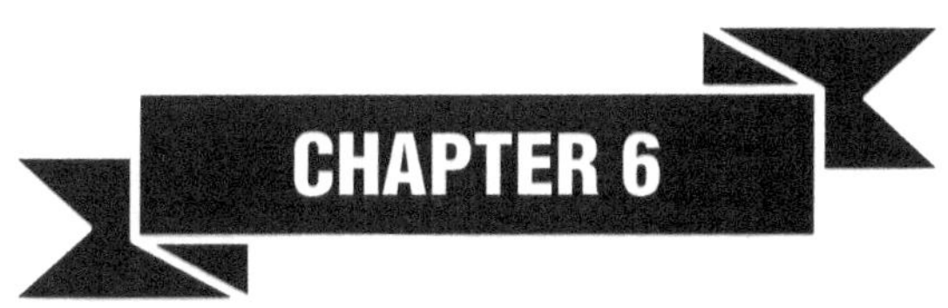

Avoiding Caregiver Burnout

THERE ARE TIMES when the caregiver role occurs over time, but it also can happen in the blink of an eye if your loved one has a sudden injury or illness that renders them unable to do anything we normally associate with everyday living (termed activities of daily living and instrumental activities of daily living). Caregiving can both be rewarding and depressing, as well as mentally and physically exhausting consecutively. It can also be one we least expect. It is one we are not trained to do, and depending upon your loved one's diagnosis or injury, you may find it one of the toughest jobs you may ever have to do. A word to the wise, caregiving is not easy for anyone. This can include both the caregiver and your loved one. There are going to be sacrifices and adjustments for everyone.

So what is caregiver burden? This refers to the problems and stress related to being a caregiver. One of the greatest burdens for most will be financial strain. This is true especially if the loved one being cared for is forced to leave the workforce, or the caregiver as well is forced to leave or reduce their work hours. Consequently, your number one task to do will be to apply for any employer benefits, as well as to apply for any state or local programs that may be available.

As a nurse case manager, I always reminded the person I was working with that Medicaid was not welfare. It is a health insurance program, so this is my reminder for anyone reading this book. The same with applications for any program offered by Medicare,

Medicaid, a managed care Medicare or Medicaid health plan, or a disease-specific agency or even the federal and your state's food assistant program, referred to as SNAP (Supplemental Nutrition Assistance Program), if your loved one is eligible for such, make use of them, as they will assist in reducing at least a portion of the financial strain. I always stressed to families that programs such as Medicaid and SNAP are not welfare since Medicaid is health insurance, and SNAP ensures those in need can have a healthy diet.

As you read this book, you will see how much it will be stressed to not ignore yourself. Too often, when one assumes the caregiver role, they are so focused on their loved one and all the tasks that must be done that they forget to take care of themselves. When you take care of yourself, this does not only mean just your physical health, eating properly, or taking care of your personal hygiene but also, equally as important, your mental and emotional health. If you ignore your own needs, this does neither you nor your loved one nor the health care team any good. If you do, the result means you may not be able to continue in your role, as you will need care yourself.

Basic Requirements

Caregiving requires not only physical strength and endurance but also mental and emotional strength, and this applies not only to the person doing the hands-on care but possibly anyone who is in a long-distance caregiver role. For the hands-on caregiver, that means also having the ability to see clearly while also performing the tasks required with good manual dexterity. You will need both initially but also possibly long-term.

Before we get further, let us now take the time to discuss long-distance caregivers since you may often have similar feelings as the one providing the physical care does. You may not feel as physically exhausted and drained as the one who is performing the actual, hands-on caregiving. However, the burden of being a caregiver can take its toll on those who perform the role from a distance. If you are a long-distance caregiver, you may have different worries since they are not on-site and must then rely on what is sent to you and what you can see if you do Facetime or any video conferences.

From speaking with a long-distance caregiver, I have learned that one of their biggest areas of guilt was not being closer and not being able to help. The worst guilt often centered around the fact that they are not close enough to help or spend time with their loved one. On top of maybe feeling guilty, they often worried about being able to take time off work, the costs of travel, or being taken away from their own family.

If you are a long-distance caregiver, you must remember that you can only do what you can do. Thus, equally as important as the caregiver doing the physical care, it is just as important you learn to take care of your health. This means physical, mental, and emotional help. This may mean joining a support group for long-distance caregivers since this might give you an opportunity to learn from others. You will find out the feelings you are feeling are probably the same as others have experienced, so you will find you are not alone! Remember that you are doing the best you can do given your circumstances.

Because the hands-on caregiver may be busy doing the physical care, possibly one way you can help will be to do any of the research on any topics that might need further clarification or those where you and the physical caregiver want to know more about a disease and its progression, as this will allow you both to know what to expect. With technology as it is, you can also join in on any care conferences as discharge plans or plans for ongoing care occur.

So what are some tips to help you?

- Do not ignore any of your limitations. If you cannot do it, it is okay to say no.
- Educate yourself on your loved one's disease or issues that may be encountered. Diseases and injuries and their complications are not going to go away. Ask your loved one's doctor to be candid about the prognosis and course of the disease and any complications that might occur. Take the time to either read online what is meant, or if you belong

to a support group, ask others who have been there with their loved one what to expect. If for example your loved one has dementia, do your research so you will understand the various stages and what to do as each stage comes into focus. For information on dementia, you may wish to contact such agencies as the following:

a. Alzheimer's Association
b. The National Council on Aging
c. The National Institute of Health and Their Institute on Aging
d. The Administration for Community Living (ACL)

- If your loved one is developmentally or intellectually challenged, again, do your research so you will understand the specifics of the disease. For information specific to the developmentally or intellectually, disabled you may want to contact the following:
- The Administration for Community Living (ACL). This agency and their website have links to a variety of topics from A-Z.
- Your region's or state's Developmental Disabilities Services (DDS) office.
- If you are a caregiver for a loved one who is LGBTQ (Lesbian, Gay, Bisexual, Transgender, Queer, or Questioning, Intersex, Asexual), you will find information and get some tips on caregiving from the LGBTQ Caregiver Center and their website. LGBTQ+ people face many barriers within health care, including discrimination, ignorance, and fear. The lack of informed care, sensitive language, research, and data prevents access to competent routine care and screening. LGBTQ+ health is emerging as a national concern due to the growing body of evidence indicating significant health care disparities experienced by the LGBTQ+ community. The LGBTQ Caregiver Center provides advocacy, education, and resources to empower LGBTQ caregivers

and those who care for LGBTQ+ people to improve their health and well-being.

- If you cannot afford to hire help, reach out to local agencies that may have a program you can use. (Several key agencies will be mentioned in the resources and help chapter.) One of the best resources to find what is available locally will be the United Way 2-1-1 phone system. Let them know what you may be looking for, and they will give you names of agencies, as well as their phone number.

- You may also want to explore any of your loved one's state websites to see what programs may be available to help keep your loved one at home, and an out-of-home placement is avoided. (More details for each of the programs listed below will be discussed in the resources and help chapter.) Those programs might be the following:

1. PACE (Program All-Inclusive Care for the Elderly), a Medicare and Medicaid waiver.

2. Any Medicaid waiver—all states have a variety of waiver programs in place—in addition to the traditional Medicaid benefits offered. Thus, no two (2) states are alike in what they offer. However, the waivers offered are based primarily on a diagnosis or a specific population (i.e., DD/ID). While you may want to apply for a state waiver, I will warn you, even if you have completed all the paperwork and your loved one is eligible, the wait list is long. For some, it is even as long as a year. This means that in the interim, you may be required to assume care at home or possibly place your loved one in a facility. Because most states are moving their Medicaid population to managed care plans, if that is your loved one's health plan, it is then key to work with that health plan to see if basically the same provisions for what would have been provided under the state's waiver can be set up. This means in

the interim of the waiver, services are provided by your loved one's Medicaid managed care plan.

There are two (2) waivers to explore.

1. The Home- and Community-Based Services (HCBS) Waiver. To find the HCBS agency to work with in your loved one's state, see the Medicaid Planning Assistance website.

2. If you have a medically fragile child who is on life-sustaining equipment and the only option for him may be placement in a long-term care facility that specializes in extremely complex care, you may want to explore the Katie Beckett Waiver, which is also known as the TEFRA waiver. At this writing, there are only twenty-four states that provide this waiver: Alaska, Arkansas, California, Connecticut, Delaware, District of Columbia, Georgia, Idaho, Nebraska, Nevada, Oklahoma, Rhode Island, South Carolina, Tennessee, Vermont, South Dakota, Massachusetts, Michigan, Minnesota, Mississippi, Maine, Louisiana, West Virginia, and Wisconsin.

If you applied for Supplemental Security Income (SSI) for your loved one, as mentioned in the resources and help chapter, and your loved one is eligible for the program, this can mean you may be able to be paid to be the in-home supportive services (IHSS) worker or personal care attendant (PCA). To approve the hours allowed, a caseworker or social worker from a state/county agency—it might be from the Department of Social Services, but again, states vary on what agency manages the IHSS or PCA program used to perform this task—will be assigned to your loved one's case.

To better understand your loved one's needs, not only must his physician submit a summary of care needs, but the social worker will also do an on-site home evaluation visit. Here they will interview both your loved one and you and then document their findings of how many minutes or hours are necessary to perform all tasks. Once the report is completed, it is sent for a review and a final determination of the number of hours per month that are approved.

If approved, some services that can be authorized through IHSS include housecleaning, meal preparation, laundry, grocery shopping, personal care services, accompaniment to medical appointments, and protective supervision for the mentally impaired. Eligibility and pay for family caregiving may vary from state to state, so it is best to reach out to the state agency that performs the needs assessment. As you develop your post-acute hospital team, be sure to add the contact information (name, phone—cell phone number or office phone number—and fax number) for the worker assigned to your loved one's case. This is critical in the event his medical condition changes, and you possibly will need more hours.

In the interim of approval, this means you and whoever is helping you must continue to perform the task until the IHSS/PCA hours are approved. This period of time may also be extended if you must hire the chore worker or PCA.

A word to the wise, the hours that are allowed are extremely limited per month and vary by state. For example, in California, the maximum hours allowed, regardless of diagnosis or care needs in a twenty-four-hour period, is 283 hours per month. Compare that to the fact that a 24-7 schedule totals 720 hours per month. As mentioned earlier, most states will allow family members to serve and be paid as the worker. However, while you can be paid as a caregiver, this does not mean you will be paid for 24 hours of care. Your hours allotted for pay will be based on the case worker's assessment and the number of hours finally approved. This means the number of hours you will be paid will vary from a few hours per week up to the 283 maximum. If you or a family member does not want to be the caregiver, you must find your own caregiver. This means you are then the employer on record, and you or your loved one will be the one who hires and supervises. If they do not perform the duties as expected, since you are the employer, you also do the firing. Payment for their work hours will be paid by the state, but you must approve their timecard before it is submitted. You also will be responsible for tracking and paying for any overtime of the worker.

Again, keep that notebook or cell phone handy as the social worker evaluates all. Ask questions and make notes.

- Even if approved for any of the foregoing, if your loved one requires 24-7 care and friends or family offer to help, accept it! Even when many of us find it hard to ask for help, do it. Accepting help does not mean you are weak in any form or fashion. Accepting help will allow you to take time for yourself, and you can relax. It also gives others a chance to better understand your needs, as well as your loved one. If you do use volunteers, make sure you set up a checklist of specific duties they will perform.
- If you do accept help, make every attempt to get a solid commitment about the days and times they are available. This allows you to develop a calendar of who will be there, what days they can work, and for how many hours. You can then plan what time you might have to take care of yourself (time for a nap, time to read or do a hobby you like, or time to go on an outing with family or a friend— any activity that will allow yourself me time).
- If you can afford to hire help, while you can hire help on your own, this often is not a wise choice, as you do not have the tools a caregiver agency may have. If you do use an agency, select possibly three in your area, as this will allow you to make an informed choice of who best may fit the needs not only of your loved one but also of the one you feel comfortable with hiring. This also means that at a minimum,

    - if you employ a caregiver without using a professional agency, you are responsible for all, such as paying taxes and keeping any bookkeeping records that are needed should you be audited by the state or Internal Revenue Services (IRS);
    - you do not have the tools to perform the background check as a professional agency has; and

○ you do not have a workers' compensation program in the event of an injury that an agency has.

A word to the wise, whether you use an agency or not, conduct your own interviews and also ask those you may be considering for references. Then call the references given to query them on their satisfaction with the person you are considering for the job—this allows you to make an informed decision. If you do use an agency, be on the alert for possible fraud and abuse from that agency since fraud and abuse are so widespread in health care. If you suspect fraud and abuse, the Centers for Medicare and Medicaid Services (CMS) has a website dedicated to the topic.

- Learn to take periods within the day to take and do some deep breathing. This is critical, as it helps relax muscles that have become tense either from physical care or worry.
- Do not be afraid to cry or grieve. This includes any of you macho men, who have been taught that real men do not cry. It is natural to grieve, and caregiving can stir up a range of complicated emotions. But if you find you are increasingly emotional or feeling emotionally fragile, there may be something more going on. Depression is a real risk for caregivers. Even if you are not clinically depressed, emotional outbursts can be an unconscious outlet for feelings of being overwhelmed, so take the time to call your physician or mental health counselor and follow their advice, which might mean setting up a respite plan or even permanent placement of your loved one. This includes knowing the signs and symptoms for caregiver burnout if you attempt to do all the care alone.
- If you must also work outside the home while also serving as a caregiver, work with your employer on completing any Family Medical Leave (FMLA) paperwork.
- Make attempts to have your loved one join in any everyday activities they may be capable of performing. Also, create a plan to do things such as dancing (even if they are in

a wheelchair), taking part in any community recreation activities, taking walks, gardening, or listening to music or looking at old photo albums—any activity that allows your loved one to join in.

- A great resource you may wish to explore for your loved one will be the National Library Service (NLS) or the Library of Congress. This is a free service for anyone who is blind or near blind or has a physical, perceptual, or reading disability. There is also an online application form you can complete to start your subscription (all services are free, delivered to your home and sent back). NLS has both talking books, books in braille, and downloadable electronic books and music.

- Join support groups for your loved one's disability (either online or local in your community). Using your computer or even you cell phone, let your fingers do the walking and search for online support groups, which have virtually exploded since the COVID pandemic and the isolation that was required to help control the outbreak. One online website might be SELF. Joining a support group will allow you to learn firsthand tips for care, help manage your stress, locate helpful resources, help reduce feelings of frustration and isolation, and provide pointers you may wish to consider, helping you take care of yourself.

If you join an online support group, this is not the same as getting professional mental health help. While a support group can be helpful, it is not a replacement for professional mental help. Keep in mind, you can do both—receive professional help while also joining a support group. If you join a support group and it does not feel like a good fit or does not provide support, look for another one. I know from personal experience, as I joined a bereavement group after my husband died. It was a horrible experience, as everyone did nothing but cry and complain. So after two meetings, I dropped out.

- If possible and available in your loved one's local town, explore any day care programs. This can include not only those for the adults, but many regions in your state may also have day programs for a child or young person offering some high-tech care (advances in medical knowledge and technique that have resulted in improved diagnostic, therapeutic, and rehabilitation procedures).

- Due to the fact that there has been for so many years stigma (negative thoughts, beliefs, or comments about an issue or topic) associated with getting mental health care, consequently, when we think of health care, we only think of our physical health. It cannot be emphasized enough that caring for ourselves means taking care of all our physical, mental, and emotional needs. Thank goodness the stigma surrounding mental health is slowly going away, so take advantage of any programs you feel can help you. Thus, if you do so, as you build your post-acute care team, include the mental health counselor you are using.

  This professional can not only help you deal with any feelings that arise but can also help you set goals or boundaries. Setting boundaries is easier said than done. It is especially hard to do if you, like many of us, are used to not saying no. You put others and their needs before your own. If this is you, work with your mental health counselor and let him serve in a teaching role so you can learn to set boundaries. Boundaries are a skill that can be learned, but it takes practice. Thus, as you talk to your physician or mental health counselor, remember your notebook so you can make notes, and you can practice between sessions.

  If needed, you can find a wealth of information on mental health and the importance of support groups as well as a wide variety of mental health topics on any number of websites such as:

  o   National Alliance on Mental Illness or NAMI
  o   Mental Health America

- o Substance Abuse Mental Health Services Administration or SAMHSA
- o Mental Health.gov and its website

- Create a patient-specific area in the home for your loved one's care. As you do this, make sure you also prepare an emergency preparedness plan. I have given you tips on both in two chapters in this book and also in the chapter on getting the home ready. Creating a specific area for care helps in the following:

  a. Your loved one will feel more secure, and for some, it helps to decrease confusion or emotional or violent outbursts.
  b. It allows you to have any caregiving supplies readily available at your fingertips.
  c. It helps to decrease frustration as you look for whatever you might need.

- As you build your patient-specific area, create a space where you can store key documents, such as copies of key medical reports, insurance handbooks, advance directives, or award letters for care. Keep them in a central file, as this will allow you and other family members to have them readily accessible should something happen to you.
- For the caregiving tasks that must be done daily, create a schedule (to-do list) of tasks to do and possibly add the time of day they must be done. By creating such, this allows you to be organized and helps keep frustration to a minimum. As you create such a schedule, include break times for yourself.
- Divide care into segments so not all is done at one time, and you get too tired. For example, perform oral care during bathing time or doing skin assessments during bath time or any changes in position or assistance with mobility.

- Try to keep a sense of humor. Laughter is one of the best medicines.
- Keep a calendar handy, and keep it updated to show not only doctor or other appointments but also when and what needs to be reordered (i.e., medications or any other supplies needed).
- Stay in contact with friends. Isolation is one of the biggest factors for caregiver burnout, so make every effort to stay in contact with friends, family, and colleagues joining in whenever possible. If you do join in, keep your focus on other things other than your caregiver duties.

Common Ailments Associated with Caregiving

If you do not make time for yourself, you may find you may have any one or several of the following ailments, many of which can lead to caregiver burnout:

1. Headache, apathy, loss of interest, anger, lack of concentration.
2. Depression is the most common psychological issue encountered by caregivers, so do not be afraid to talk to a mental health counselor or therapist.
3. Muscle fatigue from lifting or turning your loved one multiple times in a day or possibly using improper body mechanics.
4. Stomach or bowel issues, as you are not eating properly.
5. Increased weight loss or, in reverse, weight gain, again, as you are not eating properly.
6. Skin irritations, such as rash or hives, as you are a basket of nerves, and you are frustrated with all tasks required.
7. Decreased sex drive, as you are too tired, and too much is on your mind.
8. Inability to sleep due to the frequency of care or worry you did something wrong.

The American Medical Association (AMA) has a great guide on its website for physicians on how to recognize and treat patients suffering from caregiver burnout. While aimed at physicians, it has some great tips one can use to help avoid caregiver burnout. Caregiver burnout can occur when caregivers do not get the help or support they need and when the demands on a caregiver's mind, body, and emotions are overwhelming, leading to fatigue and sometimes hopelessness. Unfortunately, caregiver burnout may cause unnecessary rehospitalizations or placement in a long-term care facility.

What are the signs of caregiver stress or burnout?

1. Always feeling overwhelmed and tired due to lack of sleep or the amount and frequency of care needed daily by your loved one.
2. Starting to find that you are forgetful or that you have difficulty with concentration.
3. Losing control physically and emotionally or blowing up or losing your temper unexpectedly over little things that arise. It can also include feeing angry toward friends, family members, or even your loved one.
4. Social withdrawal from friends or even family or not participating in activities you previously enjoyed, as you feel you are too busy or tied down with the care needs.
5. No longer finding pleasure in things you have done in the past.
6. Having intense feelings of hatred or resentment toward your loved one. This does not mean you are a bad person or caregiver in any way.
7. Having intense feelings of anger, sadness, or fear of the unknown or of things that can come.
8. Drastic weight changes, as you are not eating, and you are losing weight. Or in the opposite, you are eating excessively and not exercising correctly, so the weight is piling on.
9. Changes in your own health or an increase in signs and symptoms for your own health-related issues you have ignored.

10. Starting to cope or manage your stress or painful feelings through developing an unhealthy lifestyle or use of substances—alcohol or drugs.

If you feel or see any of the foregoing as you perform your caregiver duties, you may want to do any do the following:

1. By all means, ask for help.
2. Work with your loved one's case manager to see if they are able to help get the needed information that can be used to support medical necessity from the health plan, and you can then qualify for respite care. Respite care, if approved, can let your loved one be cared for in a facility. If respite is approved, it generally will be for up to five days and will be provided in a local SNF or other care facility designed to treat your loved one's diagnosis.
3. Take a day at a time. Remember, Rome wasn't built in a day.
4. Have serious conversations (or what we health care professionals call hard conversations) with your loved one. You both must understand what to expect, and it is often when in the caregiver role that you need to say no to even your loved one. This may also mean discussing what steps are needed to avoid certain situations.
5. Discuss your feelings with other family members or friends, your physician or mental health counselor, or those from a support group you may find in your community or online.
6. If available in your area, take advantage of any day care programs that might be available. This will allow you time to hopefully have some time, if nothing else, to take a nap or a long, hot bath or perform any activity that may help you relax.
7. Take any opportunity during the day to use relaxation techniques, such as deep breathing, yoga, or other exercises.
8. Remember to eat healthy.

9. While it may not be a covered benefit of your loved one's health plan, attempt to locate and use any extra equipment that can help ease caregiving and prevent any back or muscle strains you may encounter. Such may be a patient lift system, a wheelchair or bedside commode with a removable arm, or a semi-electric bed so the bed can be at the right height for you to perform any daily tasks or move your loved one about.

10. In today's world of technology, take advantage of any apps or online information you may find either by use of your cell phone or computer. If you do not own a computer, many local libraries have one designated for community use. The same, if your health plan has a local office, they may have a designated area for members to use. So check out any such local offices and make use of the available resource.

Summary

As you can see from the above, the caregiver role (physical care and long-distance) can be overwhelming; and as such, as you plan your loved one's care and the tasks needed, you must also plan on how you can also schedule time for yourself. If not, you will be a candidate for caregiver burnout. This can lead to either yourself getting sick or injured and requiring help or even your unexpected death or your loved one placed in a long-term facility, which is what you hope to avoid.

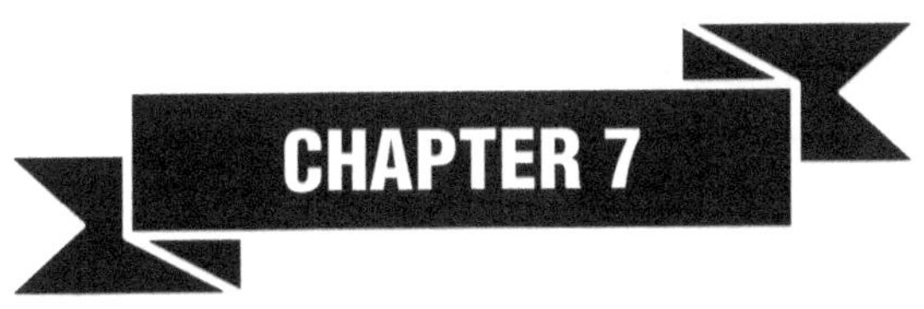

Caregiver, a Role We Least Expected, and Your Mental Health

AS YOU FIND yourself in a new role as a caregiver, the overwhelming responsibilities and multiple tasks will be overwhelming. Suddenly, the new caregiving demands will take over your own needs; and literally, it will take over your current life. As people face these new challenges, it is difficult to find balance due to new and intense responsibilities. However, if you do not find balance, eventually, it will affect your mental, emotional, and physical health. The purpose of this chapter is to give specific ideas and resources to help you cope with different aspects of this new role but most importantly to bring awareness and empower you to take priority and responsibility over your own mental, physical, and emotional health.

My heart feels special compassion for those who every day bravely and kindly answer to the call of duty—the call to take care of a child, parent, family member, or friend who has unique needs and requires special care and ongoing attention. Some of these needs can be mental, physical, or emotional; and the period of care can range from months to decades, and that can be eventually exhausting.

As you engage in this role, it is normal to prioritize the care of your loved one and forget about yourself and your own needs. Somehow, the idea of even thinking about yourself does not make any sense, and it may feel selfish. But after a certain time, your body will feel the negative effects of ignoring your own needs. The purpose of this chapter is to bring awareness to the need of taking care of yourself in a practical and simple way.

Something happened that put you in a caregiving role. It may be a role you share with family members, or it may be a personal role. However, as you engage in this new role, it is important to take time to acknowledge and grieve the personal loss you and your family members are experiencing. Grieving is an essential part of healing that we need to acknowledge.

Grieving as a Part of the Healing

To be fully functional, we need to understand what happened and how this is going to change our lives individually and collectively. There is no better way to start our emotional healing than through grieving properly. Grief is an intense emotional experience triggered by a loss.

Grieving is a process in which we try to make sense of some important losses in our life or in the life of the people we care. Therefore, we all need to be able to identify our losses and grieve them properly. I worked once with an amputee who due to a health condition lost his leg below the knee and part of his other foot. His physical loss devastated him and affected his mental health. As part of his mental and emotional healing, he went through a process of grieving. At the beginning of the process, he was angry with himself. Then he was very sad and depressed and started to lose any desire to be alive. However, after some time, he started to accept his new reality and started looking for and found solutions that helped him create a meaningful and functional life. He became an amputee advocate, and he visited amputees at their homes and shared his life experience. In doing so, he found new meaning for his life.

Five Stages of Grieving

Most likely, you have already experienced or are currently experiencing the five stages of grief. These stages are attempts to understand and process our losses; the purpose of these stages is to protect ourselves while we adapt to a new reality. They come in cycles and do not have to be in order. These five stages of lose are

- denial,
- anger,
- bargaining,
- depression,
- acceptance.

As we suddenly take the role of caregivers, you may experience feelings of anguish, confusion, distress, depression, anxiety, guilt, and emotional pain. Those feelings and emotions are normal and are associated directly with a conscious or unconscious process of grief. We usually tend to grieve not only the death of our loved ones but also their suffering and our own suffering and our own losses. As a caregiver, you may identify some of your own loses, such as the lack of time to do some of your favorite activities that give you joy. Your social interactions may have also been severed or limited, and that may be adding stress to your already demanding life.

Grieving Is a Continuous Process

It is imperative that you take note of the losses you may be experiencing or may be experiencing in your life due to your new role as a caretaker and start the process of grieving as a necessary way toward healing and adaptation of a new reality. As you grieve properly in a healthy way, you will be able to overcome the sadness and anguish. But remember, grieving is a universal process, and it is continuous.

For instance, one of my friends has a son who is twenty-five years old, and he has severe autism, which means that his son has very limited speech, is unable to be independent or safe by himself (he cannot stay alone at home or in the community, and he cannot take care of all his physical needs, like toileting), and requires ongoing care. He mentioned that he identified three times during which he grieved his son. The first one was when he was born and was told he was autistic., the second time was when he realized that his son will never be able to speak, and the third time was when he realized that he will never have grandchildren from his son.

To be effective caretakers, it is important that we understand that part of our loved one's healing is that we grieve properly and in a healthy way, and that includes the following:

- To identify and accept our losses.
- To acknowledge and express full range of feelings we experience because of the loss.
- To adjust to a life in which much will be expected from us.

To say goodbye, to ritualize, and to make peace with the loss, I recommend people to write down our negative feelings, emotions, and fears caused by our loss and, in a safe way, burn it as a ritual that symbolizes that it is time to let go.

The Benefits of Healthy Grieving

Processing your loss properly will allow you to free up the energy that is connected to the lost person (health), object, relationship, or experience so you may reinvest that energy elsewhere, like taking care of your loved ones and yourself. Until you grieve effectively, it is highly likely that you will find reinvesting that energy difficult, because a part of us remains tied to the past. Please take time to reflect in gratitude for the current opportunity you have to be of some help to your loved one. Take time every day to find things to be grateful for, and that will give you the energy and motivation to keep doing what you need to do in your new role. Focusing on gratitude during difficult times means that you intentionally choose to celebrate the positive memories of a loved one's life rather than focusing on the negative emotions of their loss.

Compassionate Care

In your new role as a caregiver, very quickly, you will come to the realization of the extent of your loved one's care needs, and it may be necessary to assess and analyze your personal, family, and community resources to help take care of those needs. Do not think that you are alone in this role. Allow and involve people to help you even if it is for a short time.

Make a daily and weekly schedule of caretaking activities that need to be done (medical, supervising, feeding, cleaning, etc.) and schedule breaks around that schedule. Even small breaks will make a difference in your mental health. But make sure that as you show compassionate care for the person you are helping, you also show care for yourself. You are an important part of this equation. Please make sure you understand that taking care of yourself is necessary and as important as taking care of your family member.

Compassion Fatigue

Be mindful and give yourself some grace, because nothing in this life could have prepared you for such an intense and demanding role. Be aware that this role is stressful, emotional, and tiresome; and it will take a toll on you if you do not find ways to balance your personal and family life in a healthy way. In my experience as a mental health professional, I have noticed that it is easy to experience compassion fatigue, which is the cost of caring for others or their emotional pain. It is easy to arrive to this point if you are neglecting your own emotional, mental, and physical needs to serve others.

Compassion fatigue is a condition characterized by emotional and physical exhaustion, leading to a diminished ability to empathize or feel compassion for others, and that others includes you. If you let yourself go, eventually, you will be burned out and will have no desire or energy to keep helping. Compassion fatigue is also referred to as secondary trauma stress, because it is the trauma you experience when trying to help others.

These are some of the most noticeable symptoms and behaviors of compassion fatigue:

- Feelings of helplessness and powerlessness in the face of the suffering individual

- Diminished ability or interest to care for others (you may feel saturated with emotional pain)
- Mental or physical exhaustion
- Feeling overwhelmed and exhausted by current caretaking demands
- Anger and irritability
- Feeling detached, numb, and emotionally disconnected (like a zombie)
- Loss of interest in activities you used to enjoy
- Anxiety or depression
- Intrusive thoughts
- Difficulty concentrating and making decisions
- Sleep problems
- Being easily startled (hypervigilant)
- Extreme preoccupation with the people you help
- Increased conflict in personal relationships (becoming overly emotional)
- Neglecting your own care (not prioritizing your own needs)
- Withdrawal and isolation (detaching from reality)
- Physical symptoms, like headaches, nausea, upset stomach, and dizziness

Remember that to be emotionally and physically present for your loved ones, first, you must take care of yourself. Only in taking care of ourselves can we make a difference in the lives of family and friends who are on a healing process or sometimes on an end-of-life journey. One way to avoid compassion fatigue is by implanting transitions and by having a self-care plan.

Implementing Transitions

Many years ago, I interviewed a mental health provider. At that time, she was working in an oncology hospital. In there, part of her job was to provide emotional support and psychotherapy for the patients and their families as they transition to the end of life. She was there with the doctors when they gave the bad news to the patients, and she was there to support their families as they tried to process that difficult news.

I remember being amazed by her willingness to do that job, and I asked her how she can perform that emotionally draining job and still be okay. She told me that early in her career, she learned to practice transitions, meaning that she learned to separate her different roles in life. At the hospital, she was a mental health provider. But at home, she was a mother, a wife, but also a human being with her own needs and emotions.

So as a part of transitioning from her role as a mental health provider to her roles at home, she took twenty to thirty minutes at her office, cleansing herself from her work emotions; and when she was ready, she moved to her home roles. Some people do that while driving (listening to music and intentionally leaving feelings and thoughts related to a previous role). Traditional Japanese people leave their shoes at the entrance of their home maybe not just to avoid bringing unclean things home but also as a symbolism of leaving their external worries outside their family life. I think we can do the same with our emotions.

As you transition temporarily from roles, you can separate the intense emotions that come with daily caretaking of a loved one. Remember, we all carry different hats, but we have only one head. As you transition from role to role, make sure you separate your emotions. When you consciously make time to be with yourself, even if it is only ten minutes, make it count. During that time, you can take a walk, watch a fun video, call a friend or supportive family member, or simply take a power nap if needed.

Self-Care

Self-care is an important principle of mental health. If you do it in the right way, you will experience a renewal of energy and peace of mind. However, to practice self-care, it may require a switch in the way you understand things. It may require that you understand that only in taking care of ourselves can we make a difference in the lives of family and friends who are on a healing process or sometimes on an end-of-life journey. So self-care is not only about you but also about the person you are taking care of.

For those who have a hard time understanding this principle, I always ask them, "If an old lady falls down on the ground in front of you, what do you do?" Immediately, all of them answer, "I will quickly pick her up and see about her." Then I ask them, "How come you do not do the same for yourself? Why do you think it is okay to run and help others, but it is okay not to do the same for yourself?"

This new role will require that you understand and accept that it is okay to love and have compassion for yourself. How do you do that? Through a series of conscious activities purposely chosen to give you peace of mind and renew your mental and physical energy. We will get into much detail in this regard in the following paragraphs.

Learning to Love Yourself

Love means different things for different people. The type of love that I am referring to is the one that is perfect and unconditional. Imagine that you deserve infinite and unconditional love. (The truth is, you really do.) What would that mean for you? How would that change your life? I want you to keep thinking on that as you continue reading this chapter.

Most people attribute love to God; others to different deities or to the universe. Regarding the source, you can become that source of perfect love for yourself as you learn how to accept and love who you are. If you believe that God or the universe is perfect and his love is perfect, then it will make sense to believe that it is okay to love yourself as he loves—with abundant, perfect, and self-compassion. But what is that?

Self-compassion is extending compassion for oneself even in instances of perceived inadequacy, failure, or general suffering. There is no self-love without self-compassion. You do not have to be perfect to love and accept yourself for who you are. You can start now by showing yourself some kindness. Make a list of negative beliefs or ideas you have developed about yourself, and next to it, I challenge you to add the opposite (write the kindest words you may find). This exercise will challenge you to develop self-kindness.

Self-kindness involves being warm toward oneself when encountering pain and personal defects rather than ignoring them or hurting oneself with criticism. As you work toward developing self-kindness, you will consciously choose to be nicer to yourself.

Give yourself the love and the value you deserve. Love yourself like nobody has ever loved you, and you will experience more love for yourself but also for the person you are caring. Have you heard that love moves the world around? That is true, but start with loving yourself.

Self-Compassion as a Caregiver

As a caregiver, it is expected of you to take care of others but also to take care of yourself. I want you to think what self-compassion means to you and how important it is for you in your new role, as well as in your other roles in life. Your family member or the person you are taking care of needs your love, not your sacrifice. He needs you alive, whole, and happy. Self-care will provide you not only with the energy but also the mental and emotional peace of mind to be present for him. Now that you are understanding this, give yourself some grace. It is never late to give yourself some love—maybe the love that you expected from parents, siblings, friends and that maybe you never received.

Self-Love as a Caregiver

Self-love is also another important concept in understanding the principle of self-care. Even if you did not experience much love in your childhood or in your life, love is available to you, and you can be the main provider of it. First, you deserve it. Give yourself unconditional love, but to do that, I want you to make a list of negative ideas that come to your mind every day that contribute to your feelings of being undeserving of love or care. (It is very common to think that love applies to others, but we tend to think that we can be okay without much love.)

I have seen my clients' list, and I have seen my own. Some of the items in this list look like "I am not enough," "You are not smart," "You are a bad person," "You are not the center of the universe," "You are not special," etc. Let me tell you if nobody has told you yet that you matter and that you are special. Taking care of yourself is not just required but of much importance not only for normal functioning but also for happiness. The moment that you start loving yourself, many things will improve in your life, even your physical and mental health.

Self-Care

There is no self-care without self-love. If you think that there is no time for self-care, you are not there yet, and this may be a great opportunity to reconsider that. You may be asking yourself, "How can I take care of myself when life is so demanding?" You may be thinking, "It sounds all good, but after taking care of my family members' needs, I do not have time or energy for that." I understand that it is difficult to take care of our own needs when we consciously place other people's needs ahead of our own, However, you will not be of much help if you do not practice self-care.

Self-care is a conscious decision that involves taking action to preserve or improve your mental, emotional, and physical health during periods of stress. There are five areas of self-care: physical, intellectual, emotional, social, and spiritual. Don't abandon yourself because you are too busy or you do not have time. Time is a human construct, and you will make time for yourself because you are as important as the person you are taking care of.

Breaking the Barriers of Self-Care

As you learn and consider implementing a self-care plan, it is important to identify the self-care barriers in your life. Are there any cultural, religious, or limiting beliefs that are interfering with the principle of taking care of yourself? Some people use the concept of self-care to spend money and time as an excuse of taking care of themselves, but that is not self-care. That is self-centered behavior, and that has nothing to do with self-care. Self-care implies growing and improving your mental, emotional, intellectual, and physical state to become the best version of yourself.

Self-Care Misconceptions

There are many misconceptions regarding self-care. For instance, it is only for rich people. No it is not. You don't need money to take care of yourself. What you need is the willingness to learn and do what is best and work for you. In this chapter, we are going to give you simple ideas and resources so you can learn how to take care of your emotions, your physical body, and your mind.

Self-Care for Caregivers

In your new role, it is important that you take priority of your physical, emotional, mental, and spiritual health. Even if you have a self-care plan, it may be necessary to adjust it to your new life's demands. Here are some ideas that you can implement in your life as a part of your care plan.

1. *Physical self-care.* Take the decision to become more physically active and improve your nutrition and sleep. Make this decision a must, not just a wish, and it will happen. Here are some examples of physical self-care.

   - Regular exercises you can do at home, as recommended by the CDC and possibly going for a walk combined with breathing exercises, even for short periods of time.
   - Getting enough sleep. If you have a hard time falling asleep, practice *progressive muscle relaxation* or PMR. If you need more information on PMR or sleep dis-

orders, you may want to visit the Mayo clinic or the Verywell Mind websites.

- Regular hydration. Carry a refillable water bottle whenever you go. If you want to make it fun, add some flavor to your water.
- Breathing exercises.
- Have alarm reminders for your medicine and supplements.
- Think on nutrition instead of just eating or dieting. Include fruits and grains in your food intake and food that you like and that is nutritious.
- Schedule regular visits to your doctor.

2. *Emotional self-care.* We are emotional beings, and our mental peace is easy to disturb. As we interact with other people and as we respond to life's multiple demands, life can be stressful, and stress, when not managed properly, will affect your mental and physical health. One of the most important life skills, in my opinion, is to learn how to manage your emotions. The opposite of that is being emotionally reactive. People who are reactive tend to not think much before acting. They just react to situations through their emotions, and those are the ones that they come across as blaming, resentful, insecure, or angry. Basically, when you are a reactive person, you do things only in response to others. Some people grew up in a highly reactive environment and learned to be reactive, and eventually, that became a behavior by default.

Emotional regulation is the acquired ability to modify or control your thoughts, emotions, actions, and words. We all have different triggers that are activated by people or life events. Learning to regulate how we respond to our triggers is a valuable life skill, because it brings you back from an emotion-altered state to a calm one. When you are calm, your brain is no longer activated by the fight, flight, and freeze state. You are back to using your frontal lobe, which oversees executive functions such as the cognitive control of behaviors, and that is what we want—to be fully conscious and aware of our actions and their consequences.

When you self-regulate your emotional state, you consciously engage your brain to stop you from saying or doing things that may hurt others. So any action that alters the intensity of an emotional experience is a way to self-regulate your emotions. Some people regulate their emotions through the following:

- Identifying their emotional triggers. What makes me angry, afraid, sad, etc.?
- Noticing what they are feeling. For instance, I am feeling offended. Why?
- Naming what they feel. You may have to increase your emotional vocabulary to be able to express a full range of emotions.
- Accepting the emotion.

3. *Practicing mindfulness.* Mindfulness is the basic human ability to be totally present with yourself. When you practice mindfulness, you learn to be aware of where you are and of your actions. This gives you power to pause and breathe instead of being reactive and overwhelmed by what is going on around you.

Emotional Triggers

As part of your learning how to regulate your emotions, be honest with yourself and make a list of your emotional triggers, those little things that quickly provoke emotions that are difficult to control. It can be anything—memories, experiences, words, etc. Develop a specific strategy for each one. For instance, if my trigger is anger when I feel people are blaming me, I will consider and challenge the story I am telling myself, and I will take a breath to calm down my physiological response before I say or do something.

As a caregiver, you will experience a roller coaster of emotions. Therefore, finding the calming coping skill that works for you will be instrumental to help you regulate your emotions. Consider going briefly to therapy specifically to learn how to regulate your emotions the same way you will go to school to learn a specific skill.

Intellectual Self-Care

Please make sure you take the conscious initiative to keep your brain active. Reading is a rewarding activity that will engage your imagination and a channel for your emotions. Make sure that you are always learning something, have a hobby, listening to a podcast, etc. Keeping your brain engaged in mindful activities will stimulate your self-esteem and your willingness to enjoy life.

What is your passion in life? Can you learn more about it? What is stopping you? In this era of much technology, the access to information is at the tip of your fingers. So yes, you are busy. But still, you can learn. It is a matter of what you want to know more about. Make a list of topics that interest you that you will be willing to explore, and listen to a podcast or watch videos about it. Also, you can get a library card and have access to thousands of books and audiobooks. As you learn more about and follow your passion, you will feel great and fulfilled. Take a decision to do something in that regard today.

Social Self-Care

We are social beings, and maintaining meaningful and healthy human connections is important to our integral well-being. Intentionally choose to be connected to others (family, friends, coworkers, or members of your community). Be intentional about scheduling regular phone calls or texts to touch base with family and friends. You don't have to have many friends, but pick who you want to have in your life whom you can be supportive of, and they can be of support to you.

In your new role as a caregiver, you are going to need supportive friends and people you can trust even if it is just to listen about your day or what you are going through. Just remember that it takes being a friend to have friends. It takes being mindful and intentional about calling, texting, and reaching out to others.

As you engage in this demanding role, remember that relationships are live entities that need care and attention; and most of the time, you get what you give or what you are willing to put into it. Now if I ask you the five more important relationships in your life, who will be in your list? (Hint: I hope you include yourself in this list, because the relationship with yourself must be a priority.) Now that you have figured it out, what are your relationship expectations with each one of them? What do you want to get out of maintaining those relationships?

Your marital relationship will greatly suffer if you are not mindful about it. The daily demands of taking care of a child, an ill parent, or family will take most of all your goodness. Therefore, it will be a smart choice to do something to nurture your relationship with your spouse. For instance, according to an article from *Psychology Today* from February 28, 2023, the divorce rate of families with a child with disabilities may be as high as 87 percent. The divorce rate of families with a child with autism is 80 percent. A common factor in these two statistics is the stress related to the caregiving task, which may apply to you as well. Therefore, learning how to manage stress.

Keeping Your Marriage Together while Being a Caregiver

Due to the intensive demands of time and energy that comes with becoming a caregiver, in order to keep a successful marriage, it is important that you understand three important components of the triangular theory of love by Robert Sternberg (1986). These three components are commitment, intimacy, and passion. Successfully married couples take the time to work in these three areas, because it helps strengthen their relationship.

Commitment. Ask yourself, in a scale from 0 to 10, where zero means "I don't want to be in this relationship" and ten means "I am 100 percent committed to this relationship," where are you at? Where is your spouse or partner at? It is common to hear in couple's therapy that each spouse is on a different level in this scale, which means that if they are willing to do the work, improvements can be made. Everyone has his own definition of commitment, and that needs to be clarified.

Commitment is a rational rather than an emotional decision and must be at 100 percent. It is not at 50-50. Commitment is not only sanctioned promises to each other but is also the decision to be engaged and faithful to each other. Working with couples, I have seen that when both say that they are equally committed, I usually see that the couple resolves their issues. As you work with your spouse or partner in recommitting to each other, your chances are high to keep the passion alive and increase intimacy in your relationship.

Intimacy. This is the sense of feeling closely connected to the person we love. Intimacy is feeling safe, valued, and supported and feeling that you can count on the other in times of need. It is a process that can never be fully completed. Sometimes, intimacy can be holding hands as we go for a walk or feeling that your spouse/partner has your back. There is not greater feeling than that in a relationship.

There are seven types of intimacy, and each one deserves and needs special attention. These seven types of intimacy are the following:

- Emotional intimacy—experiencing a feeling of closeness. Expressing love in any form (writing love notes, calling, texting, etc.) and small details will strengthen your sense of closeness.
- Social intimacy—having common friends, date nights, and spending time together and with friends will keep you intentionally away from isolation. You need friends. Keep them close.
- Intellectual intimacy—sharing ideas and respecting, valuing, and supporting each other's intellectual interests.
- Sexual intimacy—sharing affection and sex.
- Recreational intimacy—doing fun things together.
- Spiritual intimacy—sharing similar sense regarding meaning of life or religion.

- Aesthetic intimacy—sharing in the experience of sense of beauty.

Passion. Passion is the third component of the love triangle. Passion is the romance, the life, and the light of the relationship. To keep the passion alive, make the commitment to spend time together and the desire to be curious and interested in your spouse or partner. In your new role, your time is going to be limited, but consider making time to be intentionally intimate and passionate about each other. There is nothing more damaging to a relationship than the routine. In addition to that, caregiving couples with special needs family members who have successful marriages have certain things in common: accepting each other's strengths and weaknesses, seeking outside assistance, making time for each other, and practicing individual self-care. On this regard, requesting help from others will be key to have some time to invest in your relationship.

Spiritual Self-Care

Not much has been written in this subject; however, spiritual self-care is developing a sense of meaning. It is reminding yourself who you are, your worth, and your purpose. Spiritual self-care is anything that helps you develop a profound sense of meaning and understanding.

Spirituality in any form has been demonstrated to be very helpful in strengthening mental health, especially when people go into stressful and challenging times. Faith is a powerful instrument, because it is a source of hope, and having faith invites us to keep going, even when you think that you cannot anymore. Here is where meditation and pray will help you to be centered and calm. Some examples of spiritual self-care are some activities such as meditation, yoga, going to a place of worship, being in nature, dedicating time for self-reflection, etc. Choose one or two favorite spiritual activities that in the past have been useful to your spirituality. If you do not have a favorite spiritual activity, choose one and dare yourself to experiment one.

Coping Strategies

Coping strategies are skills that you can learn to manage your emotions in a healthy way. In your role as a caregiver, you are expected to go through a roller coaster of emotions and stress; therefore, knowing how to regulate your emotions and manage your stress is going to be instrumental in helping you be emotional healthy. We already talked about some of them, but I want to list the most important so you can have it in your emotional toolbox. Some of the most common coping strategies are the following:

- mindfulness
- progressive muscle relaxation for stress or stress related sleep disorders
- use of different types of relaxation techniques

Any one of these and more can be found by browsing the web or doing a YouTube search to help teach you why this is so important. The National Institute on Health and the National Center for complementary and integrative health has a great article on relaxation techniques that will be of great help as you learn why relaxation is so critical.

Listed below are some of the different types of relaxation techniques.

- *Progressive relaxation.* Also called progressive muscle relaxation, this technique involves tensing different muscles in your body and then releasing the tension.
- *Autogenic training.* Make a list of relaxation ideas and use autosuggestion to allow your body to focus on the experience of relaxation.
- *Guided imagery or visualization.* In guided imagery, focus on your favorite picture objects, scenes, or events that you associate with relaxation or calmness and challenge your mind to produce a similar feeling in your body.

- *Self-hypnosis.* Make a list of empowering, positive affirmations, affirmations that are believable, and repeat them to yourself. You can do it before falling asleep, as you wake up, or as you need self-encouragement. Repeating these positive affirmations will change your subconscious mind and will increase self-esteem and self-love.
- *Breathing exercises.* Breathing exercises will calm your physiological responses to stress. As you breathe, focus on taking slow, deep breaths—also called diaphragmatic breathing. Engage in noticing your breath, and be mentally present as you do that.

Other complementary health practices, such as massage therapy, meditation, yoga, tai chi, and qigong, can produce several beneficial effects in the body, including the relaxation response; however, these practices are not discussed in this fact sheet.

Here are other ways to help with self-care and coping.

- *Thought changing.* Remember that you will feel the emotions that you focus on. If the emotions that you are feeling are not healthy, you have the power to change them, and how fast can you change your emotions? As fast as you change your focus. As a kid, every time I wanted to change the TV channel, I must walk in front of the TV and change the channel selector. If you are feeling sad and overwhelmed, try to change your focus to a fun and happy memory, and that will make you feel happy. Don't dwell on emotions that are harmful and detrimental for your mental health.
- *Distraction.* Here, involve any action designed to decrease the intensity of our emotions by redirecting to more pleasurable activities, such as listening to music, painting, drawing, watching a video, etc. Make a list of distracting activities that you can easily do on your own and on the go.
- *Social support.* This coping mechanism is characterized by seeking resources and support provided by a social network (family, friends, community, and church members)

to help you cope with the stress of being a caregiver. This social support can be manifested as financial aid, preparing meals, having a substitute caregiver, even for short periods of time, or just somebody willing to listening to you when you need to vent. Who would you include in your list as social support?

- *Setting boundaries.* Boundaries are meant to protect you, and it is a skill that sometimes is hard to set and enforce. As a caregiver, it is expected that you separate your feelings from other people's feelings. When you set emotional boundaries, you do not let other people's feelings, thoughts, or moods affect yours. An emotional boundary is the one you set for yourself. Here are some examples of boundaries that you may consider setting.

  o Delegating chores when feel overwhelmed.
  o Avoiding overcommitting. Know and accept your physical and emotional limitations.
  o Speak up when you feel uncomfortable.
  o Request help as needed.
  o Ask for space when you need your own time.

- *Self-talk.* This is a way to engage your emotional brain and your logical brain. As both establish a dialogue, it is expected to produce more balanced and wiser thoughts. Therefore, as you talk sense into yourself, you will become wiser as you use positive self-talk and words of encouragement. In other words, make sure you become your best cheerleader.

There are many other coping skills that would take lots of space in this book; however, remember that the purpose of these coping skills is to help you be emotionally regulated, because when your brain is calm, it can function at its best. It's probable that you already have a set of coping skills that you use often. Whatever it is, choose healthy ways to cope with stress in your new role. Some people use drugs, alcohol, aggression, food, negative self-talk, etc. If you find yourself struggling to cope with your emotions, it may be necessary to seek the professional help of a therapist.

There is nothing wrong with seeing a therapist. As a clinician, I have my own therapist too. Finding a safe place to explore your emotions and learn regulatory emotional skills will be beneficial to yourself and your relationships. Your mental health is important and should be your priority. Remember that you may not be of much help if first you don't seek help for yourself.

Mental health is a very extensive topic. I hope that what we talked about in this chapter was of interest to you and a useful resource. Therapists have many therapeutic models and resources to help you if you need specific assistance in different areas of your life. In your demanding caregiving role, you definitively may need some professional assistance even if it is a monthly checkup appointment. Thirty percent of success in therapy will depend on the relationship of trust you may develop with your therapist. Forty percent will depend on your willingness to do the work required of you to make changes and improvements in your life. Therefore, to be successful in therapy, as well as in life, you may have to intentionally engage.

I wish you the best in your new role. You have so many tools and supportive people at your disposal, and as you take care of yourself and enroll people to help you, your chances to do well are great. Read enthusiastically this book, take notes, highlight what is most important to you, and make commitments to implement improvements in your life. The intention of writing this chapter was to provide some guidance for people in the caregiving role, and in no way has this been intended to substitute mental health therapy. If you need assistance for a clinician or mental health provider, please schedule an appointment as soon as possible.

Best regards in your caregiving role, with much appreciation for what you do.

Luis A. Torres, LMFT
Licensed marriage and family therapist

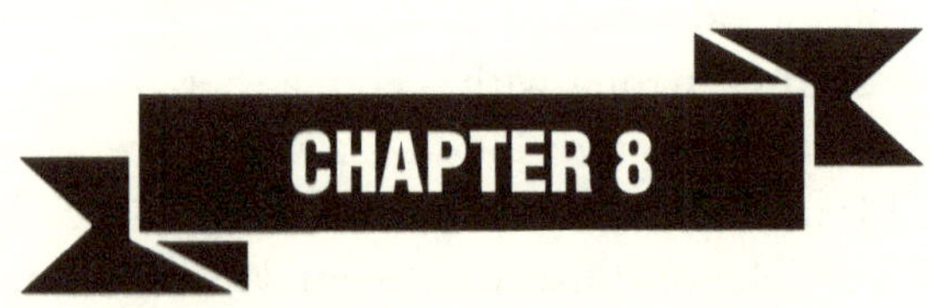

CHAPTER 8

Dealing with Challenging Behaviors

AS A CAREGIVER, you may see or experience any number of behaviors from your loved one, many of which can tax your wits as to what to do. While it is easy to snap back when you encounter a challenging behavior, this can often only set them off even more. This chapter is to offer you some examples of challenges you may face, as well as some resources you may wish to explore, to see if they will help in your situation. The key is to never to punish or restrain them. The goal is, if you have already experienced some violent ones, you can prepare for them ahead of time not only to protect your home but also, more importantly, to protect yourself or even your loved one from harming themselves.

We often think the challenging behaviors will come from our loved one suffering from substance abuse or post-traumatic stress disorder (PTSD) or the elderly with dementia, where they may be forgetful or have a tendency to wander. However, this is not always the case. Challenging behaviors can be seen in some persons with a brain injury, mental illness, or intellectual or developmental disabilities (IDD), such as autism or oppositional defiant disorder or persons suffering from chronic pain or substance abuses. It is often these categories of illnesses where we may see even more disruptive, disturbing, or violent behaviors.

I am a nurse, and while I have seen and dealt with many of the following behaviors during my career, I am not a psychiatrist or a mental health counselor. And consequently, I do not know all the various diagnoses or all the new treatment techniques used in attempts to control a challenging behavior. Thus, I will give you a wide variety of websites to use, as this will allow you to do your own research and educate yourself not only on a diagnosis but also on treatment options you may wish to explore with your loved one's mental health or developmental disabilities team.

Remember, you are often the eyes, ears, and voice of your loved one; and one of your key goals is to ensure not only that your loved one is safe but also that so are you. If you feel your loved one's physician is not listening to you or responding to the needs of your loved one, do not hesitate to change physicians. This may seem mean, but you may need to possibly make several changes until one that fits your loved one's needs is found. So plan and act wisely and accordingly.

Challenging behaviors are behaviors that are seen as problematic by others noticing the behavior. They often are those behaviors that may also involve actions that come into conflict with what is considered acceptable in one's individual community. If your loved one does have challenging behaviors, these may not only possibly isolate them from their community. But in some instances, the behaviors may also pose a barrier to the person living or remaining in a community. This could mean possibly an admission to a crisis home or psychiatric hospital or, worse yet, hospitalization in a state hospital with a forensic ward or even incarceration.

Challenging behaviors vary in seriousness and intensity and depend upon the reason and what trigger(s) that may have set off the behavior. Challenging behavior activity can include but is not limited to any of the following:

- Yelling, cursing, screaming, or threats.
- Hitting and kicking and punching.
- Talking or moving in response to hallucinations (hearing voices or seeing things).
- Physical aggression, hyperactivity, mania (overacting with great excitement or activity), and violent outbursts.

- Excessive consumption of alcohol and subsequent intoxication.
- Property damage and destruction.
- Inappropriate sexual behavior (ISB), which can occur as a potentially disruptive form of behavior in people with dementia and some persons diagnosed with IDD. ISB can include sex talk, such as using foul language or verbally expressing sexual feelings, openly reading or looking at pornographic material, or performing actual sexual acts, such as touching, grabbing, exposing, or masturbating, any of which can occur in private or in public areas.

You may want to explore this topic in more detail as you will find excellent information on such websites as the National Library of Medicine and its PubMed and the National Center for Biotechnology Information website (PubMed (nih.gov) on inappropriate sexual behavior in adolescents with autism spectrum disorder or intellectual or development disorders, or from the ABA (Applied Behavioral Analysis) Centers of America website.

Examples of Disorders That Can Cause Challenging Behaviors

Self-injurious behaviors (SIB). This could be cutting of the body or picking at skin or open areas, pulling out hair, head-banging, or poking at eyes or burning oneself. In most cases, self-injury is done in private, and it is a way to cope with emotional pain, sadness, anger, and stress. SIB is often most common in adolescent females; individuals who have a history of mental, physical, emotional, or sexual abuse; individuals who have coexisting problems of substance abuse; individuals who have an obsessive-compulsive disorder or an eating disorder; individuals who were raised in families that discouraged expression of anger; and individuals who lack skills to express their emotions and lack a good social support network.

At times, self-injury, while not intended, can cause life-threatening injuries or even death. SIB is a relatively common behavior in individuals with intellectual disabilities (ID). The National

Library of Medicine and its PubMed and the National Center for Biotechnology Information website (PubMed (nih.gov) has a great article that may give you more information on the dangers of self-injury behaviors often seen in individuals with an intellectual disability.

Severe withdrawal or depression. Per the National Institute of Mental Health and other websites, symptoms caused by major depression can vary from person to person. Depression (also known as major depression, major depressive disorder, or clinical depression) is a common but serious mood disorder. It causes severe symptoms that affect how a person feels, thinks, and handles daily activities, such as sleeping, eating, or working. To be diagnosed with depression, the symptoms must be present for at least two weeks. There are different types of depression, some of which develop due to specific circumstances.

1) Major depression includes symptoms of depressed mood or loss of interest, most of the time for at least two weeks, which interferes with daily activities.
2) Persistent depressive disorder (also called dysthymia or dysthymic disorder) consists of less severe symptoms of depression that last much longer, usually for at least two years.
3) Perinatal depression is depression that occurs during or after pregnancy. Depression that begins during pregnancy is prenatal depression, and depression that begins after the baby is born is postpartum depression.
4) Seasonal affective disorder is depression that comes and goes with the seasons, with symptoms typically starting in the late fall and early winter and going away during the spring and summer.
5) Depression with symptoms of psychosis is a severe form of depression in which a person experiences psychosis symptoms, such as delusions (disturbing, false, fixed beliefs) or hallucinations (hearing or seeing things others do not hear or see).
6) Bipolar disorder (formerly called manic depression or manic-depressive illness) also experiences depressive episodes,

during which they feel sad, indifferent, or hopeless, combined with a very low activity level. But a person with bipolar disorder also experiences manic (or less severe hypomanic) episodes or unusually elevated moods, in which they may feel very happy, irritable, or up with a marked increase in activity level.

7) Schizophrenia is a serious mental disorder in which people interpret reality abnormally. Schizophrenia may result in some combination of hallucinations, delusions, and extremely disordered thinking and behavior that impairs daily functioning and can be disabling. Schizophrenia involves a range of problems with thinking (cognition), behavior, and emotions. Signs and symptoms may vary but usually involves delusions, hallucinations, or disorganized speech and reflect an impaired ability to function.

If you want more information on any of the foregoing topics, you may want to conduct your research on such, but your research may not be limited to such websites as Verywell Mind, WebMD, *Psychology Today*, or the National Institute on Health website and its mental health websites.

Severe anxiety or panic, extreme delusions, and confusion. Again, the web can educate you on any of the conditions and the challenging behaviors you may expect. For these issues, I used information from the Mayo Clinic and the Cleveland Clinic websites. Experiencing occasional anxiety is a normal part of life. However, people with anxiety disorders frequently have intense, excessive, and persistent worry and fear about everyday situations. Often, anxiety disorders involve repeated episodes of sudden feelings of intense anxiety and fear or terror that reach a peak within minutes (panic attacks).

These feelings of anxiety and panic interfere with daily activities, are difficult to control, are out of proportion to the actual danger, and can last a long time. To help prevent these feelings and if at all possible, your loved one may need to avoid specific places and situations. Research shows symptoms may start during childhood or the teen years and continue into adulthood.

Extreme delusions. Delusional disorder is a type of mental health condition in which a person can't tell what's real from what's imagined. There are many types of delusional disorders including persecutory, jealous, and grandiose types, any one of which you can conduct your own Internet research on for tips on dealing with it by typing in your web browser "delusional disorders."

Extreme confusion. Some signs of confusion include slurring words or having long pauses during speech, abnormal or incoherent speech, lack of awareness of location or time, forgetting what a task is while it's being performed, and sudden changes in emotion, such as sudden agitation. While one of the first couple of medical conditions to think of will be a stroke or head injury, your first response, if you do suspect this, is to call 9-1-1. When dealing with a loved one with dementia or a brain disorder or a medical condition, confusion may be the result of other medical issues, such as dehydration, an infection, not taking medications appropriately, low blood sugar, malnutrition, or fever. In any case, when severe confusion arises, your first response as a caregiver will be to seek medical care.

Eating disorders. The most common are anorexia nervosa, bulimia, pica (an eating disorder involving eating items that are typically thought of as food and that do not contain significant nutritional value, such as hair, dirt, and paint chips or their own poop), compulsive eating, and laxative abuse. For your research, you can type in your web browser "eating disorders," and it should bring up various sites to use as you learn more about this disorder. One key website might be Healthline.com as this website contains a wealth of information on the topic. As you conduct your search, you may also wish to find a weblink that will offer you information on support groups in your loved one's region. One of your best resources to use as you conduct your Internet research on eating disorders will be the National Association of Anorexia Nervosa and Associated Disorders website: https://anad.org/. To find an online support group, go to the Health line website and in your web browser type in Health line best-eating-disorder-support-groups.

Oppositional defiant disorder. If you are dealing with a child or adult with oppositional defiant disorder (ODD), which is one of a group of behavioral disorders called disruptive behavior disorders (DBD), your loved one will often have trouble at home, school, or work and have difficulty making friends. ODD often occurs along with other behavioral or mental health problems, so it is critical you encourage your loved one to undergo a full medical examination. This will help determine the cause. Also, to better understand ODD, do your own Internet research on the topic, making notes so that when working with the treating medical professionals, a treatment plan can be developed. Some common symptoms associated with ODD are the following:

1. Frequent temper tantrums
2. Excessive arguing with adults
3. Habitual use of foul language
4. Never obeying an adult's request and question rules
5. Attempting to annoy adults or upset people
6. Easy provocation to anger/annoyance
7. Frequent anger/irritation
8. Spiteful attitude and revenge seeking

Some of the complications associated with ODD are the following:

1. Poor school and work performance
2. Antisocial behavior
3. Aggression and disobedient behavior
4. Impulse and rebellious behavior and issues with control of behavior, as they do not know how to control their anger
5. Substance use disorder
6. Suicide

Children with Developmental Disabilities

Most children with developmental disabilities are not any more violent or aggressive than other children. However, some children may feel a lot of frustration related to their developmental disability. This frustration is sometimes shown through aggression or even self-harming behaviors, such as banging their head or cutting their skin.

Other children have conditions that are more directly connected to aggressive behavior. For example, children with oppositional defiant disorder are often annoyed and angry, and they argue with adults in order to gain control.

There are many reasons children with developmental disabilities may have aggression problems. It is important to remember that everyone has times when they get frustrated or angry, and children should be taught that frustration is normal. However, the key is to work with your loved one's behavioral or mental health provider on what is right and wrong and tips to suggest it may be more than normal.

Dealing with Autism

Autism spectrum disorder (ASD) is a developmental disability caused by differences in the brain. People with ASD may behave, communicate, interact, and learn in ways that are different from most other people. There is often nothing about how they look that sets them apart from other people. Autism spectrum disorder (ASD) is a neurological and developmental disorder that affects how people interact with others, communicate, learn, and behave. ASD is known as a spectrum disorder because there is wide variation in the type and severity of symptoms people experience. Although autism can be diagnosed at any age, it is described as a developmental disorder because symptoms generally appear in the first two years of life.

The abilities of people with ASD can vary significantly. For example, some people with ASD may have advanced conversation skills, whereas others may be nonverbal. Some people with ASD need a lot of help in their daily lives; others can work and live with little to no support. For more detailed information on ASD, including signs and symptoms, social communication and interactive skills, restricted or repetitive behaviors or interests, and other characteristics, as well as treatment modalities, see the Centers for Disease Control and Prevention websites and the links provided under the ASD, where you can learn about ASD homepage column. Here you can do your own research on the disorder and then discuss the treatments and intervention and strategies with your loved one's mental health professional. To conduct your own Internet research on autism and the resources or treatments, you may wish to investigate might be either the Centers for Disease Control and Prevention (CDC) or the National Institute Health and its National Institute of Mental Health (NIMH » Autism Spectrum Disorder (nih.gov) websites.

Two excellent resources for you as the caregiver and parent will be the Autism Speaks (autismspeaks.org) and the National Autism Association (NAA) websites. From the Autism Speaks website, you will find a wealth of information, including the following:

- booklet called *A Parent's Guide to Autism*
- downloadable toolkit
- resource directory that will let you search your loved one's region for resources you might wish to investigate and use.

From the National Autism Association website, again you can access a wealth of information as well as the NAA's Big Red Safety Box which contains such items as:

- educational materials and tools, including NAA's BeREDy booklet
- two (2) door/window alarms including batteries
- one (1) road ID bracelet or shoe ID tag. You will receive instructions in the box to submit your custom personalization order at http://roadid.com/naa.
- five (5) laminated adhesive stop sign visual prompts for doors and windows
- two (2) safety alert window clings for car or home windows
- one (1) child ID kit from the National Center for Missing & Exploited Children

Where once you enter your state and the level of support you are seeking, a wealth of information is at your fingertips. Here you can find resources to assist you with (a) advocacy support, (b) autism-friendly services, (c) information on employment and secondary education, (d) evaluation and diagnosis, (e) health and medical, (f) housing and community living, (g) multiservice providers, (h) community recreation, (i) safety, (j) schools, (k) state services and entitlements, (l) support, (m) support groups, and (n) treatments and therapy.

Note: As you research the Autism Speaks or any of the websites referenced here, remember that I have only provided general information about a topic so as to educate you of services within a community. The information provided on any of the websites, as well as what I have written, is merely to assist you in your search for resources that can help you in your role. However, do not let any of these serve as a recommendation, referral, or endorsement of any resource, therapeutic method, or service provider, as none of what is written definitely replaces the advice of medical, legal, or educational professionals you may need to consult. You need to do your homework, discuss all with your loved one's medical team, and let them help you find the right treatment modality for your loved one's medical or mental health issue.

Individuals with autism or other mental health or developmental disorders may also suffer from numerous comorbid medical conditions, which may include allergies, asthma, epilepsy, digestive disorders, persistent viral infections, feeding disorders, sensory integration dysfunction, sleeping disorders, and a wide array of challenging behaviors. Often, you are not only dealing with a mental or developmental disability but also what may be called a comorbid condition. Comorbid conditions often include Fragile X, allergies, asthma, epilepsy, bowel disease, gastrointestinal/digestive disorders, persistent viral infections, PANDAS (pediatric acute-onset neuropsychiatric syndrome, commonly called PANS), feeding disorders, anxiety disorder, bipolar disorder, ADHD (attention deficit hyperactivity disorder), Tourette syndrome, OCD (obsessive-compulsive disorder), sensory integration dysfunction, sleeping disorders, immune disorders, autoimmune disorders, and neuroinflammation. So your research must include finding and educating yourself on these diagnoses as well.

Wandering

While we often associate wandering with the elderly, it is not limited to that diagnosis, as it is very common in children. Regardless of age, wandering or elopement is the tendency for an individual to leave the safety of a responsible person's care or safe area, which may result in potential harm or injury. For children, this may include running off from adults at school or in the community, leaving the classroom without permission, or exiting the house when the family is not aware. This behavior is considered common and short-lived in toddlers but may persist or reemerge in those with autism.

According to research, nearly half of children with autism and six out of ten adults with Alzheimer's disease are at risk for wandering away from a safe setting. People who wander are vulnerable to dangerous situations, including drowning, traffic incidents, becoming trapped in hot cars, etc. It's important to take critical precautions. For both, a leading cause of death can be from a fall or traffic injury; and for children with autism, one of the biggest will be from drowning.

Wandering/elopement is typically a form of communication, often occurring to get to something of interest or away from something bothersome, usually noise, commotion, fears/phobias, and demands. These impulses and incidents can increase with added anxiety and stress, especially if the individual has challenges with coping, calming, or regulating their emotions.

Early signs of exit-seeking behavior can start in toddlerhood. They include social/demand avoidance, moving to a different area of building or home unnoticed, bolting when upset, and seeking out quiet places.

Quick Facts about Autism

- According to a study in pediatrics, nearly half of children with autism have a tendency to wander/bolt from safe settings.
- More than one-third of children with autism who wander/elope are never or rarely able to communicate their name, address, or phone number.
- According to a study by NAA (National Autism Association), accidental drowning accounts for 71 percent of lethal outcomes, followed by traffic injuries at 18 percent.
- Other dangers include dehydration, heat stroke, hypothermia, falls, physical restraint, and encounters with strangers.
- Increased risks are associated with autism severity.

Here is a prevention checklist.

- Secure home, outdoor gates, and garage door.
- Use simple window/door alarms or baby monitors.
- Identify and address triggers.
- Teach safety/coping and pursue forms of communication.
- Enroll in swimming lessons.
- Provide safe space escape alternatives, such as a tent or quiet nook or area within the home.
- Secure wearable identification or locative technology.
- Alert relatives, school, and neighbors.
- Alert local first responders.
- Speak with your loved one's health care team of other techniques to use.
- Create an emergency plan.
- Stay extra vigilant during transitions, parties, vacations, new moves, visits, and noise/stress/commotion.

The National Autism Association (NAA) is committed to those with an autism spectrum disorder (ASD) and warns if a person with ASD may be prone to wandering off or eloping from a safe environment and may be unable to recognize danger or how to stay safe. Wandering, elopement, running, or fleeing behaviors among those within our community not only present unique safety risks but also create extraordinary worry and stress among caregivers. Drowning fatalities following wandering incidents remain a leading cause of death among those with ASD, so my research pointed out that one thing you may need to do is sign your child up for swimming lessons.

As you will see on their website, the NAA provides direct assistance to caregivers, educators, and first responders. NAA's Big Red Safety Box includes the following resources:

1. Their Be REDy Booklet contains the following educational materials and tools:

   - A caregiver checklist
   - A family wandering emergency plan
   - A first responder profile form
   - A wandering-prevention brochure
   - A sample IEP letter
   - A student profile form
   - Emotion identification cards
   - Wandering quick tips

2. Two GE wireless door/window alarms with batteries.
3. One ROAD iD bracelet or shoe ID tag, which is customized with personal information on your loved one and engraved and mailed to you free of charge.
4. Four adhesive stop sign visual prompts for doors and windows.
5. One safety alert window cling for car or home windows.
6. One child ID kit from the National Center for Missing and Exploited Children.

As you will see when you use the NAA website, you will find a wealth of information; and by all means, you will want to obtain their Big Red Safety Box, as well as view and educate yourself on many of the topics found under their link labeled Autism and Safety.

Another website you may wish to explore to see if it offers the information you are seeking will be the Autism 360 website. This is a parent-led organization where you can work one-on-one with a multidisciplinary team of health care professionals.

Dealing with Dementia

In a newsletter published by the National Institutes of Health (NIH) and their publication, *News in Health*, you can find a great article called "Dealing with Dementia" that contains a wealth of information that may be useful to you and your caregiving role. Dementia is a brain disorder that most often affects the elderly. It's caused by the failure or death of nerve cells in the brain. Alzheimer's disease is the most common cause. By some estimates, about one-third of people ages eighty-five and older may have Alzheimer's. Although age is the greatest risk factor for dementia, it isn't a normal part of aging. Some people live into their nineties and beyond with no signs of dementia at all.

In the later stages of dementia, Verywell Health indicates some people with dementia will develop what's known as behavioral and psychological symptoms of dementia (BPSD).

The symptoms of BPSD can include the following:

- increased agitation
- aggression (shouting or screaming, verbal abuse, and sometimes physical abuse)
- delusions (unusual beliefs not based on reality)
- hallucinations (hearing or seeing things that do not exist)

While these types of behaviors can be distressing, as such, it is important to ensure you have your loved one examined to help rule out or treat any underlying causes, such as

- uncontrolled pain,
- untreated depression,

- infection (especially a urinary tract infection),
- side effects of any medicines.

Persons with dementia often develop restless behaviors, such as pacing up and down, wandering out of the home, and agitated fidgeting or picking at objects or even their own skin. Some tips to try if such behavior arises will be to ensure your loved one has a daily routine you follow, and if they fidget, give them something thing to occupy their hands. This may be a ball or doll to hold or even towels or other simple laundry items to fold.

People living with dementia often exhibit challenging behaviors, as they are trying to communicate, and they often do it in ways that seem odd to us who do not have dementia. For example, common behavioral problems for people living with dementia include the following:

1. Overreaction to trivial matters; this may result in weeping, screaming, wildly moving arms about, or other unreasonable accusations or movements.
2. Compulsive behavior. Repeating what is said, following you around, asking the same question over and over.
3. Hoarding all sorts of items for safekeeping and often accusing others of stealing their precious possessions.
4. Loss of inhibitions and the consequent lack of awareness of the rules of appropriate behavior.
5. Physical (pushing or hitting) or verbal (abusive language) abuse.
6. Suspicious of others, including neighbors, or feelings of others plotting against them.
7. Aimless or purposeful wandering that can result in getting lost, leaving a safe environment, or intruding in inappropriate places.
8. Pacing and fidgeting. This could be due to thirst, pain, medication side effects, or even boredom, stress, noise, or lack of exercise.

9. Calling out continuously or weeping and whimpering for extended periods of time.
10. A common behavior found in many with dementia will be, confusion and restlessness may become even more apparent when dusk approaches. This is termed sundowning.

If your loved one has been tested and the results validate the diagnosis is dementia and it is known it cannot be treated, slowed, or reversed, your loved one's physician may then focus on possible medication management to make it easier to live with dementia and make it more manageable. Treatments can vary, and it will depend upon the stages your loved one is in the course of their disease.

So what are some examples of things that may help? One key will be to make attempts to anticipate concerning behaviors and then use guidance or reassurance as you implement and guide your loved one. Other dos might include the following:

1.	Implement a routine and do specific tasks at the same or about the same time each day. This may be such activities as getting up at the same time each day, having meals at the same time, doing personal care at the same time, maybe taking a walk, or even doing nontiring exercises each day.
2.	Spend time talking with your loved one about family outings or key family events or even hobbies they enjoyed. Maybe while doing so, hold their hand and speak softly and gently to them.
3.	Serve healthy meals at the same time each day and also offer snacks at set times during midmorning and afternoon and even just before bedtime.
4.	Schedule activities that promote creativity and satisfaction—maybe looking at old photo albums or reading books or listening to their favorite music, which can be by use of audiobooks or music you can download from the Library of Congress. Activities may include taking a walk or drive or, if they like to dance, maybe even dancing. It could be any activity that will help them stay in the moment.

5. If medications are to be given, give them at the right time and as directed by the physician. At times, your loved one may refuse to take a pill. This means you will have to be creative in how you give it, and it may mean you will need to disguise them in other food, liquids, or other favorite soft food your loved one may like. As some time-released pills cannot be opened or crushed, check with the pharmacist on how best to give such pills.

Prevention of Injuries, Wandering, and Home Safety Checklist for Persons with Dementia

As we have discussed earlier in this book, you must prepare your home and surrounding garage, carport, or yard. It is critical to remove or lock up any items that can be used as a weapon or a product that can poison or cause other serious injuries for your loved one. Just to remind you, this might be one of the following:

1. Placing deadbolts out of the line of sight, either high or low, on exterior doors.
2. Use night-lights throughout the home.
3. Cover doorknobs with cloth the same color as the door or use safety covers.
4. Camouflage doors by painting them the same color as the walls or covering them with removable curtains or screens or adding Stop or Do Not Enter signs near or on the doors.
5. Install warning bells above doors or use a monitoring device that signals when a door is opened.
6. Place a pressure-sensitive mat in front of the door or at the person's bedside to alert you to movement.
7. Put a fence around the patio, yard, or other outside common areas.
8. Use safety gates or brightly colored netting to prevent access to stairs or the outdoors.
9. Monitor noise levels to help reduce excessive stimulation.

10. Create indoor and outdoor common areas that can be safely explored.
11. Label all doors with signs or symbols to explain the purpose of each room.
12. Store items that may trigger a person's instinct to leave, such as coats, hats, pocketbooks, keys, and wallets, out of sight.
13. Do not leave the person alone in a car.

Other tips, also discussed in a precious chapter on preparing your home for caregiving but worth repeating here, include the following:

- If you have sliding glass doors, place stickers on the glass to help your loved one see them and not walk into the glass, possibly breaking and causing serious injuries.
- If you have a swimming pool and your loved one has dementia or is a child, fence in the pool area and add locks to the gate.
- If your barbecue grill is a concern, lock the cover and access to gas tanks and remove all fire starters.
- Check the garage and back or side yards for safety hazards, like gasoline, tools, or ladders, and block access if they pose a danger for your loved one.
- If you have a golf cart or riding lawn mower and your loved one has dementia or another brain disorder that makes him an unsafe driver, place the keys in a safe place; otherwise, they may try to use this as a means of transportation.
- Ensure you keep cleaning and laundry supplies in a central area, and it has a lock on the door where such is stored.
- Install locks on all fence gates to help prevent wandering.
- If your loved one is one who has a brain disorder of any sort and tends to wander, take the time to sew in and label all clothing with tags where you can write in washable ink their name and address, at a minimum. Also, make every attempt to write identifying information on glass cases or

their wallet and shoes. If they will wear it, have them wear a medical alert bracelet or necklace; or better yet, if they will wear a watch, invest in one of the GPS watches now on the market.

- As you prepare the home, ensure smoke and carbon monoxide detectors are working, and the batteries are fresh. (They should be replaced twice yearly; a good habit to follow will be to replace them on January 1 and June 1. If you do this, make sure you add the information to a calendar you keep for all your reminders.) You will also want to ensure you have a fire extinguisher, you know how to use it, and it is working properly.
- If there are guns in the home, consider removing them or other weapons; and if not, store them in a locked cabinet.
- Make sure all medications, even yours and any over-the-counter medications, such as aspirin, are in a locked drawer or cabinet.
- As you ready the house, ensure all razors, safety pins, and other sharp objects are locked up.

Dealing with Trauma-Informed Care

Trauma-informed care (TIC) or at times referred to as adverse childhood experiences (ACEs) is a fairly new concept, where research is showing that trauma experienced by a child under the age of eighteen has lasting effects on how an individual functions physically, socially, emotionally, or spiritually. TIC or ACE also has an impact in later life, especially if there was not any professional help given after the event occurred. The medical and psychological conditions most seen are cardiovascular disease, chronic obstructive pulmonary disease, autoimmune diseases, substance abuse, and depression.

The Centers for Disease Control and Prevention in collaboration with the Substance Abuse and Mental Health Services Administration (SAMHSA) developed six strategies or guidelines that are used when training emergency response personnel, with the training aimed at increasing first responders, the impact that trauma can have. The principles are (1) safety; (2) trustworthiness and transparency; (3) peer support; (4) collaboration and mutuality; (5) empowerment, voice, and choice; and (6) cultural, historical, and gender issues.

As you conduct your research and learn more on trauma informed care or Adverse Childhood Experiences (ACEs), you may wish to explore such websites as:

- Centers for Disease Control and Prevention at CDC.gov and trauma informed care and approaches.
- Wikipedia
- SAMSHA and its article on Concept of Trauma and Guidance for a Trauma-Informed Approach

Educating Yourself

As stated multiple times so far in this book, keep your notebook or cell phone handy so you can make or record notes on your loved one's behavioral outbursts or challenging behavioral events. It is these notes that will help serve as your guide as you discuss all with your loved one's medical professional. This is critical since some behaviors may be controllable with medications or alternative techniques the team may teach you. For your notes, you will want to record such things as the following:

- Time of the behavior
- Frequency
- Intensity
- Duration

Other things to consider as you make your notes will be these:

- Were any big changes occurring in the home at that time?
- Did you move, or did anyone move in or out?
- Did you make any changes in caregiving arrangements?

- Has your loved one started any new drugs or changed drug dosage?
- Has your loved one suffered a recent injury?

Observation of any body language (pacing, grinding of their teeth, frowning or furrowing of their brow, clenching of their fists, or other body positions) may help you identify an oncoming outburst of the behavior. An event may also be triggered by changes in the environment, such as chaos, odd or different noises, or sounds or lights. They can also be triggered by the following:

- Anxiety
- Rapid mood swings
- Feeling frightened
- Fatigue
- Frustration
- Not sleeping
- Depression
- Discomfort and pain

It is critical that if your loved one has a challenging behavior, you educate yourself on it. This step is critical, as the more you know about it, the more likely you will know what to do. Often, mental illness or an intellectual or developmental disability (IDD) is not the only thing going on in your loved one's life. Other medical conditions may also be present, which may complicate the issues created by your loved one's mental illness or IDD. Conditions such as these are referred to as co-occurring, comorbid conditions or dual diagnosis, meaning there is more than one condition causing the difficulties. One of your best tools will be to ensure your loved one has had both a complete and through medical and psychological examination, including any imaging (X-rays or scanning via an MRI or CT scanner) and blood testing, and a treatment plan has been developed.

Some Dos and Don'ts

Unfortunately, while today's medical care does include what is called an electronic medical record (EMR), if the medical and psychological examinations are completed by differing physicians or medical professionals, both types may order differing medications, and they may not be using the same company for their EMR. As a result, notes from other physician(s) are not reviewed. Thus, it will be critical to ensure any medications ordered are ordered from the same pharmacy. This will allow the pharmacist to alert the ordering physician of a conflict, especially if the medications are not compatible with the medications your loved one is already taking. As was stated earlier in this book, one of the key team members you will want to use will be the pharmacist. They can alert you and the ordering physician if there are issues that can arise from the medication prescribed.

Almost always, there are warning signs that a person's behavior is moving toward a crisis. It is critical to look for tips that can help you recognize when a crisis is coming and use any training you may have had to take any early interventional steps to help you to de-escalate an incident before it can become dangerous.

Sometimes, despite our best efforts, the person's behavior will escalate, and it will become even more challenging. In these circumstances, here are some important dos and don'ts, which may be helpful to consider. In an article on the crisis prevention website they offer the following Dos and Don'ts.

Do This	Do Not Do This
Stay calm. Approach in a calm manner. Move and speak slowly and quietly and project confidence. Watch your own body language, voice pattern, facial expressions, and rate of speech. Talk in a consoling and empathetic manner, and do not touch the person.	Don't touch the person if the person is not harming himself or someone else. Touching can escalate the behaviors.

Maintain a relaxed posture. Make sure there are at least three to six feet between you and the person with whom you are speaking. A good measure will be staying at least an arm's length away.	Don't invade another person's personal space. Don't stand directly face-to-face, hands on hips, crossing your arms, pointing your finger, or staring at them. These are very challenging behavioral messages and will in most cases increase the behavior.
Adjust your position so you are communicating with the person at the level of their physical height so their eyes can look at your eyes without difficulty. By all means, do not turn your back on them.	Don't tower over a shorter person or a person in a chair or wheelchair.
Acknowledge the other person's feelings even if you disagree. Let them know it is clear that what they are saying is important to them. Avoid arguing; remember, the person is not deliberately trying to upset you. Their logic and reasoning are impaired by the illness, and it is up to you to comfort and reassure them. So be clear, direct, and respectful in what you say.	Don't challenge, threaten, or dare the other person. Never belittle or make fun of them.
When acknowledging a person's feelings, use words like *frustrated*, *upset*, or other words that describe a softer version of the emotion displayed.	Don't use words that are emotionally charged, like *angry* or *pissed off*. If the emotion that you named is not on target, allow the individual the control of naming the emotion.
Maintain a pleasant, open, and accepting attitude and try not to overreact. Be flexible and offer an alternative.	Don't argue back to or over the person. Don't try to change their mind about something. If the behavior is about a task they don't want to do or have done, leave this task for later when they have calmed down.

Ask for small, specific responses from them, such as moving to a quieter area or lowering their voice. Focus on small requests.	Don't position yourself where you are blocked by the person from having access to an exit if need be.

The National Alliance on Mental Illness (NAMI) has a great booklet online that outlines what can contribute to a mental health crisis, warning signs that a crisis is emerging, strategies to help de-escalate a crisis, and resources that may be available for those affected. It also includes information about advocating for a person in crisis, along with a sample crisis plan. Thus, this booklet may offer you tips on how to avoid a mental health issue from moving to a crisis. Because it is critical to know the signs of an approaching mental health crisis and those tips that may help avoid a future event. In your research one on the topic, the National Alliance on Mental Health (nami. org) website has a great booklet you can download. This booklet is titled *Navigating a Mental Health Crisis*, and it contains some great information you may find useful.

Calling for Help

If the situation escalates and you feel you or your loved one is in danger, any of us in health care will recommend you call 9-1-1, as taking your loved one to an emergency department will be the best option. Be aware that if they are transported in a law enforcement vehicle, usual policy is to use handcuffs; and if taken by ambulance, your loved one may be in full restraints. This can be upsetting for everyone involved but may be the only option available if the transporting personnel are to be kept safe during the transport.

Once first responders arrive, you are not in control of any decisions. As you speak with the emergency response team, it is important to also alert them of your loved one's

- mental health history and diagnosis,
- medications and, at a minimum, those taken currently and possibly when the last dose was taken,

- suicide attempts and any current threats,
- prior history of violence and what may have triggered the current threat,
- any substance abuse and treatment history, and
- any other medical conditions.

If the episode has escalated to the point of a crisis requiring emergent help, the most important thing will be to get to stay as safe as you can and to get your loved one to a medical facility for evaluation and treatment as soon as possible. If your loved one is taken to the hospital and doesn't communicate, do not forget the emergency kit (as described in the chapter or section on emergency preparedness) you prepared. Remember to take it with you.

A visit to the emergency department doesn't guarantee admission, and often, due to the overcrowding in an emergency room, the wait may be long and drawn out. However, while a visit to an emergency room may not result in an admission, hospitals with an emergency room are required by law (the Emergency Medical Treatment and Labor Act) to do a medical screening of an individual regardless of their ability to pay. This screening helps determine if a person can safely be discharged and, if not, if they should be admitted to either that hospital or transferred to a hospital that can meet the medical needs of the individual being seen.

Because of EMTALA, if your loved one is taken to an emergency department, do not be alarmed if your loved one encounters a long delay in getting seen or treated. Delays are often encountered due to the emergency room's clients awaiting treatment. Or if seen and the decision is to admit your loved one, this may mean your loved one will be held in a holding area, as finding an appropriate facility to treat him is not immediately available. If the decision is that your loved one will require an admission, the stay in the emergency room may be long not only due to finding a bed but also since criterion for admission varies. All depends upon the medical necessity of the treatment and level of care ordered by the attending physician, as well as an approval for the admission from your loved one's health plan.

What Can You Do?

There is no single way to reduce aggression and violence in a child or adult. But there is no excuse for behavior from your loved one that turns to abuse (domestic or parental). Even if your child or teenager or loved one is older and has a developmentally disabled diagnosis and is going through a tough time, this type of behavior is never acceptable. If violent and aggressive behavior is happening in your home, it's important to learn effective strategies to keep everyone safe, help your loved one learn more appropriate means of solving problems, and hold them accountable for the choice to become abusive. If you are the target of parental abuse (which is a form of domestic abuse), you're probably living in fear every day of what your loved one will do next, always waiting for what will set off a volcanic eruption.

Parental abuse occurs when a child, usually a teenager but sometimes a preteen, engages in behavior that is abusive toward a parent. The abuse may be a onetime incident, or it may escalate in frequency, even to the point of a daily occurrence. It may arise with explosive anger or rage, or it may be a quiet, deliberate act, often used to show power over a parent. Parental abuse can range from verbal abuse to threatening a parent, intimidation, to outright physical assault.

As with other violent behaviors, parental abuse and the child or teen often expresses behavior that can show warning signs before the attack. None of these should ever be minimized or ignored. Behaviors to watch for include the following:

- Frequent periods of intense anger or extreme irritability
- Frequent loss of temper or blowups
- Periods of extreme impulsiveness or becoming easily frustrated

There's a lot of debate about whether violent media is harmful, and parents should do what they think is best. But if violence or abuse is a problem in your home, while it may be hard to do in our world of technology, work with your loved one's health care team to find possible solutions to eliminate any violence media.

Is It Roughhousing or Abuse?

If you are not sure if the behavior displayed is really roughhousing or violence, you need to step in, especially if it is known one of the persons involved has a tendency for violence. If you suspect it, step in immediately when you see or hear any of the following:

- One child wants it to stop, and the other child doesn't stop.
- Someone gets hurt even if both parties want it to continue.
- The roughhousing is in retaliation for something.
- The roughhousing is designed to dominate a younger or smaller child.
- It's done at the wrong time or in the wrong place.

You may notice that in rough play, kids are smiling and having a good time, and kids will take turns attacking and being attacked. In contrast, in real fights, one or both may be angry or crying, and one kid is trying to hurt the other.

As you deal with violence, some key things to consider will be your child's age and of course their disability or diagnosis. As you work with the health care team, they may not only teach you some techniques you may wish to use but also encourage you to create an environment in which violence and aggression can be minimized. To do this, tips might include actions such as the following:

- Do your best to keep your home life calm, supportive, and respectful; and be sure to praise your child often when good behavior is displayed.
- Have a safe play area with lots of pillows or soft items they can throw.
- Let your loved one talk about his feelings and why or what is causing such behavior.
- As you work with the mental health team, they will teach you how to work with your loved one to help develop calming strategies you can use when an episode of anger or frustration arises.

Resources and References

The Challenging Behaviors Tool Kit from Autism Speaks provides strategies and resources to address challenging behaviors and to help support you and your loved one with autism during these difficult situations. To find the autism speaks tool kits, you can find a full list of what is available by typing "autism speaks tool kits" in your web browser. Here, you will find they offer several tool kits any one of which you can double click on the name of the kit and the information you might need will be at your fingertips.

This tool and other resources you may want to conduct research on for your own use can be found by searching such websites as:

- autism speaks and their Challenging Behaviors' Tool Kit.
- American Academy of Child and Adolescent Psychiatry (AACAP), the booklet they offer on "medications to use to help control outburst" with this one a booklet you may wish to explore with your loved one's treating mental health professional.
- If your loved one has a diagnosis of Alzheimer's or dementia, there are several websites that offer online tools you may wish to review and use. To access such information, you can type in your web browser "dementia and challenging behavior," and this will bring up a wide variety of resources you may wish to explore.

Keeping Your Loved One Safe

One of the best ways to manage challenging behaviors is to keep them from developing in the first place. Key is to discuss all with your loved one's treating mental health professional, as he may prescribe either medication or treatment modalities you may wish to try. Addressing common behaviors early and getting family therapy will be one mechanism to use, as this can help prepare you to help keep a challenging behavior from escalating.

Understanding what may be causing the challenging behavior and learning how to respond to it will enable you as the caregiver to take better control of situations when they arise and diminish the occurrence of the behavior. Thus, if you find a tactic that works, write it down so you or others can use it again, if the behavior returns.

As mentioned earlier, there are ways to set up the home to be safe for your loved one if they have an outburst. However, it is critical it be repeated in this chapter as well. Technology is here, so investigate what might work in your situation, should it be any variety of alarms, cameras, programmable door locks, sensors, or any devices that can alert you of movement. By all means, if your loved one is total care with or without a variety of equipment and you will be sleeping in another room, invest in a baby monitor, one with both a camera and also audio features.

To protect the home from damage if your loved one is violent and tends to damage walls and other areas of the home, modifications to consider will be the following:

- Installation of plywood or plastic panels over all walls, and as needed, painting them to match other areas.
- Installation of protective film over any mirrors or windows, if you have not already installed plexiglass, tempered glass, or impact-resistant windows.
- Installation of steel or metal doors.
- Anchor china hutches, TVs, dressers, bookshelves, and other tall furniture to the walls to prevent pulling them over in a fit of rage.
- Anchoring the refrigerator to the wall.
- Cover any exposed wires with either baseboards or other hollow covers that can be used or designed to hide such. You may also want to consider bundling them together with tape or wire and pinning them to the backs of furniture or hiding them under furniture.
- Cover any electric outlets not used with a full protective plate.
- Removal of breakable objects, if not already destroyed.

Other Ways for Safety

Your motto must be safety first not only for your loved one but also for you and other family members as well. Your role of caregiver does not include allowing yourself to be physically hurt. As is repeated numerous times in this book, for all aspects of caregiving, don't ignore your own needs and feelings. Definitely dealing with aggression or violence can frighten and exhaust you and you may feel any number of emotions ranging from anger to depression to guilt. However, try to keep in mind that these problems are not happening because you are a poor caregiver; the problems are part of the disease itself.

So what are some ways to keep yourself safe?

1. If you have long hair, keep it pinned back and away from your face, and don't let it dangle as you render care to your loved one or approach him.
2. Avoid hooded garments with ties around the neck area.
3. Avoid wearing dangling necklaces, chains, or earrings.
4. If your loved one bites, pinches, or hits, you may want to invest in some garments that, while designed for health care workers, might be ones you will want to consider.
5. Trust your gut. Your instincts are often better at recognizing danger than your rational mind is.
6. Always have access to an exit. If you're inside with a potentially violent person, make sure you can get to the door easily.
7. Avoid dealing with a violent person alone.
8. Learn basic self-defense.
9. Keep children away from the person.
10. Have an emergency plan.
11. Approach your loved one from the front and maintain your composure and be aware of your own emotions, body position, and tone of voice.
12. Maintain eye contact, keep arms at your sides, and maintain a safe distance if the potential for violence exists.

13. Do not initiate physical contact if your loved one's behavior is escalating.
14. Hide a key to the house and car in the yard so that if you are locked out or need to escape you have a way to do so.

Safety Items to Prevent Potential Injury

During their fit of rage, your loved one may be at risk of serious injury, which can lead to broken bones, internal injuries, or head trauma or other trauma. If this is so, check with your loved one's mental health physician as to what may be the right protective garments; many may be padded or of a hard device to form a splint or guard. Or to prevent a head injury from a fall or head-banging, a helmet may be the device to obtain. The key? Get what may be needed. In many cases, these items will be covered by your loved one's health plan, as they can be authorized in lieu of hospitalization or emergency room costs, as they will be the cheaper alternative. To help protect yourself, if your loved one is violent and bites or hits, it might help to discuss this with his physician if he will help you obtain protective clothing to help protect you from injury. Such garments are available from such online vendors as BitePRO or stealthwear.

Restraints Are a No-No

A restraint is anything that hinders movement or restricts freedom. Years ago, restraint use was much more common and included extremely restrictive restraints, such as straitjackets and vests. While these restraints aren't used today, it is important to recognize that other equipment can act as a restraint even if the goal in its use is to keep someone safe. What are the different kinds of restraints, and when may restraints be needed?

- Restraints may be needed when behavior is out of control, and there is a likelihood your loved one can hurt themselves or others. Restraints or seclusion should never be used to punish your loved one or to make it easier for you to take care of them.

- Restraints may be used for medical or surgical reasons, and restraints may be so your loved one cannot pull out any tubes or pull at stiches or bandages, or they may be needed to administer a medication.
- Restraints may be used to keep a person in proper position and prevent movement or falling during surgery or while on a stretcher.
- Restraints can also be used to control or prevent harmful behavior or harm others.

What Are the Dangers Associated with the Use of Restraints?

Restraints can be very dangerous if not used correctly. However, some of the following can assist to ensure safety when your loved one is up in a wheelchair or recliner. The types of restraints below are simple, safe, and successful.

- *Lap buddies.* A lap buddy is a cushioned device that fits in a wheelchair and assists with reminding a person not to get up by himself. Lap buddies can also be used to help with positioning if a person tends to lean forward in his wheel-chair and is in danger of falling out of the chair.
- *Seat belts.* Seat belts have been used in wheelchairs to protect your loved one from falling out or from getting up without assistance. However, a seat belt is used as a restraint and can pose a danger to the person if your loved one tried to get out of the chair by either falling forward with the wheelchair or by pushing and falling backward. An alternative is a seat belt that comes loose easily but sounds an alarm when it's removed to alert someone for assistance.
- *Recliner chairs.* While a recliner chair can be used for comfort and positioning, it also can be a restraint for some people if they can't get out of it independently.

- *Side rails.* Side rails, while important for you as a caregiver and can help you to ease turning and repositioning, can be a dangerous restraint. Typically used to prevent someone from rolling or falling out of his bed, side rails can also be used to keep someone from getting out of the bed, thus making them a restraint. They can also cause your loved one to become entrapped in them or go over the top of them, causing a greater injury or even death.
- *Tucking in sheets tightly.* If sheets in a bed are tucked too tightly so your loved one can't get out of bed or move freely, this serves as a restraint.
- *Positioning at a table.* Pushing someone in a wheelchair up to a table and locking the chair in position can also be used as a restraint since it prevents your loved one from freely moving. A locked wheelchair can be quite dangerous, as your loved one can push backward and tip the wheelchair (and themselves) over.
- *Seat trays.* Placing a locking tray in front of your loved one, even if its purpose is for use as a writing or feeding tray, is considered a restraint if your loved one tries to remove it, and they are unable to get up.

Per Verywell Health, there are many negative consequences of restraints.

- Bruises
- Decubitus ulcers
- Respiratory complications
- Urinary incontinence and constipation
- Poor nutrition
- Increased dependence in activities of daily living
- Impaired muscle strength and balance
- Decreased cardiovascular endurance
- Increased agitation

- Increased risk for mortality caused by strangulation or as a consequence of serious injuries—for example, fracture or head trauma

In addition to those physical consequences, restraints are frequently ineffective and don't prevent falls. Rather, research has shown that injuries are escalated because of the force the person needs to use to escape from the restraint. To help educate yourself on the use of restraints and the potential dangers of their use, this is the time you will want to have a discussion with your loved one's treating therapist and ensure they teach you the proper way for the restraints to be applied.

What May Be Some Alternatives to Restraints?

As you are preparing your home and the area for your loved one to live and move about, some alternatives to use of restraints might be the following:

- Bed alarms, chair alarms, and door alarms can provide freedom for the person with dementia while still alerting you of their need for assistance.
- Develop some meaningful activities to distract your loved one and help prevent some behaviors such as restlessness, combativeness with care, and wandering.

Summary

Dealing with your loved one if they present challenging behaviors is going to be possibly one of your hardest tasks as a caregiver. Critical will be to educate yourself on your loved one's diagnosis and potential options you may wish to explore with your loved one's medical and mental health professionals. If a treatment option is suggested, try it; after all, nothing ventured, nothing gained.

Learn to do your own research of various topics, including therapeutic approaches on ways to control the behavior. This will allow you to discuss in detail what may help in your situation. By all means, do not blame yourself; and if the behavior escalates and you feel threatened or in harm's way, call for emergency response help.

This will also be the time to reach out to support groups so you can learn firsthand what may have worked versus what has not. This also allows you to take a breather during the day so you can talk with someone who understands and can offer empathy. Remember, keep notes of actions so you can follow up with professionals. Equally and just as important, remember to find times during the day to take care of yourself.

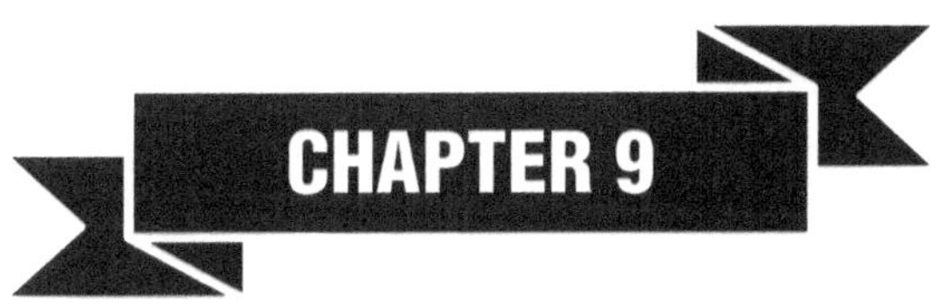

Final Tips and Tidbits to Help in Your Role

THIS CHAPTER WILL be to provide you with additional information you may need on a wide variety of topics, many of which you can use to help make your role easier. Remember, the goals of this book are the following:

- Help you learn to be your loved one's case manager.
- Give you as many tips as possible where you can have some online resources at your fingertips, any one of which can help you educate yourself on your loved one's diagnosis or lead you to resources that can help with his care.
- Help ease the burden of caregiving since it can be overwhelming, tiring, and frustrating. Many health care professionals are unaware of what is available outside their own area of health care in which they work. Consequently, you are never taught what may be needed so that care can continue after discharge or as ordered.
- Help you find ways not only to provide care for your loved one but also, equally as important, give you tips on taking care of yourself mentally, physically, and spiritually and the importance of keeping yourself healthy.

- Help you understand how important it is to work with mental health professionals not only for therapy for yourself and your loved one, but also, if your loved one is one with challenging behaviors, you can explore and learn techniques that can assist you in their care.

It is critical in today's world that you learn to use any of the technological resources that may be available. If you are afraid to learn or are technology challenged, recruit a friend or relative to help you do it. In the past, in order to access some of the resources, one needed a computer. However, this is not the case today. A handheld cell phone is worth its weight in gold and is basically a mini computer. Not only can you record information, but you can also quickly, in many cases, find what you might want to know by the touch of typing in what information you want your command to take you to. So learn to make use of it.

Another critical key is, learn to say yes and no at the right times. Say no when you feel or your gut tells you, you cannot do it or when you dislike what you see and smell or when you know you cannot continue in the role. Similarly, you want to learn to say yes when family or friends ask if they can help. Keep your notes, to-do task list, phone number listing, and other key documents current, updated, filed, and organized. Then if you are not available, your volunteers or family can find them.

If the care your loved one requires is complex, insist on training, and do not let it happen as you are walking out the door. Have the staff spend the time needed to teach you, and when completed, you should thoroughly understand how to do it. The best way to learn is by what is termed the teach-back method. Here the teacher will show you how to do it, and then you must demonstrate back what was taught. For some of the care, this will not be a onetime session. So until you feel you can do it, don't let the discharge occur, and this may be one of those times you will learn when to say no and yes appropriately.

Not all care is safe outside the hospital, or in some instances, care is very extensive and will require care beyond what can be provided or supervised by a hospital outside the acute hospital or, at times, certainly by a home health agency. This may mean your loved one may have a longer inpatient stay than planned, or it may mean he will require placement between the acute hospital stay and going home.

This chapter will cover a variety of topics that may help you in your role. As such, it will cover the following:

- Importance of learning CPR and the Heimlich method
- Making use of technology
- Your role as your loved one's advocate
- Understanding the appeals process and how to write an effective letter of appeal
- Changing health plans or primary care physicians and requesting second opinions
- Bullying
- Dental care
- Foot care
- Diabetic care
- Managing or, as needed, performing your loved one's hygiene and helping them with their activities of daily living (ADLs)
- Cutting hair for a person who is bedbound or with challenging behaviors
- Recreation and its importance
- Special equipment and rent versus purchase
- Wound care
- Importance of vaccinations and preventive health
- Caregiving and intimacy

Cardiopulmonary resuscitation (CPR) and Heimlich

If your loved one is on life-sustaining equipment, you must be taught, prior to discharge, how to perform, at a minimum, CPR. However, as this is taught, also ensure they teach you how to perform the Heimlich method should your loved one choke as they eat.

While learning CPR and the Heimlich method may only seem necessary if your loved one is on life-sustaining devices, this is not true. You never know when within a nanosecond something can happen. Your loved one can stop breathing, or their heart can stop. Or they can easily choke, and you may be the only person in attendance when such an event occurs. Thus, you want to be prepared.

Several things can cause choking, including a severe allergic reaction, accidentally inhaling a foreign object, a near-drowning incident, or a medical disorder that affects nerve and muscle functions. CPR is performed when a person is not conscious while in contrast Heimlich is performed when a person is conscious. Even if your loved one is not on life-sustaining devices, it is wise to take a class on how to perform both techniques. Your loved one's local Red Cross office will be your best resource from which to take a class. To find a class near you, your best resource will be to use the 2-1-1 telephone system.

Making use of technology, including teletherapy
and telehealth and video visits

In the old days, the only way to see a doctor or health care provider was to see them in person; and often, one of the challenges of doing this was to get to their office location. This is especially true when transportation is an issue. Either none is available, there are long waits or rides, or you have to make many changes to get to your destination. Technology and subsequent laws have now made getting seen by a health care provider (not only a doctor but also even therapy and other key appointments) possible. This new technology is known as telehealth or telepsychiatry.

Telehealth or telepsychiatry is a visit with a provider who uses a telecommunication system between the provider and you or your loved one. The Centers for Medicare and Medicaid Services (CMS) now considers these visits the same as ones where you would see the provider in person. CMS considers these as real-time communications that occur between the provider and patient, as it uses both audio and video techniques. Because CMS now allows such, health plans have followed as well, allowing a visit without leaving home. This liberalization of teletherapy and telepsychiatry coverage in many health plans means professionals can now provide many treatments virtually.

The literature strongly suggests that the quality of teletherapy care is as effective as in-person sessions for most people with most conditions. Telehealth may be particularly helpful for older adults with limited mobility and for those living in rural areas, as they will have the opportunity to see and talk with their doctor from their home. For older adults, talking with their doctor online or through a phone, tablet, or other electronic device can often be easier, faster, and less expensive than making a trip to an office. Telehealth can also help support family caregivers who are taking care of their loved ones either close by or from afar. If a caregiver needs to ask the doctor a question, they can do so through an online health portal rather than waiting for and traveling to an in-person appointment. However, it is not always ideal for everyone and for some persons, especially with autism spectrum disorder, so discuss what may be best in this instance with the provider.

Another technology resource you may wish to consider, especially if you want to learn more of a care technique, will be to use any of the online YouTube videos. These videos can show you how to perform any care your loved one possibly needs. To access, merely type in the browser the name YouTube followed by what topic you wish to explore—bathing, body mechanics, feeding tips for challenging behaviors, mobility training, or whatever topic you may want to learn more on.

Advocacy

Families, not institutions, provide the majority of care to chronically ill and disabled persons, so remember, as stated many times in this book, you may be the eyes, ears, and voice of your loved one. So learn to use them. As the caregiver, you know firsthand the enormity of the burden in caring for someone with any variety of illnesses, diagnoses, or injury that has resulted in long-term conditions where your loved one needs help. Not only have you maybe struggled with their care; often, the greatest challenge(s) will be in finding appropriate advice and services and how and where to get help that is within your income range, as well as respite.

Your own experiences in dealing with your loved one's health plan, community agencies, round-the-clock care, and financial hardships means you know firsthand what the important issues are. As a result, you are in a perfect position to help advocate for change for them and, possibly, for others. Let what you have learned be your guide, and you can then educate elected officials charged with development of public policy and funding priorities of what needs to be changed.

There are some great tips on how and what you can do to help advocate on the Family Caregiver Alliance website. You can also use the American Association of Retired Persons (AARP) website to learn of some of the advocacy projects AARP is involved in. This same website allows you to share your story and reasons needed for change. On the Family Caregiver Alliance website, you will find tips on who to write to and tips on what you may wish to include in your letter or email.

Understanding the Appeals Process and Writing
Effective Letters for an Appeal or Arbitration

We discussed earlier in this book the importance of keeping your and your loved one's Evidence of Coverage (EOC) booklet— the booklet produced by a health plan—handy, as this booklet can serve for more than one purpose. For example, it will help serve as a guide as to what is covered versus what is not, as well as what has limitations. Equally as important, it will tell you how and when to file an appeal if a service is denied. If a denial is issued, you will receive not only the denial in writing but also the letter, as the EOC will tell you how to file an appeal and the time frame allowed to file the appeal.

Most health plans only offer two (2) internal levels of appeal while in contrast Medicare allows five (5) levels of appeal, and if you or your loved one has Kaiser Permanente, Kaiser only allows for arbitration. The five levels of appeal allowed by Medicare are the following:

- Level 1: reconsideration from your plan
- Level 2: review by an independent review entity (IRE)
- Level 3: decision by the Office of Medicare Hearings and Appeals (OMHA)
- Level 4: review by the Medicare Appeals Council
- Level 5: judicial review by a federal district court

The key is, if your loved one's health plan denies coverage and what was denied is a service that is considered medically necessary, you always have the right to file an appeal or request arbitration. If a claim or service is denied, it is often due to the following:

- The treatment or service is not deemed medically necessary or appropriate.
- The plan does not cover the treatment, service, medication, or goods.
- The health care provider is not in your loved one's provider network, and there is no letter of agreement between the health plan and the provider submitting the claim.
- Your loved one's health plan requires preauthorization or a referral from their primary care physician.
- The treatment is considered investigational or experimental.
- Your loved one's health plan coverage has lapsed, or they are not enrolled with the insurer any longer.
- A paperwork or data entry error (often a diagnosis or procedure code is missing) and prevented the claim from being processed correctly.
- The claim was not filed on time.

There are two ways to appeal a health plan decision.

- *Internal appeal.* If your claim is denied or your health insurance coverage is canceled, you have the right to an internal appeal. You may ask your insurance company to conduct a full and fair review of its decision. If the case is urgent, your insurance company must speed up this process.

- *External review.* You have the right to take your appeal to an independent third party for review. This is called external review. External review means that the insurance company no longer gets the final say over whether to pay a claim.

Internal appeals. The internal appeals process will guarantee a venue where you can present information the health plan may not have been aware of, giving you and your loved one a way to ensure they have all the facts. The Affordable Care Act and new regulations established by the Departments of Health and Human Services, Labor, and the Treasury require health plans to have an internal appeals process that

- allows consumers to appeal when a health plan denies a claim for a covered service or rescinds coverage;
- gives consumers detailed information about the grounds for the denial of claims or coverage;
- requires plans to notify consumers about their right to appeal and instructs them on how to begin the appeals process;
- ensures a full and fair review of the denial; and
- provides consumers with an expedited appeals process in urgent cases.

The timelines for an internal appeals process are the following:

- Internal appeal must be completed within thirty days if the appeal is for a service your loved one has not received yet.
- If your appeal is for a service your loved one has already received, the appeal must be completed within sixty days.
- You can file an expedited appeal if the timeline for the standard appeal process would seriously jeopardize your loved one's life or their ability to regain maximum function. An

expedited appeal is used when you need urgent medical care. In this case, the decision must be made within seventy-two hours. The expedited appeal process can be used if you are hospitalized, and if your health plan is a Medicare plan, you will be given a letter called the Important Message from Medicare that you are to be discharged. Yet if you feel you or your loved one is not ready, you can appeal and be allowed to stay in the hospital while awaiting a decision.

At the end of the internal appeals process, your health plan must provide you with a written decision. If your insurance company still denies you the service or payment for a service, you can ask for an external review. The insurance company's final determination must tell you how to ask for an external review.

External appeals. If your loved one's internal appeal is denied and he is in a new health plan, they—meaning you—have the right to appeal all denied claims to an independent reviewer not employed by the health plan. While forty-four states provide some form of external appeal, the laws governing these processes vary greatly and fail to cover millions of Americans. The new rules will ensure that consumers with new health coverage in all states have access to a standard external appeals process that meets high standards for full and fair review.

These standards were established by the National Association of Insurance Commissioners (NAIC). The NAIC standards call for the following:

- External review of plan decisions to deny coverage for care based on medical necessity, appropriateness, health care setting, level of care, or effectiveness of a covered benefit.
- Clear information for consumers about their right to both internal and external appeals, both in the standard plan materials and at the time the company denies a claim.
- Expedited access to external review in some cases, including emergency situations or cases where their health plan did not follow the rules in the internal appeal.

- Health plans must pay the cost of the external appeal under state law, and states may not require consumers to pay more than a nominal fee.
- Review by an independent body assigned by the state. The state must also ensure that the reviewers meet certain standards, keep written records, and are not affected by conflicts of interest.
- Emergency processes for urgent claims and a process for experimental or investigational treatment.
- Final decisions must be binding, so if the consumer wins, the health plan is expected to pay for the benefit that was previously denied.

(Reference: https://content.naic.org/.)

If state laws don't meet these standards, consumers in those states will be protected by comparable federal external appeals standards. In addition, people in health plans who are not subject to state law, including new self-insured employer plans, will be protected by the new federal standards.

Writing the Letter of Appeal

As you write the letter of appeal, the following is critical:

1. Use a business format for the letter. This means you will

   a. add the date of your letter;
   b. add the address of the health plan and to whom the letter is to be sent;
   c. your address;
   d. your loved one's (a) full name (generally referred to as the member of beneficiary name), (b) the insurance identification number, (c) the plan number, and (d) the date of birth; and
   e. the name of the subscriber for the health plan—you or your loved one.

2. Write the body of the letter.

    a. Keep your letter factual and to the point.
    b. Clearly explain the situation or event with facts only and include what has worked versus not.
    c. Cite any specific information or literature you can find on the medical issue you are appealing. If you have supporting evidence of what worked, include it, and attach copies of any documents you have. If you had a second opinion, include that doctor's recommendations. The National Library of Medicine website gives you detailed information on how to conduct a literature search that may help you gather any facts you may need for your letter of appeal.
    d. Explain or focus the point of your letter on what you want and why it should be approved. Clearly state the outcome(s) you expect. This makes it clear, and there is no confusion about what you expect the outcome to be.
    e. Once you have written your letter, proofread it (you want it grammatically accurate) and maybe even read it aloud. Or better yet, have a friend or family member read it as well.
    f. The critical factor here is to keep your letter objective and to keep emotions out of it. State only facts; if not, your letter will not serve the purpose you want.

3. End with an appropriate closing and your signature.

If you type in your web browser "Centers for Medicare and Medicaid Services (CMS.gov) and appealing health plan decisions," you will find some tips that may help you as you appeal a health plan denial.

Changing Health Plans or Primary Care Physicians
and Requesting Second Opinions

The primary time to make changes to your loved one's health plan is generally during the annual open enrollment period. This is annually from November 1 to December 15 to start coverage for a new year after January 1, and you pay the premiums. However, this isn't the only time you can update or change your own or your loved one's health plan coverage. You can make changes if you or your loved one has a new or qualifying event occur in your life. These qualifying events allow you the ability to make changes in health plan coverage when the date occurs after January 15, and you meet a special event definition. These qualifying events might be the following:

- ✓ Your loved one is a child who is neither disabled nor dependent upon you or your spouse for income and living expenses. However, if not disabled, then he will meet the health plan's term "aging out." This means (a) he has turned the age of twenty-six and has then aged out of a parents' health plan and (b) must then obtain their own health plan.
- ✓ Death of your spouse and you were covered under his or her employer's health plan. Upon the death of your spouse, you and any dependents are no longer eligible to remain on the policy. The same will be true if you should divorce. This means you must apply for your own health plan coverage or enroll in your state's Medicaid plan.
- ✓ You and your spouse move out of the health plan's service area, or you change zip codes or counties or even move to another state.
- ✓ You or our loved one exhausts any COBRA coverage.
- ✓ If you or your loved one enroll in a Medicare Advantage plan and there is not a qualifying event and for some reason you want to disenroll before open enrollment, you can do so. However, coverage reverts back to the original Medicare plan, which means if you do not have a secondary plan,

you or your loved one is responsible for a 2 percent co-payment for Medicare Part B services you use. This also means you can then not sign up for another Medicare Advantage plan until the next open enrollment period rolls around.

Once enrolled in a health plan and you have selected a primary care physician and for some reason you do not like him or you feel you cannot talk to him or they do not listen to you or for whatever reason you want to change physicians, you can do that. You can even make this change multiple times within the enrollment period until you find a primary care physician you like.

Second Opinions

Sometimes, your health problems are straightforward, but there are other times when a diagnosis and treatment are less clear. Getting a second opinion may be helpful.

- Your loved one's diagnosis isn't clear, or you are not satisfied with what the other doctor said.
- Your loved one has a wide variety of medical conditions.
- The treatment proposed may be considered experimental.
- Your loved one has a rare or life-threatening medical condition.
- Your loved one is not responding to treatment.
- Your loved one's doctor says they can't help your loved one and won't treat him, or they give you a poor prognosis and yet offer treatments for a cure.
- Your loved one's doctor doesn't specialize in your loved one's medical condition.
- You want peace of mind, so you consider all options.

The best place to start the process is working with the treating physician and asking for a referral. If your loved one has not seen a specialist, ask for a referral; and if your loved one is already seeing a specialist, ask to see another who has the same level of training and expertise and who isn't their close peer. If you feel you can't ask your current doctor, there are other ways to get a second opinion. You can try the following:

- Asking your insurance provider to recommend a specialist
- Asking a local clinic for a recommendation
- Asking a local hospital for a recommendation
- Searching a medical association for a specialist near you

Also, check with your loved one's health plan to make sure your second opinion is covered. If not, this means you and your loved one will be responsible for any costs associated with the second opinion. You will also want to know if there are any special instructions you must follow. While getting a second opinion outside the health plan is ideal, to be covered, your loved one's health plan may require him to be seen by another specialist within that health plan.

For the second opinion, you need to ensure your loved one's medical records are sent to the new doctor. This means you or he will need to sign a release of information so the records can be made available before the visit. By law, your loved one's treating doctor must give you or send a copy on to the second opinion doctor. However, be advised, they will more than likely charge you or your loved one a fee.

As you prepare to take your loved one to the second opinion doctor, start thinking of the questions you will want to ask and write them down, and definitely do not forget them when you go. Some questions you may want to consider might be the following:

- What are our choices?
- What are the pros, cons, and risks if we go with your advice?
- If we do nothing or wait, what might be the results?
- Do you agree with my loved one's diagnosis?
- What does this condition mean, and why did it occur?
- Do you agree with the prognosis?
- What do you suggest for treatment?

Bullying

Bullying is unwanted, aggressive behavior among school-age children that involves a real or perceived power imbalance. The behavior is repeated or has the potential to be repeated over time. Both persons who are bullied and who bully others may have serious, lasting problems. In order to be considered bullying, the behavior must be aggressive and include the following:

- *An imbalance of power.* Kids who bully use their power, such as physical strength, access to embarrassing information, or popularity, to control or harm others. Power imbalances can change over time and in different situations even if they involve the same people.
- *Repetition.* Bullying behaviors happen more than once or have the potential to happen more than once.

There are three types of bullying.

- Verbal bullying is saying or writing mean things. Verbal bullying includes:

  o Teasing
  o Name-calling
  o Inappropriate sexual comments
  o Taunting
  o Threatening to cause harm

- Social bullying, sometimes referred to as relational bullying, involves hurting someone's reputation or relationships. Social bullying includes:

  o Leaving someone out on purpose
  o Telling other children not to be friends with someone
  o Spreading rumors about someone
  o Embarrassing someone in public

- Physical bullying involves hurting a person's body or possessions. Physical bullying includes:

  - Hitting/kicking/pinching
  - Spitting
  - Tripping/pushing
  - Taking or breaking someone's things
  - Making mean or rude hand gestures

To find more information that may be of help to you, you may want to search the websites Stopbulling.gov and the National Institute of Child Health and Human Development—Eunice Kennedy Shriver. Here you will find several articles on the topic that may assist you in techniques you may be able to use.

Having special health care needs due to neurological, developmental, physical, and mental health conditions can add to the challenges children and young people face as they learn to navigate social situations in school and in their personal life. Persons with special health care needs often have difficulty getting around the school or in a work environment and have trouble communicating and navigating social interactions by showing signs of vulnerability or emotional distress. These challenges can make them be perceived as different; this then increases their risk of aggression and bullying from peers.

Children and youth with special needs are impacted by their conditions in a variety of ways. Every person is unique, and so are the ways their health condition affects them. Some impairments, such as brain injuries or neurological conditions, can impact a person's understanding of social interactions, and they may not even know when they are being bullied. Here are a few ways that disabilities affect a child or person with a neurological or mental health disorder.

- Children and youth with cerebral palsy, spina bifida, or other neurological or physical conditions can struggle with physical coordination and speech.
- Brain injuries can impair speech, movement, comprehension, and cognitive abilities or any combination of these.

A person with a brain injury may have trouble with body movements or speaking in a way that others can understand. It could take them longer to understand what is being said or to respond.

- Children and persons with autism spectrum disorder, attention deficit hyperactivity disorder, and Tourette's syndrome may have difficulties with social interactions, sensitivities, impulsivity, and self-regulating their behavior or effectively communicating.
- A child or person who experiences anxiety or depression or who has a mental health condition may be withdrawn, quiet, fearful, anxious, or vulnerable. They may exhibit intense social awkwardness or have difficulty speaking.
- Children or a person with epilepsy or behavioral disorders may exhibit erratic or unusual behavior that makes them stand out among their peers.

Another category of persons who are subjected to bullying include persons who are a lesbian, gay, bisexual, transgender, queer, intersex, nonbinary, or otherwise gender nonconforming (LGBTQI+) youth; those perceived as LGBTQI+ are at an increased risk of being bullied.

You may visit the following for references:

- stopbullying.gov
- psychologytoday.com/us/basics/bullying
- psychologytoday.com/us/therapists/child-or-adolescent
- stopbullying.gov/bullying/lgbtq

The National Institute for Child Health and Development offers some tips on supporting a person who is bullied, as well as ways to address the behavior. This same web page also gives a guide of what to do and who to call if the bullying is not being addressed and maybe not followed up on or if bullying continues even after steps are taken.

Dental Care

People with disabilities face greater challenges than people who don't have disabilities in finding access to affordable dental care. One of the reasons is that many people with disabilities have coverage through Medicaid. Dentists are often less willing to accept dental insurance for disabled adults with Medicaid because it means that they will earn less money. There's also the fact that many dental offices simply aren't prepared to treat people with disabilities, either because of lack of equipment or lack of training.

There's also the fact that many dental offices simply aren't prepared to treat people with disabilities, either because of lack of equipment or lack of training. In the not-so-distant past, many patients with disabilities were simply turned away by dentists. Patients often turned away are those with a developmental or intellectual disability, and they will include those who have the following:

- Mental capabilities vary from person to person, and if present, these may have an impact upon how well someone can follow directions in a dental office and at home.
- Behavior problems often complicate oral health care, as anxiety often makes a patient uncooperative.
- Mobility problems, and a patient requires the use of a wheelchair or a walker to move around may then make access to and from the dental chair difficult, and there are even more problems if the patient requires physical assistance to get into the chair.
- Neuromuscular or gastroesophageal reflux problems can affect the mouth, and they may have trouble with drooling, gagging, and swallowing problems that complicate oral care.
- Uncontrolled body movements can jeopardize safety and the ability to deliver oral care.
- Cardiac disorders, particularly mitral valve prolapse and heart valve damage, are common in people with developmental disabilities such as Down syndrome. When a car-

diac issue is known, you will need to consult your loved one's cardiologist prior to the dental care to determine if there is a need for pretreatment antibiotics.
- Seizures—if your loved one has seizures, this may complicate the procedure, as any undue stress may trigger a seizure.

In 2018, the American Dental Association changed their code of ethics to prohibit dental care providers from denying care to patients with disabilities. If a dentist doesn't have the skills, knowledge, equipment, or expertise to treat a person with a disability, then they must refer that patient to a dentist who can provide the right care. Sadly, even if so, it can still be difficult to find a dentist who will treat people with disabilities (physical, developmental, or intellectual); and if you can find one, they may be hours away, or getting an appointment may be months away. It is partly because of these reasons people with intellectual and developmental disabilities have poorer oral health on average than people without disabilities. People with physical disabilities can also have a more difficult time caring for their oral health because oral hygiene practices may be more difficult, they may have a sensory issue, and it may be more difficult to get to dentist visits for routine cleanings.

As a caregiver of a totally dependent person, one of your tasks will be to ensure they have daily mouth and teeth care. To assist you in doing mouth care for your loved one, the National Institute for Health has a booklet you can download that shows tips on how to brush someone's teeth. The National Institute of Dental and Craniofacial Research offers several booklets online you can download that are designed for any number of dental health care you might wish information on. For example, you can finds a booklet titled *Dental Care Every Day a Caregiver's Guide*; another called *Chemotherapy and Your Mouth*, and under their tab "Order Free Publications," you will find a full listing of the many booklets available to you.

The following are some common oral health problems seen in persons with disabilities:

- Tooth decay is common in people with developmental disabilities, as they often do not allow any one or thing to touch their mouth.
- Periodontal (gum) disease occurs more often and at a younger age in people with developmental disabilities. Difficulty performing effective brushing and flossing may be an obstacle to successful treatment and outcomes.
- Malocclusion occurs in many people with developmental disabilities, which can make chewing and speaking difficult and increase the risk of periodontal (gum) disease, dental caries, and oral trauma.
- Damaging oral habits, such as teeth grinding and clenching, food pouching, mouth breathing, and tongue thrusting, can be a problem for people with developmental disabilities.
- Oral malformations may cause enamel defects, high lip lines with dry gums, and variations in the number, size, and shape of teeth.
- Delayed tooth eruption may occur in children with developmental disabilities such as Down Syndrome. Children may not get their first baby tooth until they are two years old.
- Trauma and injury to the mouth from falls or accidents may occur in people with seizure disorders or cerebral palsy.

The National Institute of Dental and Craniofacial Research offers information you may find useful on its website and its article on "Developmental Disabilities and Oral Health."

Coverage for Dental Work

If your loved one has basic health plan coverage and has an aversion to having any work done in the mouth, the dentist in most

260

cases will or can only provide the dental care in a hospital with your loved one given an anesthesia. This type of care is often referred to as adjunctive dental care and is a medically necessary covered benefit, and it can be allowed, if a prior authorization is issued by the health plan. Adjunctive dental care is medically necessary dental care that is

- for the treatment of an otherwise covered medical (not dental) condition;
- an integral part of the treatment of such medical condition; or
- required in preparation for or as the result of dental trauma, which may be or is caused by medically necessary treatment of an injury or disease.

Here are examples.

- Removal of teeth and tooth fragments to repair a fractured jaw
- Tooth restoration, if the trauma was directly related to treating a covered medical condition
- Complete or partial ankyloglossia (tongue-tie) to alleviate difficulty swallowing or speaking
- Dental care directly related to surgical correction of a severe congenital anomaly
- Dental care in preparation for or as a result of radiation therapy for oral or facial cancer
- Anesthesia and facility fees to safeguard the life of the patient

If your loved one does not have dental coverage, you can also investigate what is available for dental care under the basic Social Security Disability Insurance (SSDI). Another option will be to explore what is available under a state's Medicaid disability dental coverage for adults with disabilities who are younger than sixty-five. You can also have a look at the different dental insurance plans available in your state by typing in your web browser "Medicaid benefits by state."

If your loved one is a child and their health coverage is provided by the state Medicaid, they are eligible for dental care under the EPSDT program. Medicaid covers dental services for all child enrollees as part of a comprehensive set of benefits, referred to as the Early and Periodic Screening, Diagnostic and Treatment (EPSDT) benefit. Though oral screening may be part of a physical exam, but it does not substitute for a dental examination performed by a dentist. A referral to a dentist is required for every child in accordance with the periodicity schedule set by a state. Dental services for children must minimally include:

- Relief of pain and infections
- Restoration of teeth
- Maintenance of dental health

The EPSDT benefit requires that all services must be provided if they are determined to be medically necessary. States determine medical necessity. If a condition requiring treatment is discovered during a screening, the state must provide the necessary services to treat that condition, whether or not such services are included in a state's Medicaid plan.

Each state is required to develop a dental periodicity schedule in consultation with recognized dental organizations involved in child health care. Dental services may not be limited to emergency services for children entitled to EPSDT.

Dental services must be provided at intervals that meet reasonable standards of dental practice and at such other intervals, as indicated by medical necessity, to determine the existence of a suspected illness or condition. States must consult with recognized dental organizations involved in child health care to establish those intervals. A referral to a dentist is required for every child in accordance with each state's periodicity schedule and at other intervals as medically necessary. The periodicity schedule for other EPSDT services may not govern the schedule for dental services.

Dental Benefits for Children with CHIP

States that provide CHIP coverage to children through a Medicaid expansion program are required to provide the EPSDT benefit. Dental coverage in separate CHIP programs is required to include coverage for dental services "necessary to prevent disease and promote oral health, restore oral structures to health and function, and treat emergency conditions."

States with a separate CHIP program may choose from two options for providing dental coverage: a package of dental benefits that meets the CHIP requirements or a benchmark dental benefit package. The benchmark dental package must be substantially equal to the (1) the most popular federal employee dental plan for dependents, (2) the most popular plan selected for dependents in the state's employee dental plan, or (3) dental coverage offered through the most popular commercial insurer in the state. For more information on dental care for children, you can type in your web browser "Insure Kids Now.gov." This will allow you to research a variety of health coverage options for children.

Dental Benefits for Adults in Medicaid

As a rule, health plans do not cover routine dental care, but some Medicare Advantage plans or managed care plans may offer dental plans as part of a benefit package they offer. If not, you may need to search your local area to find a dental plan that is offered at a lower cost. Per the US Department of Health and Human Services, you may want to search your loved one's community to see what is available from local community health centers or dental schools or if there are any low-cost dental clinics around. States have flexibility to determine what dental benefits are provided to adult Medicaid enrollees. While most states provide at least emergency dental services for adults, less than half of the states currently provide comprehensive dental care. There are no minimum requirements for adult dental coverage.

PEGGY A. ROSSI, BSN, MPA RETIRED RN AND CASE MANAGER
AND CASE MANAGEMENT ADMINISTRATOR CERTIFIED

Donated Dental Services

Donated Dental Services (DDS) is the flagship program of the Dental Lifeline Network, a nonprofit organization that provides access to dental care and education for people who can't afford it and who

- have a permanent disability,
- are age sixty-five or older, and
- are medically fragile.

DDS is a nationwide program with a network of 15,000 volunteer dentists and 3,700 volunteer laboratories. The program itself has a staff of 60 permanent members. The staff work as program coordinators who put patients in touch with the volunteers who can provide them the care they need. DDS provides free, comprehensive care for patients with disabilities who can't afford standard treatment fees. To find out if your loved one qualifies for donated dental services (DDS), you can type "donated dental services" in your web browser, and this will allow you to complete an application for possible acceptance into a program. From this same site, you will then find a full listing of dental partners they work with.

Another donated dental health link will be the Aspen Dental's Healthy Mouth Movement. This helps people with barriers to access to dental care around the country, whether for lack of funding, disabilities, or both. One of their main focal points is dental care for disabled veterans. Veterans with disabilities may have a particularly difficult time finding affordable dental care. For disabled veterans to qualify for dental insurance through the Department of Veterans Affairs (VA), they have to meet very specific standards, including having a service-related mouth injury or having been a POW. In response to the lack of VA dental care for disabled veterans, Aspen also has a MouthMobile, a dentist office on wheels, which travels the country to give free care to veterans in isolated communities. The MouthMobile is handicap-accessible and has operation rooms and digital X-ray capabilities. Aspen also has a day of service every year where they provide veterans with free pain relief and connect them with other free resources for oral health care.

Helping Your Loved One with Brushing Their Teeth

Taking care of someone with a developmental disability requires patience and skill. As a caregiver, you know this as well as anyone does. You also know how challenging it is to help that person with oral health care. It takes planning, time, and the ability to manage physical, mental, and behavioral problems. Oral care isn't always easy, but you can make it work for you and the person you help.

- Brush every day. Depending on whether the person you care for is able to brush his or her teeth, you may need to take on the job of brushing their teeth yourself or modify the toothbrush to accommodate physical limitations to allow the person to continue brushing his or her own teeth.
- Floss regularly. Some people with developmental disabilities may find flossing a real challenge. As the caregiver, you may need to do the flossing yourself, using aids such as floss holders or floss picks.
- Visit a dentist regularly. Professional cleanings are an important part of maintaining good oral health. It may take time for the person you care for to become comfortable at the dental office. A get-acquainted visit with no treatment provided might help to familiarize them with the office and the exam routine before a real visit. Depending on where your loved one resides, you may be able to find a dentist or dental hygienist that can make home visits, if going to the office is too difficult.

Many persons with aversions (a strong dislike) to mouth care require a special toothbrush. Thus, to help you in finding the right adaptive toothbrush for your loved one, there are several websites you may wish to explore.

For information on special toothbrushes for the disabled, you may find information for:

- A child or loved one with autism spectrum disorder, you can find toothbrushes and other products if your loved one has sensory issues on the Bright Autism website.
- An elderly loved one, you can find information on six different types of toothbrushes on the Graying with Grace website.

A loved one with a spinal cord injury or quadriplegia, you can find information on a hands-free toothbrush that may be right for your loved one on spinalcord.com website and view their blog on the Top Four Hands-free Toothbrushes.

Foot care

As a caregiver of someone who is diabetic, has diabetic neuropathy, peripheral vascular issues, or any major foot injury, proper foot care is vital and essential. This will be essential if you are to help prevent any open areas from developing on your loved one's lower extremities, which if not properly cared for can lead to an infection or, worse yet, an amputation. It is absolutely critical you educate yourself on how critical this task "good foot care for a person with diabetes or any neurological medical condition that prevents healthy feet" is. Thus, you need to do as much research as possible so you can find the tips you need to include in your daily caregiving routine.

While routine foot care for persons without diabetes or another neurological or medical foot condition is not a benefit of any health plans or Medicare, this does not mean your loved one, if unable to do their own foot care, is not needed. For health plans, routine foot care includes such services and treatments for flat feet or any service that is considered not medically necessary, but it does mean good foot hygiene, which can be provided either by you the caregiver or a person who specializes in pedicures and can provide.

- nail trimming
- treatment of calluses
- removal of dead skin
- foot soaks
- application of lotions

However, if your loved one has diabetes, diabetic neuropathy, or nerve damage to their foot or feet or they have a hammer toe, bunion deformities, or heel spurs, Medicare Part B and most health plans will cover a podiatrist to do routine foot exams and provide the necessary treatments that help prevent further damage to the toes, feet, or legs. This care can include

- nail care,
- removal of calluses and corns,
- specialized shoes and inserts,
- any medically necessary treatments required.

To have care provided by a health plan or Medicare (original Medicare and Part B or a Medicare Advantage plan), your loved one will need a diagnosis of diabetes, diabetic neuropathy or nerve damage or bunions, hammer toes, or heel spurs to their foot or feet to have podiatry and foot care services covered.

If your loved one is a diabetic and a podiatrist recommends it, your loved one can be allowed coverage for one pair of custom-molded or extra-depth shoes each year, with this to include any appointments needed to fit the shoes. Medicare and health plans will also pay for inserts to help regular shoes your loved one wears, as these will help provide the right support and potentially help prevent any sores developing. If your loved one prefers inserts instead of therapeutic shoes, coverage is allowed for two pairs of custom-molded inserts or three pairs of extra-depth inserts each year. But to ensure the actual number of shoes or inserts or such, you will want to either contact your loved one's health care insurer or explore any information you can find online by typing in your web browser "footwear coverage for diabetes or neuropathy."

Tips for Healthy Feet

If your loved one has diabetes or any neurological disorder of the feet or lower legs, meticulous (careful or thorough) foot care is a must. This means your loved one must wear the right shoes and socks, and you will need to ensure to take steps daily to prevent any damage to their feet. Thus, it is critical you check your loved one's feet daily. Here you will be looking for any cuts, redness, swelling, sores, blisters, corns, calluses, or any other change to the skin or nails that may indicate he or she needs to be seen by a podiatrist. Other care includes the following:

1) Washing their feet daily with warm (never hot) water, and as you do so, do not soak their feet. It is also important that you dry their feet (especially between the toes) completely and apply a lotion to both the top and bottom of their feet. However, never apply lotion between their toes, as this can lead to moisture and may cause an infection.

2) Do not let your loved one go barefoot, and when putting their shoes on, always check for pebbles or other objects inside their shoes, making sure any linings are smooth and not wrinkled.

3) If your loved one sits for long periods of time, encourage them to wiggle their toes several times per day and, if they can, even stand periodically. This helps to keep the blood flowing.

4) If your loved one is a diabetic it is critical to consider the fact that not all socks are created equal. Thus, try to choose socks that

- are white or light-colored, as this makes it easier to spot any bleeding or drainage (for example, if they have a cut or an ingrown toenail);

- fit well and aren't too tight, especially around the ankle area or above;
- are made of a synthetic fabric or wool so that moisture is not collected since moisture can lead to skin break down and infections;
- have no seams; and
- have some padding if your loved one needs more cushion on the bottom of their feet.

As my husband was a diabetic and we fought leg and foot problems on a regular basis and while not covered by his health plan, I insisted he only wear special diabetic socks that I was able to purchase at a local store where we purchased his shoes. Thus, you may want to discuss with your loved one's doctor what type of socks you should purchase. The main thing with diabetic socks is that they have an elastic area in and around the ankle so they are not too constricting. With technology today, some socks even have smart sensors that can monitor temperature and detect early signs of infection. So who knows what we can expect in the future for something as simple as a pair of socks!

Diabetic Care

If your loved one has diabetes, this means you must learn all you can on the disease and take even more steps with their care than possibly with any of the other care you perform. Why? Diabetes is one of the diseases that, if not controlled, can lead to a whole host of medical issues that can affect almost every body organ and can be life-threatening. Complications can include the following:

- Heart disease such as heart failure, high blood pressure, high cholesterol, narrowed or blocked arteries (those that supply blood to the heart, brain, or extremities), and irregular heartbeat
- Stroke

- Kidney disease, including end-stage kidney failure requiring dialysis or a transplant
- Nerve damage (numbness, tingling, especially of the hands and feet and legs)
- Eye disease, including blindness
- Digestion problems
- Erectile dysfunction, impotence, or sexual problems
- Skin problems and infections
- Dental problems

Diabetes, also known as diabetes mellitus, is a group of common endocrine diseases characterized by sustained high blood sugar levels. Diabetes is due to either the pancreas not producing enough insulin or the cells of the body not responding properly to the insulin produced. There are three main types of diabetes: type 1, type 2, and gestational diabetes (diabetes while pregnant).

- Type I diabetes often develops quickly, and it is usually diagnosed in children, teens, and young adults. If your loved one has type 1 diabetes, they will need to take insulin every day to survive. This also means you will need to be diligent with their care and diet and watch their activity to ensure their blood glucose is monitored closely, and their insulin is adjusted accordingly to their activity.
- Type 2 diabetes is when your loved one's body doesn't use insulin well, and they cannot keep their blood sugar at normal levels. Type 2 diabetes develops over many years and is usually diagnosed in adults (but more and more in children, teens, and young adults).
- Gestational diabetes develops in pregnant women who have never had diabetes. If your loved one has gestational diabetes, their baby could be at higher risk for health problems. Gestational diabetes usually goes away after the baby's birth. However, for your loved one, it increases their risk for type 2 diabetes later in life; and for their baby, the baby

is more likely to have obesity as a child or teen and develop type 2 diabetes later in life.

As with any of your loved one's care and they are a diabetic, it is critical you are taught how to perform the glucose monitoring he or she will need, as well as to administer their medications and prepare a healthy diet. These are necessary, as you will need to perform the following:

1) Blood sugar checks several times per day or as directed by your loved one's doctor. This also means you should have been taught how to use the glucometer and do the testing. As you do the checks, this also means you should record the numbers so you can share them with the doctor on the next visit.

2) Administer the medications as prescribed by your loved one's doctor, and if they are taking insulin, you should have been trained on hot to do these as well before you assumed such care. Any medications administered must also be recorded so you can share these as well with the doctor on the next visit.

3) Cook and provide your loved one, following the diet prescribed. Healthy eating is important, as it helps keep your loved one's blood sugar in the target range his or her doctor feels is right for them.

4) In addition to this care, you will want to ensure your loved one has the following follow-up visits and testing done at the frequency prescribed by their doctor:

- A1c testing (a test that shows your loved one's average blood sugar level over the past two to three months)
- Cholesterol testing
- Dilated eye exam
- Hearing check
- Complete foot check

As your loved one's caregiver, you should have been trained on what to look for when it comes to high or low blood sugar. However, the following is a guide:

- Feeling very thirsty
- Frequent urination
- Fatigue
- Feeling very hungry
- Unexplained weight loss
- Blurred vision
- Slow healing of cuts or sores

If your loved one has any of these symptoms in addition to vomiting, deep, labored breathing, or confusion, it is critical you call 9-1-1 or go to the nearest emergency room as soon as possible. This step is critical, as your loved one may have what is called diabetes-related ketoacidosis, which is a life-threatening condition.

Symptoms of low blood sugar include:

- Shaking or trembling
- Sweating and chills
- Dizziness or lightheadedness
- Faster heart rate
- Intense hunger
- Anxiousness or irritability

If your loved one is a diabetic, you as the caregiver must educate yourself on as much as you can on the disease. Some of the best websites to do this will be use: American Diabetes Association (ADA); Centers for Disease Control and Prevention (CDC.gov) and Medicare.gov/publications.

Helping Your Loved One with Activities and Instrumental Activities of Daily Living

When it becomes clear that a loved one can't get through their daily routines without assistance, the logical next step is that you as their caregiver must assume such tasks that will provide the support they need. So what are activities of daily living (ADLs)? These are the basic skills we use every day to properly care for ourselves. This type of care is classified as custodial care (care that is nonmedical in nature but care that is needed to help a person perform on a daily basis); custodial care differs from skilled care, which is care that can only be provided by or under the supervision of a license and trained medical professional, whether it's a nurse or a rehabilitation professional, such as a physical therapist.

ADLs include the following:

1. Eating—the ability to move food and drink successfully to one's mouth.
2. Dressing—the ability to select appropriate clothing and put it on.
3. Bathing—the ability to maintain good personal hygiene practices, including taking a bath or shower, caring for our nails and hair, and performing oral hygiene.
4. Toileting—the ability to use the toilet and cleanse ourselves.
5. Continence—the ability to control our bladder and bowel function.
6. Ambulating—the ability to walk and transfer to and from a bed or chair.

On top of ADLs, if you are a caregiver, this means you also will assume many activities that are classified normally as instrumental activities of daily living (IADLs). IADLs are the more complex tasks we take for granted and yet are the one's necessary if we are to live and function independently.

IADLs include the following:

- Cooking—the ability to plan, prepare, and serve adequate meals.
- Managing medications—the ability to take correct doses of medications at the right times.
- Shopping—the ability to shop for all one's needs, including clothing, personal care items, and groceries.
- Communicating—the ability to use a phone, computer, or other methods of communication.
- Managing money—the ability to make and follow a budget, write checks, pay bills on time, make trips to the bank, and monitor one's income and expenses.
- Housekeeping—the ability to clean and maintain one's home.
- Transportation—the ability to drive, use public transportation, or arrange other means of transport.
- Laundering clothing—the ability to wash and dry personal laundry.

In each area, ADLs or IADLs, this means a person may and each may be classified in a rehabilitation professional's notes as

- Totally independent (I)
- Requiring prompting, reminders, or supervision (A)
- Relying on durable medical equipment (DME) or other assistive devices (AD)
- Requiring moderate hands-on assistance (mod A)
- Contact guard assistance (CGA)
- Completely dependent on another person (D)

Functional status and the ability to care for oneself have a significant impact on one's quality of life. Changes in ADLs and IADLs can be caused by underlying medical conditions, but failing to recognize these growing needs can also contribute to a cycle of physical and mental health problems. Unmet needs for help with activities of daily living may contribute to the following:

- Malnutrition
- Poor personal hygiene
- Isolation
- Illnesses like urinary tract infections (UTIs)
- Falls

Bathing

Getting a person with a developmental or intellectual disability or an aging loved one to bathe can be a major battle that many caregivers experience. When you are a caregiver of a person with autism or other developmental or intellectual disability or with dementia, you may find your loved one may refuse to bathe for any number of reasons. Understanding why they resist can help family caregivers navigate these issues and keep their loved ones as clean, healthy, and comfortable as possible.

Because this can be such a difficult task, one important consideration is how often your loved one truly needs to bathe. If your loved one will not shower or bathe daily, in most cases, this will not be a serious issue to consider. However, if your loved one is bed confined or one who perspires profusely, is incontinent of bowel or bladder, has skin issues, or is active, a daily bath is reasonable to consider. The key purpose of a bath or shower is critical for helping to prevent infections.

A full bath or shower isn't always needed every single day, but there are certain areas of the body that warrant more frequent attention. This area is you must ensure your loved one's perineal area (what some call their privates) are cleaned thoroughly each day. This can be done by using a peri bottle (a bottle you can fill with water and squirt onto your loved one's privates). The bottle is filled with warm water, and you can use it to clean your loved one up after they have a bowel movement or pee. Keeping a loved one's private areas clean and dry is of utmost importance. So try to focus on this task above all, as a urinary tract infection can occur if the area is not kept clean and if not treated can lead to a serious infection called sepsis.

For the developmentally or intellectually disabled or persons with some mental or dementia issues, sensory sensitivities make it difficult to take a bath or shower. While you or I may not think about it, both a shower and a bath involve a lot of sensory sensitivities. These can include the fact the room may be too cool or hot; the same goes with water or merely the sound of the water or the echoes water makes as it hits tiles, as water goes down the drain, or even lighting being too bright, any or all of which can be overwhelming for a person with sensory issues.

Once in the shower, water touching the face, skin, or head and hair can be scary; and for some, just the touch of the water on the skin, may feel odd. Even drying with a towel may be difficult and can be overwhelming and cause sensory overload. Thus, you may want to prepare the area ahead of time and think of ways to take the stress out of bath time. For example, you may want to fill the bathtub or start the shower ahead of time, and you may want to put towels on the floor on the tub or shower to help dull the sounds or prevent your loved one seeing water go down the drain. You may also want to dim the lights and maybe even turn on their favorite music if that can help. Once you have a calm environment, you can then help your loved one with their bathing. In some cases, you may even want to think of a prize you can give your loved one once the task is done.

If a shower is the best option for your loved one, be sure to install grab bars for extra stability. A comfortable shower chair and a handheld showerhead are worthwhile investments as well. The chair allows your loved one to rest as needed. Meanwhile, the showerhead keeps the water from continually coming down on their head and allows you to carefully direct where the stream goes, minimizing discomfort and fear.

As you help your loved one you may find you need to talk through each step if needed and verbally tell them what will happen next. Your loved one may not understand exactly what you're saying, but it will help them remain calm and included in the process. Surprises can lead to agitation, anger, and confusion. Describe each move in a low, soothing voice. For example, say "I'm going to wipe your face with this warm cloth, okay?" or "I'm going to lift your arm and wash under your arm." Some kids—and you may find even your older loved one with dementia—may enjoy a countdown so they know what is going to happen next.

As you wash and rinse them try to find a rinse routine that fits, and as with washing, try to make if a fun event. Rinsing suds out of hair is a common trigger for a freak-out, as your loved one may have fears and anxiety with soap or water going into their eyes or ears or nose, any one of which can be painful. Most of us, as we rinse, find leaning forward much more comfortable than leaning backward where we can lose our balance. If soap suds are an issue, try a visor or swim goggles. Key is to try different methods to get the job done and ways your loved one feels comfortable and safe.

As you bathe or help them shower, stick to preferred textures and pressures—foamy soap versus slimy soap, loofah versus washrag, or gentle towel drying versus a vigorous rub. Any one of these can take time to try to see what works. Key is to learn your loved one's needs and sensitivities and, once found, sticking to them will help tremendously.

here are other tips to use for bathing or showering

> A soap dispenser, as dropping the soap can cause slipping or falls as they try to pick it up
> Ear plugs if water noises are an issue
> Dry shampoo
> Try a soft sponge to help wash hair or even the body in place of a washrag
> Face or body wipes in place of a washrag
> A warm towel to dry off
> Having them go into a shower backwards to avoid any water hitting the face
> Dimmed lights, and if light bulbs are starting to go out and flicker, change them immediately

If unsure on how to give a bath or shower or control behavior when this event occurs and regardless of whether they are a child, adolescent, or an elderly, you will find many resources on the Internet that may be of help. Here, you can find tips on how to shower or bathe your loved one who might be autistic, with a mobility issue or dementia. In my research, I also found one that will actually provide a step-by-step guide on how to give a bed bath. So let the Internet help give you the information you may need to use as you perform this task.

For a teenage girl or young woman with developmental or intellectual disabilities, you will want to investigate how to teach her (if teachable) hygiene and use of menstrual pads. For this, it may include use of a picture book, which includes images of important hygiene products, such as soap, deodorant, and pads.

What to Do if Your Loved One Refuses to Stop Driving

When you realize it is time to have your loved one (parent or spouse) to stop driving, this will be one of the times when you will want to have that difficult discussion with them. Believe me, this in most cases will be a heated discussion, but you must do it. Unsafe drivers are a huge and serious issue.

So what might be some warning signs your loved one is no longer safe behind the wheel and is a danger not only to their selves but equally as important a danger to others? I know for my mom, who was declared legally blind and she continued to drive, her way to get to and from the store was to count the stop signs! Probably some of the biggest clues you will want to look out for will be the following:

- Forgetting how to drive to familiar stores or even how to get to a friend's or family's home
- Failing to observe traffic signs, making slow decisions in traffic, or driving at erratic or unsafe speeds
- Hitting curbs or dividers or unsafe lane changes
- Becoming angry or confused while driving and screaming and cursing

Like my mom, many older adults stubbornly refuse to give up the keys or continue driving despite the fact you and possibly other family members have had repeated discussions with them about the issue. Even with my mom, we had made arrangements for Uber to take her places, but she refused to use it, always saying, "I know how to drive. Why should I have this unnecessary expense?" So my brother and I had no other option, and as guilty as we felt, we had to again have one more really serious and difficult conversation with her. This time, we demanded she give up her keys and her car; and despite her crying and sobbing, she finally did!

What might you need to do when your own situation regarding an unsafe driver needs attention?

1) If your loved one's doctor has not made the referral, you can anonymously call and report your loved one to the local DMV office. Each state has different procedures to follow, but in most, even if it is not time to renew their license, the unsafe driver you can call and alert the DMV of your concern. In most cases, they will alert your loved one of the needs to be retested.

2) For an example of what a form might look like, for either you or your loved one's doctor to complete, see the CA DMV website where you can search their portal for what information is required.

3) If your loved one is forgetful or has dementia, an effective way to stop him or her from driving will be to remove the car and the hide keys or any reminders of what might be needed to drive.

4) You can have a friend or other family member borrow the car or pretend it is in the shop or even park it out of sight. Thus, the old saying "Out of sight, out of mind" might help deter them from their demands to drive.

5) You can also hide the keys and pretend they are lost, or better yet, work with a family member or friend and disable the car.

Losing the ability to drive can be difficult, but driving is only one form of transportation. Consider finding other ways your loved one can travel safely on their own. Some suggestions will be to see what is needed to sign your loved one up for any community Handicapped bus or other transportation services. Your best option will be to call your loved one's local bus services and make an application for their handicapped program. If unfamiliar with what number to call, make use of the 2-1-1 phone service now available in communities. If your loved one is elderly, a good resource will be your loved one's local Area Agency on Aging. They can help you find local services that may include free or low-cost buses, taxis, or carpools for older people. Many communities have a wide variety of bus services for the disabled, so explore those. So investigate what is available, and your best way will be to use the 2-1-1 phone directory.

Cutting Hair for a Person who Is Bedbound
or with Challenging Behaviors

Children with autism spectrum disorder (ASD) and persons with sensory processing issues may react negatively to personal hygiene and grooming routines because they become overwhelmed by certain types of touch and smell. Although persons with sensory challenges are often upset by day-to-day tasks, such as brushing teeth, many caregivers report that one of the most distressing activities is going for a haircut.

So what might be tips to help you with your loved one when a haircut is needed?

- Consider hiring a mobile hairdresser/barber who can cut your loved one's hair in your own home, a familiar environment. Alternatively, you may also want to learn to cut their hair yourself.
- Use safety scissors and pretend to cut your loved one's hair prior to their actual haircut. You can also allow them to do this to you.

- Look into purchasing quiet clippers or asking your loved one's hairdresser/barber to use the least noisy equipment they have.
- Give your loved one something to play with or fidget with during the haircut, such as an iPad or fidget toy. You could also talk to them about something they are interested in.
- Plan something fun after the haircut so that they have something to look forward to.

Recreation and Its Importance

If your loved one has been injured or ill or has a chronic disability and they have difficulty performing everyday activities and as such they remain fairly inactive, it is critical you make every effort to get them involved, and they remain as active as possible. They may benefit from taking part in any community local or regional recreational activities or working with a recreational therapist.

Recreational therapy, also known as therapeutic recreation, is not a game. A recreational therapist uses activities to help your loved one to move better and feel better. While a physical or occupational therapist may use exercises to improve functional mobility, a recreational therapist uses recreational activities to help him or her regain their mobility and improve well-being. Activities may include doing puzzles and playing games, cooking, or outdoor activities, like horseback riding or hiking. Therapeutic recreation is not all about playing games. It involves using specific activities to help your loved one regain your independence. Examples of activities that a recreational therapist may perform may include art, cooking, community outings, participating in sport events, exercise classes, music, and dancing.

Who Pays for Recreational Therapy?

If your loved one has a prescription from their physician and it contains the medical necessity reason for recreational therapy, Medicare and the VA will cover this service for some diagnoses and in certain settings, so do your homework and investigate what is needed. It may also be a benefit of the following:

- ✓ Some private health plans, but you will need to research this with your loved one's health plan.
- ✓ If your loved one has a developmental or intellectual disability (DD and ID) and they are followed by his or her state's agency that serves such diagnoses, work closely with your loved one's assigned case manager.
- ✓ Recreational therapy may be provided by your loved one's local Easterseals or United Cerebral Palsy agency, as these offices work closely with your loved one's agency that provides services for the DD and ID population.
- ✓ It can also be provided by the agency called Faces, as they have a camp for kids with craniofacial deformities.

As you search the Internet for recreation services for your loved one, you will find at a minimum the following offer such as the following:

- Verywell Health
- United Cerebral Palsy
- Easterseals
- The National Craniofacial Association
- Autism Speaks
- Veteran's Administration
- Wounded Warriors and their adapted sports and recreation programs

Physical activity plays an important role for any of us in maintaining health, well-being, and quality of life; and it helps use to control our weight and improve our overall health. This is even more important for persons with disabilities as physical activity can help support daily living activities and independence. Per the CDC, one in four US adults living with a disability is more likely to have obesity, heart disease, stroke, diabetes, and cancer. Thus, key as you provide care for your loved one will be to explore what activities might be the best for them and ones that may be available within their region. This can include merely taking your loved one on a walk around the neighborhood or a local park, seeking camps or adaptive sports programs for persons with a specific disease or disorder, or possibly participating in Special Olympics or the Paralympics.

Adaptive sports are similar to typical sports, such as basketball, biking, softball, tennis, skiing, kayaking, and more. They are adapted for people with disabilities, allowing many more people to participate with increased independence, comfort, and confidence. Sometimes, special equipment is needed to make participation possible, such as sit-skis that allow athletes to sit rather than stand when they ski or specially designed wheelchairs for sports like basketball, rugby, or lacrosse. These sports can be purely recreational or highly competitive.

Many camps for people with developmental and intellectual disabilities utilize therapeutic horseback riding. Additional outdoor recreational activities include hiking, boating, fishing, swimming, and participating in outdoor team sports. When it comes to outdoor activities for adults with disabilities, the possibilities are endless.

Park and recreation departments across the country are establishing inclusive recreation programs and participation opportunities to give all citizens—from toddlers to seniors—an equal opportunity to participate in local activities, classes, and athletic events. Such programs are helping communities to foster cultures of social inclusion and acceptance and are helping young people develop into confident, capable adults no matter their learning or development challenges. If you are ready to incorporate such programming into your activities, it will be critical that you understand the fundamentals of a successful implementation.

You may also want to investigate program designed for persons with intellectual and developmental disabilities that involve music therapy. This category of persons with disabilities typically responds well to music activities because it motivates action, captivates attention, brings joy, and offers success. In particular, music can be helpful because it is processed in both the right and left hemispheres of the brain. Music is a multisensory activity that incorporates auditory, visual, tactical systems, and kinesthetic systems.

At the same time, music is a wonderful way to for your loved one to connect and express oneself, which can be especially helpful for those who struggle with language or are nonverbal. Whether it's singing along or playing an instrument like the tambourines, music activities accomplish the following goals:

- *Academics.* Here you can translate virtually anything into a song to improve recall.
- *Communication and speech.* Creating custom songs can help increase repetition without monotony while isolating sounds.
- *Gross and fine motor skills.* Implementing adaptive and traditional percussion instruments (such as hand drums) can help address gross and fine motor skills.
- *Behavioral.* You can create musical stories and songs to reinforce appropriate behavior.
- *Emotional-social.* Songs can be used to help persons with disabilities to identify feelings and utilize coping strategies anytime they feel overwhelmed.
- *Quality of life and self-esteem.* Successful and positive experiences can be commemorated through song and musical experiences.

Paralympics and Special Olympics

The Special Olympics differ from the Paralympics in three main areas: (1) the structure of their organizations, (2) the disability categories of the athletes, and (3) the criteria and philosophy under which they participate.

The Special Olympics provides training and competition year-round and holds world games every two years (alternating with summer and winter events). The Special Olympics welcomes all athletes with intellectual disabilities of all ability levels ages eight and up.

Specialized Durable Medical Equipment and Rent versus Purchase

Depending upon your loved one's diagnosis or disability, if they require specialized durable medical equipment (DME) and they are hospitalized, it is critical you do not allow the discharge until the equipment is made for them and available for use. This type of equipment will be custom-made and designed to fit and provide the support and ability to control it specifically by your loved one. Specialized equipment if never rented but must be purchased, which means it must be prior authorized by your loved one's health plan. While the original Medicare does not require prior authorization, any claim submitted is subject to retrospective review (review after the fact) to ensure it meets criteria and is medically necessary for the reason for its use.

Durable medical equipment (DME) is defined as a medically necessary supply or device that can be used over and over again. To qualify as DME, the item must

- Primarily serve a medical purpose
- Be prescribed by or ordered by a medical provider
- Be able to be used again and again
- Generally have an expected lifetime of at least three years
- Be used in the home
- Only be useful to patients who have an injury or disability

The most common examples of durable medical equipment (and if related supplies are needed, these will be covered as well) used outside a hospital include the following:

- Kidney machines
- Traction equipment
- Oxygen concentrators, humidifiers, nebulizers, CPAPS or BiPaps, ventilators
- Suction equipment
- Infusion equipment
- Personal care aids, like commodes and lifts

- Mobility aids, such as walkers, canes, crutches, wheelchairs, and scooters
- Gait trainers or standing frames
- Diabetes blood sugar meters, blood sugar test strips, lancets, and lancing devices
- Bed equipment, like hospital beds, pressure mattresses, Bili lights, and blankets (a Bili light is a light therapy tool that treats newborn jaundice [hyperbilirubinemia or bilirubin] that, if not treated, can cause brain damage [kernicterus], leading to cerebral palsy)

For any of the foregoing and any other devices, it may not be wise to have such purchased. If the item is purchased and is one considered a life-sustaining device that runs 24-7, the manufacturer will require it to be sent to them for refurbishment on a regular schedule. This means in the interim of the servicing, your loved one will need a second device; and if the original item was purchased, you will be responsible for both the servicing and rental of the item to be used in the interim. So discuss your options ahead of time so an extra outlay of money is unexpected.

If your loved one will be wheelchair bound, they must have a wheelchair made specifically for them (this means they must be measured and fitted for it). Included with the wheelchair, they may also need what is termed a seating system, leg or armrests, or control devices or other specifically designed products to allow them as much mobility as possible. If your loved one will be wheelchair bound, it is critical you or he or she fully discuss the type that will be best for your loved one's diagnosis and use and even the activities they may want to perform. I am sure if your loved one is to be wheelchair bound, his or her therapist will recommend a tilt in space type of chair. This type of chair will be specific of course for your loved one, but by having such a chair, the chair can recline some and is useful in helping to reduce pressure on specific areas of the body.

When such equipment is obtained, it will be purchased; and when this occurs, another similar device will not be available for another purchase for three years. For children, as they will grow, their wheelchair or mobility device will be designed to be what is termed growable. This means, at any given time when their height or weight changes, changes to the chair or seating system will be required.

Coverage for any durable medical equipment is a benefit of Medicare and most health plans, but double-check if your loved one's health plan is other than original Medicare or a Medicare Advantage plan to see what is covered versus what is not and what might be your loved one's co-payment and what requirements or rules you must follow.

If your loved one requires a scooter or power chair for better mobility, there are very specific requirements by Medicare, Medicaid, the VA, and even health plans for such. Thus, it is imperative you do not purchase a mobility device first and then expect your loved one's health plan to reimburse you or your loved one for the device. To obtain such a device, the following conditions must be met:

- Your loved one's doctor and the supplier of the mobility scooter must both be enrolled in Medicare.
- Your loved one's doctor must have conducted a face to face (F2F) examination of your loved one prior to ordering the device.
- Your loved one must be unable to perform activities of daily living (ADLs), such as bathing, dressing, or moving in or out of a chair or bed or using the bathroom, even with the use of a cane, a crutch, or walker.
- Your loved one is able to use the scooter within the home, which means that it is not too large to fit between doorways or anything in its path.
- Your loved one does not have the upper body strength or ability to use a standard wheelchair.
- Your loved one can safely operate the device and get on and off the scooter or have someone who will always be available to help them safely use it.
- Your loved one must also be able to sit up on the scooter, and to operate the steering system.

Rent versus Purchase

Depending on the type of durable medical equipment (DME) your loved one needs, Medicare and/or your loved one's health plan may require it to be either rented or purchased (as a rule, it is to be purchased if the cost is less than $150). Most equipment is initially rented, including many manual and power wheelchairs.

- Original Medicare covers 80 percent of the cost of a monthly rental fee for thirteen months. Your loved one is then responsible for a 20 percent co-payment.
- After thirteen months, ownership is typically given to your loved one automatically.

If your loved one has a Medicare Advantage Plan or private health plan, make sure to follow the plan's coverage rules. One of your best sources for information for coverage and qualifying criteria for durable medical equipment cover, including electric wheelchairs and scooters, will be to review the Medicare.gov/publication site. Once in this site, you can use the search bar and type in durable medical equipment or wheelchair or scooter benefit, and you will have the information you will need.

Specialized Items for a Person with DD or ID

If your loved one has an intellectual or developmental disability (IDD) and is a client of their state's agency that provides care for this, ensure you work with your loved one's assigned case manager so see if you are able to get possibly any type of specialized equipment your loved one's occupational or physical therapist indicates is needed. To obtain any of the following, you will need to first ascertain if it is considered a covered device by your loved one's health plan. If it is, that health plan will serve as the primary payer; and if not, you will need a formal letter of denial from the health plan for any alternate funding agency to pick up the costs. Specialty equipment for a child with developmental or intellectual disabilities includes such items as the following:

1) Seating and positioning.

- Pediatric specialty chairs. Designed to support comfort and posture in a range of environments, these unique chairs are perfect for any setting and any child's needs.
- Adaptive chairs. These modified chairs are designed to provide safety, support, and comfort for children with special needs who need more assistance than traditional chairs can provide.
- Pediatric seating. Ideal for children in any setting with any range of needs, pediatric seating includes a variety of chairs, cushions, couches, and stools for perfect comfort whether during tasks or play.
- Pediatric corner chairs. Perfect for supporting comfortable seating in corners, especially in classrooms and reading nooks; these corner chairs are great for a wide variety of settings.
- Pediatric high-low chairs. Targeted toward special needs children with more complex support needs, these chairs offer exceptional support and comfort while still keeping kids comfortable and able to be at eye level with their peers.
- Pediatric modular chairs. Great for classrooms, modular chairs are designed to be easy to adjust, easy to customize, and easy to maintain, making them the perfect addition for a range of needs.
- Pediatric sitters. Keeping kids at eye level with their peers, sitters help support the posture and alignment of the body while allowing children to remain low to the ground to engage in various activities.
- Pediatric sitter accessories. Offering additional adaptation and customization options for pediatric sitters,

these accessories make it easy for any child to get the perfect fit and experience out of their furniture.

- Pediatric therapeutic chairs. Ideal for therapy, special needs children, or kids who are recovering from injury or illness, these chairs provide optimal comfort and support while facilitating proper posture and better mobility.
- Pediatric tumble forms Carrie seating system. The Carrie system is one of the biggest names in the special needs seating industry. Mix and match components in this easily accessible category.
- Pediatric tables and chairs. Great for classrooms, day cares, and home play areas, tables and chairs designed especially for children help provide proper support for all sorts of tasks from tea parties to homework.
- Pediatric positioning. Perfect for a range of children's needs, these positioning tools help to ensure that kids are always properly supported in ideal posture and alignment for maximum comfort and health.
- Pediatric soft strapping materials. These strapping materials are great for a variety of splinting and positioning needs, helping to provide support without compromising on comfort.

2) Sensory motor

- Pediatric indoor gym. Providing all the benefits of an outdoor play center or fitness area, an indoor gym doubles as exercise and play while allowing children to remain active indoors. Perfect for areas with harsh weather or children sensitive to sun, this equipment is great in any setting.
- Pediatric motor activity centers. Perfect for helping kids to develop gross motor skills, and promote physical health, these activity centers are great for both exercise and play for children of all ages.

- Pediatric tents and tunnels. Often used in a variety of indoor playtime activities, these tents and tunnels promote creativity and physical health by helping encourage kids to engage with each other and their environments.
- Adaptive toys. Designed to provide exceptional play equipment for children with special needs, these toys are accessible for kids who may not be able to engage with traditional toys.
- Pediatric fine motor. Ideal for helping to promote fine motor skills and dexterity, often in the hands and fingers, these devices are perfect for both therapy and play and are equally as great for helping children who are delayed as they are for those in recovery.
- Pediatric manipulatives. Perfect for kids working on sensory stimulation and awareness, as well as those trying to work on fine motor skills. These toys and devices are the ideal addition to both therapy and playtime alike.
- Pediatric massage and relaxation. For children who have anxiety or a lot of nervous energy, massage and relaxation tools are a great solution for helping these children to calm down and release excess energy.
- Pediatric oral motor. These products are designed to be used in speech therapy to help promote oral motor strength and dexterity, which aids in eating, drinking, and speech skills both in therapy and development.
- Pediatric peg boards. Great for hand therapy and fine motor development, these pegboards are perfect for both play and therapy, serving dual purposes for children with a range of needs.
- Pediatric puzzles. Designed to help engage the mind and promote problem-solving skills, these puzzles are both fun and functional. They facilitate the development of important mental skills while also helping children engage.

- Pediatric sensory motor developmental toys. These toys are perfect for helping children to develop sensory motor skills. They work great for both therapy and for playtime by doubling as both developmental tools and toys all at once.
- Pediatric tactile stimulation. Great for children who have sensory issues or who are developing tactile skills, these tools and toys are designed to assist in the development of appropriate tactile sensory skills.
- Swing seats. Designed to provide more adaptive solutions for children and adults who want to play on swings, these seats offer better support and comfort while still facilitating the fun and vestibular stimulation that a swing provides.
- Pediatric mats. Ideal for exercise and floor play, these mats offer comfort and support for children on the floor, helping to make exercises, playtime, or other tasks more enjoyable.
- Pediatric mirrors. These mirrors are child-sized and designed to be used for a wide variety of tasks including therapy, exercise, play, and more!
- Pediatric scooter boards. Perfect for motor development and fun exercise, scooter boards help kids stay active and play while also encouraging the development of gross motor skills, including strength and dexterity.

Note: The foregoing listing was from the RehabMart website. Again, as I have stated, neither I nor my publisher want you to think we are endorsing this company. I merely added their listing of specialty devices here as it was one of the most complete I could find. There are certainly other companies out there that offer the same or similar products, so do your own research as you work with the therapist.

Wound Care

If your loved one is one with any type of wound when they are discharged or develop one in the course of their care, it is imperative (crucial, vital, or necessary) you take meticulous care of the wound. In most cases, your loved one's wound care will be managed initially by the home health agency with you trained on what do in if there is leakage or the dressing comes lose. If at some point when it is decided you are the one to do the actual wound care, before you take over this task, ensure you have been thoroughly trained. Again, if training is needed, request they train you using the teach-back method. Wounds are very complicated in many cases and if not cared for properly can become extensive with sepsis setting in any possible death. Consequently, the notes in this section are only a brief overview of some key points for you to be aware of. Key is to learn all you can; this could be an area where the care can be too overwhelming for you. Thus, a time when you might need to say no and have your loved one placed in a facility that can do the care needed.

As you care for your loved one, a critical factor will be to make every effort to prevent any pressure on bony areas of your loved one's body. Once a pressure sore develops, it can quickly change stages and go from merely red skin to deep and an ugly open sore.

As I did my research on wound care, two of the best resources I found that might help educate you on wounds and wound care were at Healthline and their articles on stages of pressure ulcers and then another on the four stages of wound healing.

The following is a quick summary of what the articles pointed out: Pressure ulcers are also known as bedsores and decubitus ulcers. They range from closed to open wounds and are classified into a series of four stages based on how deep the wound is.

- Stage 1 ulcers have not yet broken through the skin.
- Stage 2 ulcers have a break in the top two layers of skin.
- Stage 3 ulcers affect the top two layers of skin, as well as fatty tissue.

- Stage 4 ulcers are deep wounds that may impact muscle, tendons, ligaments, and bone.

Bedsores occur most often after a person sits or lies in one position for too long. The immobility cuts off blood circulation to specific parts of your body, damaging surrounding tissues. Pressure ulcers form mainly on any skin that covers bony areas of the body. Common places for bedsores to develop include

- butt
- tailbone
- heels
- ankles
- hips
- back
- elbows
- shoulder blades
- back of the head

Two kinds of more severe pressure ulcers do not fit into one of the four stages:

- suspected deep pressure injury
- unstageable sores

These are the stages of pressure ulcers and treatment

Stage 1. The first stage is the mildest and affects the upper layer of your skin. In this stage, the wound has not yet opened. The affected area has no surface breaks or tears but may

- appear red in people with lighter skin and blue or purple in people with darker skin,
- remain red or darker for more than thirty minutes after pressure is removed,
- not turn pale if pressed firmly,
- be sore to the touch,

- have a warmer temperature from the surrounding normal tissues,
- feel firmer than surrounding tissues, or
- cause mild burning or itching.

The first step to treating a stage 1 bedsore is to remove pressure from the area. Any added or excess pressure can cause the ulcer to break through the skin surface. If you're lying down, adjust your position or use pillows and blankets as extra padding. It's also important to keep the affected area clean and dry to reduce tissue damage. Ensure your loved one stays well hydrated, and you add foods high in calcium, protein, and iron to their diet. These foods help with skin health. If treated early, developing stage 1 pressure ulcers can heal in about three days.

Stage 2. In the second stage, the sore area of your skin has broken through the top layer of skin (epidermis) and some of the layer below (dermis). The break typically creates a shallow, open wound. A stage 2 bedsore may appear as

- a shallow, crater-like wound, or
- a serum-filled (clear to yellowish fluid) blister that may or may not have burst.

It may also cause the following symptoms:

- some drainage or pus at the ulcer
- pain
- swollen, sore, or red tissue around the sore, which indicates tissue death or damage

Similar to treating stage 1 pressure ulcers, you should treat stage 2 sores by removing pressure from your loved one's wound; and if not seen, seek medical attention for proper treatment. Your loved one's doctor will advise you on what treatment and wound dressings you will need to keep the area dry and clean. This helps prevent the wound from becoming more severe or infected. As you care for the wound, it is important to monitor the wound for any signs of infection, including

- worsening pain,
- pus,
- red skin,
- fever.

Healing from this stage can last anywhere from three days to three weeks.

Stage 3. Sores that have progressed to the third stage have broken completely through the top two layers of the skin and into the fatty tissue below. An ulcer in this stage may resemble a hole or crater. You'll likely notice visible fat tissue but should not be able to see muscle or bone. In this stage, it's important to look for signs of infection. These include

- foul odor,
- pus,
- redness,
- discolored drainage.

These sores need special attention, and your loved one's doctor may remove any dead tissue to promote healing and to prevent or treat the infection and may also order a home health wound nurse to assist you in the care of such wounds. If your loved one is deconfined, his or her doctor may recommend a special mattress or bed to relieve pressure from the affected areas. Ulcers in this stage usually need at least one to four months to heal.

Stage 4. Stage 4 pressure ulcers are the most serious. These sores extend below the subcutaneous fat into your deep tissues, including muscle, tendons, and ligaments. In more severe cases, they can extend as far down as the cartilage or bone. There's a high risk of infection at this stage.

You may notice the following symptoms in a stage 4 bedsore:

- extreme pain
- drainage
- dead tissue, which may appear black
- visible muscles and sometimes bone
- common signs of infection, like a foul smell and pus
- a dark, hard substance known as eschar (hardened dead wound tissue)

If not previously hospitalized for the stage 4 pressure ulcers, if such should develop while your loved one is being cared for at home, your loved one will require hospitalization and possibly surgery. Recovery for this ulcer can take anywhere from three months to two years to completely heal.

Additional Types

In addition to the four main stages of pressure ulcer formation, there are two other categories: unstageable pressure ulcers and suspected deep tissue injury.

Unstageable pressure ulcers are also hard to diagnose because the bottom of the sore is covered by the following:

- slough: debris that appears tan, yellow, green, or brown in color
- eschar: hard plaque that's tan, brown, or black in color

Ulcers that form from suspected deep tissue injury can be difficult to diagnose. On the surface, it may resemble a stage 1 or 2 sore. Underneath the discolored surface, this ulcer could be as deep as a stage 3 or stage 4 wound. This pressure ulcer may also form as a blood blister or be covered with eschar.

Prevention of Pressure Ulcers

Preventative strategies can help reduce the risk of bedsores. These include but are not limited to the following:

- changing positions every two to three hours in bed or every fifteen minutes in a wheelchair
- reducing pressure on areas that may be susceptible to pressure ulcers by using the following:

  - a special air or gel mattress
  - padding that protects bony areas, like the elbows or ankles
  - a wheel chair cushion

- skin care as recommended by your practitioner for incontinence
- regularly checking for bedsores, if you're immobilized

For patients who meet certain criteria and have health insurance, insurers may cover preventative supplies, so do not be afraid to ask what all can be covered, especially if you can have a home health wound nurse assist with your loved one's wound care. If the home health agency wound nurse is to stop providing the care, you will receive a letter that indicates such care will end. This letter is termed notice of noncoverage. If you feel you cannot assume the care and yet your loved one continues in need of the wound care, you can file an appeal. The website Center for Medicare Advocacy offers a self-help packet you can use as you file the appeal. To find the self-help packet to help you file your appeal, it is available on the Center for Medicare Advocacy website.

Getting Trained

If you are to assume the wound care, ensure you are trained and your training includes any and all tasks needed for not only changing of the bandages. But if devices like a wound vac is needed, how to operate and troubleshoot and decide if it is not operating correctly. Critical in your training will also be what all you need to do to document what you did, see, and smell as you did the dressing and wound care. This will allow you to keep your loved one's physician in the loop on the care and progress, and he or she can make changes in the routine or type of care to provide. For your documentation, this means as you provide the care, you must look and record the following:

1. The size and depth of the wound
2. Coloring of the skin around the wound
3. Color of any drainage
4. Consistency of the drainage

   a. Serous—thin, watery, clear
   b. Sanguineous—thin, bright red, with fresh bleeding
   c. Serosanguineous—thin, watery, pale red to pink
   d. Purulent—thick or thin, opaque tan to yellow

5. Amount of any drainage

   a. None—wound tissue dry
   b. Scant—wound tissue moist with no measurable drainage
   c. Minimal—wound tissue moist with less than 25 percent of the dressing saturated over twenty-four hours
   d. Moderate—wound tissue wet with 25 percent to 75 percent of the dressing saturated over twenty-four hours
   e. Large—wound tissue filled with fluid, with greater than 75 percent of the dressing saturated within twenty-four hours

6. Smell of the wound or drainage smell
7. Loved one's level of pain

How long it takes to heal a wound depends on how large or deep the cut is. It may take up to a few years to completely heal. An open wound may take longer to heal than a closed wound.

Risk Factors

There are several reasons why a wound may not heal properly. Age can affect how you heal. Elderly adults may have slower healing wounds. Some health conditions may lead to poor blood circulation. These conditions can cause poor wound healing:

- diabetes
- obesity
- high blood pressure (hypertension)
- vascular disease

Not all wounds heal at the same pace. Some factors affect the way how a wound heals.

- *Age.* The inflammatory response of the body generally decreases with aging. This may slow the process of wound healing.
- *Type of wound.* Deeper and longer wounds take time to heal. Also, irregular or contaminated wounds may take longer to heal as compared with clean-cut wounds.
- *Infection.* Invasion of the open wound by microbes such as bacteria hampers the wound healing process.
- *Poor nutrition.* Lack of proteins and other nutrients in the diet can delay wound healing.
- *Skin moisture.* Moisture at the wound is an essential factor necessary for the proliferative phase of wound healing. Hence, it is necessary to drink lots of water during the healing process that will hydrate the wound.
- *Poor blood circulation.* As the blood supplies all the essential nutrients to the wound required for its healing, poor blood circulation can lead to delayed wound healing.

- *Health issues.* Diabetes and obesity may delay wound healing.
- Certain medications may affect wound healing.
- Stress may retard wound healing.
- Smoking may decrease blood flow, thus retarding wound healing.
- Alcohol abuse harms general health and can delay wound healing.
- Weakened immunity such as in AIDS may slow the wound healing process.

Signs of Infection

A wound may heal slowly if it's infected. This is because your loved one's body is busy cleaning and protecting the wound and can't get to the rebuilding stage properly. An infection happens when bacteria, fungi, and other germs get into the wound before it fully heals. Signs of an infection include the following:

- slow healing or doesn't seem to be healing at all
- swelling
- redness
- pain or tenderness
- hot or warm to touch
- oozing pus or liquid

Treatment for an infected wound includes the following:

- cleaning the wound
- removing dead or damaged tissue around the wound
- antibiotic medications
- antibiotic skin ointments for the wound

Vaccinations

Vaccination is one of the safest and most convenient ways to protect not only your health but also that of your loved one. Vaccines offer protection in different ways, but they all help your body remember how to fight a specific infection in the future. It typically takes a few weeks after vaccination for the body to build up that protection.

Onetime and on-time vaccinations throughout childhood is essential because it helps to provide immunity before a child is exposed to potentially life-threatening diseases. Adults then need to keep their vaccinations up to date as immunity from childhood vaccines can wear off over time.

If your loved one has a fear of needles you may wish to follow some of the tips found on the CDC website.

Annually, the CDC publishes their recommendations for vaccinations and preventive services, and this can be found on their website. You can also find on this same website an online toolkit you can use to remind you of the importance of ensuring your disabled loved one has vaccinations as recommended. This tool kit also gives tips on ensuring the sites for the vaccine are accessible for persons with a disability and follow the ADA act of 1973.

Caregiving and Intimacy
Luis A. Torres, LMFT

In a previous chapter, we talked about how important it is to take care of yourself in order to bring balance to your life. In this chapter, I would like to bring to your attention other complementary relationships to your happiness. But first of all, I want you to identify the most important relationship in your life after yourself. For some people, it may be their spouse; for others, their children or that special someone or that friend that you love so much. Now that you identified that person, I want you to keep them in mind as you read the rest of the chapter.

At this point, you already know how important it is to love and take care of yourself. Let's say that you are making sure that you are not neglecting yourself (which is very easy to do due to the demand of being a caregiver). Then it is time to talk about maintaining and consciously improving the relationship with your partner or spouse or that special someone in your life. In this chapter, we are going to elaborate how you can maintain emotional and physical connection with your loved ones through building intimacy.

Who you consider important or special in your life may depend on what stage of life you are at—for example, if you are single, married, if you have kids, if you are an empty nester, etc. However, regardless of where you are in your life, it is important that you identify those significant relationships and make a list of who you consider the two main ones and work to build and maintain intimacy. When people face the challenge of becoming a caregiver, there is an unconscious tendency to neglect their needs and the needs of their relationships. We don't want that to happen to you.

In my clinical practice, I have seen how easily people can get disconnected and unconsciously distant from each other. It seems that we focus some much on our caregiving role that we leave behind the other important people in your life. I want you to think that your relationship with your loved one as a dependent entity and, therefore, may need attention and care from your loved one; and in order to keep it alive and improving, both of you will need to work on ways to be intimately connected. However, what comes to your mind when you heard the word *intimacy*? What value do you assign to that word? What does it mean for you individually and for your relationship with your loved one? What is the correlation between intimacy and happiness?

There are many different conceptualizations about intimacy, but what comes to your mind when you hear the word *intimacy*? For many people, especially men, intimacy has a physical-sexual connotation, but intimacy is more than that. According to Sternberg (1986, 1997, 2006), intimacy is "the sense of feeling close, connected, or bonded, having a sense of welfare for the other in times of need, experiencing mutual understanding, sharing oneself and other possessions, talking intimately, giving emotional support, valuing the other, expressing empathy for the other, communicating honestly, and finding the other person predictable [trustworthy]. These feelings give rise to the experience of warmth in a loving relationship."

In my understanding, one way to increase intimacy is to provide constant opportunities for positive experiences in order to increase the level of connection because intimacy is a process that can never be fulfilled completely. The question is, what are you willing to do to stay connected and build intimacy? Keep that in mind, as I will give you some ideas according to the seven types of intimacy. You read it right. There are seven types of intimacy—some you may already be doing. If not, it's time to take notes and feel excited about it. Here are these seven types of intimacy.

1. Emotional intimacy
2. Social intimacy
3. Intellectual intimacy
4. Sexual intimacy
5. Recreational intimacy
6. Spiritual intimacy
7. Aesthetic intimacy

Please take a piece of paper and a pen and write down some ideas or preferred activities that you can implement in each type of intimacy. Even in the cases where due to age or any medical condition that make sexual physical intimacy difficult or impossible, there are many ways to keep connected and intimate. True love is more than a physical expression; love is connection, and that can be expressed and you can feel it by the way you look or talk to a loved one. However, when the connection is missing, it creates feelings of abandonment and distance that eventually bring unnecessary distress to the relationship. If disability affects sex, please consider a sex therapist to help you to find ways to make your interaction equally fulfilling.

What you can work on your own every day as a priority is working in creating emotional intimacy, which involves the feeling of closeness, even when your partner or your loved one may be bedridden or may experience any physical, emotional, or intellectual disability. Please make sure that you find ways to express your love and positive emotions because that will enhance your emotional connection.

Do not forget the power of nonverbal communication—eye contact, smiling, and hand gestures—as they heavily influence how people interpret and react to the information you share. As we interact with people, about 90 percent of the time, we use nonverbal language to communicate; therefore, be mindful of your nonverbal communication and make it consciously fun and intentional.

Explore your social intimacy; dare yourself to connect to friends and family; and as you do, connect with them in an intellectual level, sharing what you learn in a podcast or in your book reading. When possible, set time for recreation intimacy. Your spouse, partner, that meaningful person in your life, wants to know you, wants to connect with you in intimate levels; provide those opportunities for them, taking the initiative today. Even for those who have different religion or faith still can find a common ground and identify spiritual connection that can lead to spiritual intimacy.

Finally, being intimate is a conscious choice, it is intentional and very satisfactory. Living by design and choosing today the level of intimacy do you want to have will provide vision and additional purpose to your life. The happiness and peace of mind that comes from knowing that you are in an intimate relationship, and it provides the energy to continue serving others in your important role as a caregiver.

Summary

Oh my goodness, so much to think about and do if you are a caregiver of a loved one, especially if they are total care, one on life-sustaining equipment, one with a developmental or intellectual disability, or one with challenging behaviors. It is the goal of this book to give you some resources to use in your role so as to help lift the burden of caregiving and to help ease your mind of what to do next or what might work versus not. You are not alone in this journey, so learn to use the resources available to possibly assist you.

Remember, your role is actually two-fold—taking care of your loved one and caring for yourself during this often very stressful and exhausting time. So do what is needed to reduce your stress and exhaustion. Good luck.

CHAPTER 10

Helpful Resources— Community and Finances

AS YOU START your caregiving role or as your role continues and evolves, take advantage of the technology available. Often, this is merely learning how to use a handheld cell phone and any apps you put on it. The same works with a computer. Unfortunately, if you are like many of us who grew up in the age where we did not have computers and you are afraid to work one or struggle to learn, as you have so much on your mind, you say, "Forget it!" Do not do that. Let a friend or relative or someone from your church help you. Enlist their help and let them do any research you may wish or feel should be done to try to make your role easier. If you do not have a computer or smartphone, check with your local library, as many have computers you can use for the research you may wish to complete.

In this book, you will find some basic information on various topics, but it will be up to you to do the own research on a topic and decide what best fits your situation and the plan for care you are developing. There are no two plans for care alike. Each plan of care must be individualized, and there is no one-plan-fits-all.

Also, as caregiving is not a one day or a week role, it may change and last months or years. This means you may not have your original plan or team you started when your role began. When you started in your role, your initial health care team might have included some of the case managers and social workers, and they were there to help advocate for the services your loved one needed. They were there initially, but as things settled in, they went on to other cases.

This book is written not only to give you the basics of what you need to know but also to allow you to develop the skills needed so you can advocate for your loved one and serve as their case manager. You as a caregiver are often the eyes, ears, and voice of your loved one. Some keys to help you advocate for your loved one will be the following:

- If meetings are needed to help set up services, come prepared with the documents they request you bring; and if more are needed, try to obtain them as soon as possible. Otherwise, your application could be delayed or denied.
- If English is not your native language or you have difficulty hearing or understanding, bring a family member or friend who can help.
- Learn all you can of your loved one's diagnosis or disability.
- Be a good listener. Ask questions. Listen to what other people say about your loved one. And if you joined a support group, tap into what others have learned works versus not as they cared for their loved one.
- Share what you know about your loved one. In many cases, you are the expert in their care and needs, and what worked for you may work for someone else who is struggling.
- When you don't agree, talk about it. Look for compromise (finding a middle ground) in ways that will be the right thing for your situation. By all means, don't get angry and blow up.
- If your loved one is denied, learn to write effective letters of appeal.
- Know your rights, and if you don't know what they are, seek help. This may come from your buddies in your support group, a legal center for the disabled or elderly, or merely through your own research.
- Keep good records of all meetings, and make notes on critical conversation points and date them.

- While you may discuss a request, put it in writing and keep a copy.
- If the agency is one that may offer specific services (i.e., your loved one's health plan or Social Security Disability Insurance) and you must obtain a prior authorization but the request is denied, learn to write effective letters of appeal.
- Join a support group for your loved one's diagnosis, as this will help you learn firsthand what maybe works versus not.
- Use a support group to help you cope. However, a support group is not a substitute when you need professional mental health counseling or treatment.

This chapter is designed to give you a variety of resources you may wish to explore to see if they can provide the services you are seeking. Many of the resources listed in this book are ones I would give to patients and families I worked with, but as I did research for this book, I found many, many more I felt might be needed as you start or continue in your role as a caregiver. Unfortunately, some of the financial resources, especially Medicaid, are for low-income individuals. If you are like so many of us who are in that middle income group and fall into that gray area where we have too much to qualify but too little to pay privately, you may be required to make some lifestyle changes or make choices you may not have if money were not an issue.

The websites listed in this book are to serve as a reference for you, and many also may contain a link you can click on to allow you to learn more. For other links, you may find you are able to download an application or brochure, a checklist, or a tool kit you may feel is useful. From the websites, you can also find contact information such as an address or phone number should you desire even more information.

I do not know if you remember, but in the past, the old phone companies had a jingle that went, "Let your fingers do the walking." I have done the same with this book. I want it to allow you to let your fingers do the walking and clicking on your computer or cell phone. The key is to click on any number of tabs to see if it offers the specific information you are seeking. I have also tried to include as many as I could find that will allow you to search for state-specific agencies or departments you can then go to for the assistance you are looking for.

I must warn you, many of the applications for some services are complicated and difficult. Thus, many families give up after encountering one roadblock after another, or a denial is issued due to a slight error. However, do not give up. The resource could be one to assist with any number of valuable resources that can assist you in your role. If you get a denial, learn to write effective letters of appeal, or seek the help of an advocate to help you, possibly from your loved one's state agency, designed to help the elderly and disabled. You may find such by using the Administration for Community Living website. Another resource will be to use the United Way 2-1-1 phone system to see what legal services for the elderly or disabled are available in your loved one's region.

If your loved one has a diagnosis of developmental disabilities (DD) or intellectual disabilities (ID), work closely with your loved one's state or regional office, designed to assist with finding the right resources and services. I must warn you that all states vary in the services they provide for the ID and DD population. Not only that, they have differing age limits for eligibility determination. To find your loved one's state office, use the locator found on the National Association of State Directors of Developmental Disabilities Services (NASDDDS). If your loved one is eligible, not only will the state DDS office help find the right resources. In many cases, they will actually also pay for the services or products required, as their goal is to keep your loved one at the right level of care in the least restrictive environment (LRE) and as independent as possible.

Another organization that serves primarily the DD and ID population will be the ARC. The ARC was formed back in 1953, and at that time, it was referred to as the National Association for Retarded Children (NARC). But by 1993, the acronym was shortened to merely the ARC, when the *r* for *retarded* was changed to *respect*. The ARC promotes and protects the human rights of people with intellectual or development disabilities and actually supports their full inclusion and participation in the community throughout their lifetimes. The ARC also serves as a leader in promoting access, equality, and inclusion (AEI) to ensure that the intellectually and developmentally disabled are represented and that social justice is served for this population. You can find more on the ARC at their website. The top header for this website will direct you to find a chapter in or near your loved one's community.

All or any resources mentioned in this book are merely suggestions to assist you in your role. However, be advised, under no circumstances do I or my publisher endorse any that are listed or included as this book was written. The material in this book is merely for informational purposes and should never be a substitute for legal, financial, professional, or medical advice on any diagnosis or treatment or steps you must take. They are resources, many of which are state or federal resources and are listed here as a convenience to help you in your role.

As a case manager and discharge planner, I rarely, if ever, made recommendations for privately owned companies. If you do use such, do your research. This is necessary, as many are there for the profits they make. Consequently, they hire strong marketing representatives to help sell you on their services. If you do use an agency to help locate care or services, always take the time to do your own interviewing, and make every attempt to interview, if possible, a minimum of three agencies.

If you are looking at placement, another tool to use to help narrow your search will be the Centers for Medicare and Medicaid Services (CMS) compare website. This website allows you to compare providers in your loved one's region, and their recommendations are based on the annual review they do. To better help you in your choice, they provide a five-star rating for any Medicare provider, with five stars being the highest.

I have always encouraged families to use such tools and to tour at least three facilities and to not only take the tour offered by the administrator or marketing representative but also to return after hours, usually around dinnertime. This allows you to see and hear for yourself the interactions of staff with the patients and what the activity is like. In the end, your instincts on what you see, hear, or even smell can help you narrow your search.

Good luck in your role.

Key Resources

If you are at a point where you are thinking about harming yourself, you can call anytime, day or night, the following:

- 911, or go to nearest emergency room
- 988, which is a suicide or crisis hotline
- National Suicide Prevention Line at 1-800-273-TALK (8255)

If you are hearing impaired, you can dial 711, then 988. If you are a veteran, you can call 988 and select 1 or text 838255. Or if you have hearing loss, call TTY: 800-799-4889.

Possible One-Stop Shop for Finding Local Agencies

One of your best tools for searching local resources will be using your phone and dialing the United Way phone system.2-1-1

2-1-1 is an online resource established by the Federal Communications in 2000 as a resource for consumers to locate local health care and other services within a local region. Another way is to use the United Way website: https://www.211.org/about-us/your-local-211. You then type in your zip code to search online for a variety of resources specific to your local area.

Disability Help for Independent Living

Each state has their own agencies that can provide information, help, and services if your loved one is disabled. However, such agencies are overseen by the Federal Administration on Disabilities (AoD) and must meet specific standards, as outlined by the AoD. You can find information on various topics and independent services within a community that serves the disabled, whether from a physical or developmental or intellectual disability, at the Administration on Disabilities and their Administration for Community Living website.

The main disability and information phone number is 888-677-1199.

The main weblinks you may want to explore as you search for disability information are the following:

- Administration on Disabilities and their Administration on Community Living website as well as searching this area for a state by state locator

Another key website you will find in the AoD or ACL websites will be a link to the Eldercare Locator. The Eldercare Locator is a public service offered by the US administration on aging, and it will connect you to services for older adults and their families. You can reach them by phone at 1-800-677-1116 or visit them on their website.

The USA Contact Center

Another great resource you may want to explore to find programs that may be able to help either in caring for your loved one or finding programs that may help ease the financial strain will be the USA Contact Center and their website at https://www.usa.gov/#all-topics-header. This website offers a wealth of information—both weblinks and the ability to speak with someone. For example, if you click on Health, you will find links to topics such as the following:

- Getting help on insurance
- How to get help with medical expenses
- Finding help for mental illness
- Finding help for substance abuse
- Getting reliable health information from MedlinePlus
- Contacting a state department

Finding Information on Specific Diseases

Due to the fact that there are thousands of diseases, it is impossible to list all the links one may use to see what is available in your local area. As a result, as I have suggested earlier in this book, keep a notebook available so you can ask questions and make notes.

You may also want to know more about the disease, so to do your research, you must know how to spell it. This means you probably will need the doctor to spell it out so you can write it down in your notebook and then do your research.

These are the major websites you may want to explore for a diagnosis or possible resources that may help you.

1. The National Organization Rare Disorders (NORD) website.
2. Centers for Disease Control and Prevention (CDC) and under its Diseases and Conditions A–Z tab, you can look up any disease topic.
3. National Institute on Health (NIH) and its listing of institutes and centers on health (there are twenty-seven institutes listed. You can then click on a box called Quick Link, and it will take you to a downloadable/printable booklet that lists all the NIH centers; and from there, you can possibly find the one you may want to use.
4. National Library of Medicine and Gender-Affirming Care for Transgender Patients website.
5. Centers for Disease Control and Prevention (CDC) for information on transgender medical care at their website.
6. National Institute on Health Intellectual and Developmental Disabilities (IDDs).
7. To better understand congenital disorders, the World Health Organization has an A–Z listing you can click on to help educate yourself on a wide variety of disorders.
8. If your loved one has a genetic disorder, very simply, this means at the time of conception something went wrong in whole or part with how normal DNA occurs within cells. A good reference to better understand a genetic disorder is on the Cleveland Clinic website.
9. Many of the disease-specific organizations listed below in the section called Other Agencies to Explore will not only offer brochures and education material to help you, but many will also provide you a listing of support groups and transportation to and from medical appointments, as well as other resources within your loved one's region.

Mental Health Resources
To better understand coverage and treatment for mental health, the following websites may help you: • The Healthcare.gov website   • Information on mental health and substance abuse and treatment choices at the US Department of Health and Human Services and the Substance Abuse and Mental Health Service Administration (SAMHSA) website.   • National Alliance on Mental Illness (NAMI) website.   • National Institute of Mental Health website.   • Mental Health America.   • Centers for Disease Control and Prevention (CDC) and prevention of violence in youth website.   • Centers for Disease Control and Prevention CDC) website on Safety and Children with Disabilities website.

While not all of us are tech savvy, an easy way to find a topic as you do your research and find more information on any of the topics listed below, merely type in your web browser any of the names listed in column one (Name of organization and acronym). In your caregiver role, it is critical to know as much as you can about the disease or injury as well as what tips you might find to help in your role.

Name of organization and acronym	Types of services offered
AccessText Network	The AccessText Network is a partnership between publishers of educational materials and educational institutions. Publishers offer materials in accessible formats through the network for students with disabilities. The materials are shared through the student's college or university. A student with a qualifying disability can request a book in accessible format from the disability services coordinator in their educational institution. That coordinator has login credentials to the AccessText Network and is able to download the item in a format that the student can read. Bookshare provides digital books free to all US students with qualifying me disabilities. Books are available for download in audio and braille formats.

Administration for Children and Families (ACF)	ACF has an important role in helping domestic violence survivors, runaway and homeless youth, and trafficking survivors. ACL has a variety of hotlines/helplines to serve people in need. The following are AFC regional offices: • Region 1: Boston—Connecticut, Maine, Massachusetts, New Hampshire, Rhode Island, and Vermont • Region 2: New York—New Jersey, New York, Puerto Rico, and the Virgin Islands • Region 3: Philadelphia—Delaware, District of Columbia, Maryland, Pennsylvania, Virginia, and West Virginia • Region 4: Atlanta—Alabama, Florida, Georgia, Kentucky, Mississippi, North Carolina, South Carolina, and Tennessee • Region 5: Chicago—Illinois, Indiana, Michigan, Minnesota, Ohio, and Wisconsin • Region 6: Dallas—Arkansas, Louisiana, New Mexico, Oklahoma, and Texas • Region 7: Kansas City—Iowa, Kansas, Missouri, and Nebraska • Region 8: Denver—Colorado, Montana, North Dakota, South Dakota, Utah, and Wyoming • Region 9: San Francisco—Arizona, California, Hawaii, Nevada, American Samoa, Commonwealth of the Northern Mariana Islands, Federated States of Micronesia, Guam, Marshall Islands, and Republic of Palau • Region 10: Seattle—Alaska, Idaho, Oregon, and Washington (Reference: https://www.acf.hhs.gov/about/contact-us.) Reference phone numbers:

	• National Domestic Violence hotline: 1-800-799-SAFE (7233) or TTY 1-800-787-3224 • National Human Trafficking hotline: 1-888-373-7888 or text BeFree (233733) • National Runaway toll-free phone number: 1-800-RUNAWAY Here are state and local agency contacts. • Child Care and Development Fund state and territory contacts • Child Support and Tribal Child Support Agencies • Community Services Block Grant (CSBG) • Eldercare Locator • Energy Assistance Program • Head Start Center Locator • health insurance (HealthCare.gov) • National Foster Care and Adoption Directory • public health departments (states and territories)
Administration on Disabilities (AoD)	AoD collaborates with states and its territories, communities, and partners in the disability network to equip individuals with disabilities of all ages with opportunities, tools, and supports to lead lives of their choice in their community. Under the provisions established through various authorizing statutes, the goal of the AoD is to continually seek to improve opportunities for people with disabilities while also giving you information and how to access quality community services and supports; achieve economic self-sufficiency; and experience equality, equity, and inclusion in all facets of community life. This office also oversees the following offices: 1) Office of Independent Living Programs (OILP) 2) Office of Intellectual and Developmental Disability (OIDD) 3) Office of Disability Services Innovation (ODSI)

	AoD also maintains a disability and access line and weblink that allows you to be connected to services you might need. (Call, text, or videophone 888-677-1199.) This system also encourages you to call, text, or do a video visit; or their email is DIAL@usaginganddisability.org.
Adult Protective Services (APS)	The national office is a nonprofit agency with members in all fifty states. Its mission is to effectively and efficiently recognize, report, and respond to the needs of the disabled and elderly who are the victims of abuse, exploitation, and neglect and to prevent it. To find an agency within your loved one's region, you can use the United Way 2-1-1 phone system, or you can use the National website to locate one in your loved one's region.
adverse childhood experiences (ACE)	ACEs are potentially traumatic experiences, such as neglect, experiencing or witnessing violence, and having a family member attempt or die by suicide, that occur in childhood (birth to seventeen) that can affect children for years. It can then impact their life opportunities and cause chronic health problems, mental illness, and substance use in adulthood. American Society for the Positive Care of Children (American SPCC) offers a wide range of resources for parents to use for parenting to create positive environments for children. You may also want to see if your loved one's local agency that serves the developmentally disabled can assist with locating resources or programs you may wish to explore.
Alcoholic Anonymous (AA) and Al-Anon Narcotics Anonymous (NA)	AA has been helping persons who wish to stop drinking for greater than eighty years. Their website offers a wealth of information and also a hyperlink to find an AA meeting site near your or your loved one's home. Similar to AA, if your loved one is one who wishes to stop using narcotics, he can find information on the Narcotics Anonymous (na.org) website. Your best resource to find a meeting site in your area for either AA or NA will be to use the phone directory services at 2-1-1.

Alzheimer's Association	Under the first tab, you will find links that will describe Alzheimer's disease, as well as dementia. Under the tab Help and Support, you will find a variety of key and critical information on dealing with Alzheimer's disease and dementia and some caregiving tips. Under the local resources tab, you can type in your loved one's state, and it will bring up the resources in his or her local community. Please visit the Alzheimer's website as it offers a wealth of information you may find useful for your situation and aid you in your caregiver role.
American Burn Association	Under the Resources tab, you can find a burn center near you and your loved one and also contains information on what standards they have in place for health care professionals who render care. While this may be a resource for you to use, if your loved one has a private health plan or one linked to a managed care organization (MCO), double-check as to what burn center the health plan is contracted with; if not and you make the move to one recommended on this website, any claims will be denied. (References: 312-642-9260. To explore information on burns and find support groups or tips on care visit the American Burn Association website.)
American Cancer Society (ACS)	Nationwide community-based voluntary health organization dedicated to eliminating cancer as a major health problem by preventing cancer, saving lives, and diminishing suffering from cancer. Offers multiple brochures and information on cancer and caregiving, lodging during treatment, and other resources you can explore. You can also find support groups in your area. Dependent upon your community, you may find they also provide volunteers to transport patients to and from any cancer treatments required. (References: 800-227-2245 or explore the American Cancer Society web link.)

American Chronic Pain Association (ACPA)	Provides self-help coping skills and peer support to people with chronic pain. Sponsors local support groups throughout the US. (References: 913-991-4740; or explore the American Chronic pain Association website for more information you can use to find support groups or resources you might use in the struggle to control chronic pain.)
American Diabetes Association (ADA)	In addition to offering brochures/pamphlets on a variety of diabetes topics, they will also do the following: • Refer you to an ADA-recognized providers and educational seminars and classes in your area and will assist in connecting you with the appropriate local resources in your area. • Assist people who face discrimination based on diabetes. • Inform you of local association events and programs and volunteer opportunities (References: 800-342-2383. As diabetes can lead to a wide variety of complications, it is critical you know as much as you can on the disease - so learn as much as you can and use the ADA and other websites on diabetes for your research.)
American Heart Association (AHA)	The AHA is the leader in resuscitation science, education, and training, and publisher of the official Guidelines for Cardio Pulmonary Resuscitation (CPR) and Emergency Cardiovascular Care (ECC). On the ECC website, they offer an ECC Digital Digest, which serves as their hub for podcasts, videos, blogs, and additional resources featuring industry experts sharing insights and updates on the latest scientific research and breakthroughs. You can also find support groups in your area. (References: 1-800-242-8721)
American Lung Association (ALA)	This organization offers information on various lung diseases and support groups in your area. (References: 1-800-586-4872)

American Red Cross	The American Red Cross website offers a wealth of information on caregiving and training programs all related to its Family Caregiving Program. At a minimum, the Red Cross website offers the following educational topics for caregivers: • Home safety—provide a safe environment, fire safety, infection control, and medication safety emergency preparedness. • General elderly caregiver skills—reading and recording vital signs, sudden illness, giving medication, communication and organization, and time-saving ideas. • Body mechanics positioning and helping a loved one move—prevent strains, prevent pressure ulcers, positioning your loved one in bed, getting from the bed to a chair, moving into the car, and helping your loved one walk. • Assisting with personal care—grooming, mouth care, dressing, bathing, showering, and shampooing assisting with toileting. • Healthy eating—nutrition, preparing for a meal, helping your loved one eat, how to respond to choking, fluids are important, keep food safe to eat, and dietary concerns. • Caring for the caregiver—caregiver stress, depression, dealing with depression, and end of life issues. • Legal and financial issues—gathering important documents, advance directives, last will and testament, and facts about funerals. • Caring for a loved one with Alzheimer's disease or dementia—how to deal with difficult behaviors and comforting a loved one with dementia. • Caregiver resources—local and national organizations, vital signs record, daily medication log, medication list, and emergency contact card.

	Main phone number: 1 800 RED CROSS (1-800-733-2767). National headquarters department directory: 202-303-5214.
American Spinal Injury Association (ASIA)	From this site, you can click on the resource and the find support, and you will find a wealth of information, as well as how to find a support group in your area, all of which will be available at your fingertips. Because it is critical your loved one has the right durable medical equipment (DME), their DME guide allows you to scroll down; and under the table of contents, you will find information on a variety of topics that might be able to help serve as your guide as DME is ordered. You can also find information on spinal cord injuries at the National Institute of Health and their neurological website. (References: 718-803-3782) You can also find information on spinal cord injuries at the following: • Christopher and Dana Reeve Foundation (phone: 973-379-2690 or 800-225-0292) • National Institute on Disability, Independent Living, and Rehabilitation Research (NIDILRR) (phone: 202-401-4634 or 202-245-7316) • National Rehabilitation Information Center (NARIC) (phone: 301-459-5900 or 800-346-2742) • Paralyzed Veterans of America (PVA) (phone: 800-424-8200) • United Spinal Association (phone: 718-803-3782 or 800-962-9629)

American Stroke Association	American Stroke Association offers information on strokes, tips on healthy eating and living, and importance of exercising. They also list a link to find a support group in your loved one's local area and a guide on caregiving you may find very useful in your role. In addition to multiple brochures and tips, you can also download a guide on caregiving at https://www.stroke.org/-/media/Stroke-Files/Caregiver-Support/Caregivers-Guide-to-Stroke/CaregiverGuideToStroke_2020.pdf and https://www.stroke.org/en/.)
amyotrophic lateral sclerosis (ALS)	Amyotrophic lateral sclerosis (ALS), also known as Lou Gehrig's disease, is a rare neurological disease that affects motor neurons—those nerve cells in the brain and spinal cord that control voluntary muscle movement. Voluntary muscles are those we choose to move to produce movements, like chewing, walking, and talking. The disease is progressive, meaning the symptoms get worse over time. ALS has no cure, and there is no effective treatment to reverse its progression. As you conduct your research, you may want to visit the National Institute of Health and its National Institute of Neurological Disorders and Stroke or even such sites as those maintained by major medical centers and their clinics (i.e., Mayo Clinic, Cleveland Clinic) for information on the topic.
Angel Flight Network	Volunteer pilots that provide free air and arrange for ground transportation for children or adults and their families to medical care across the nation so they can access lifesaving medical care (references: 978-794-6868).
Area Agencies on Aging	An area agency on aging (AAA) is a public or private nonprofit agency designated by a state to address the needs and concerns of all older persons at the regional and local levels. AAA is a general term; names of local AAAs may vary. AAAs are primarily responsible for a geographic area, also known as a planning and service area (PSA), that is either a city, a single county, or a multicounty district. AAAs may be categorized as a county, city, regional planning council, or council of governments, private, or nonprofit.

	AAAs coordinate and offer services that help older adults remain in their homes, if that is their preference, aided by services such as home-delivered meals, home-maker assistance, and whatever else it may take to make independent living a viable option. By making a range of supports available, AAAs make it possible for older individuals to choose the services and living arrangements that suit them best. (References: 1-800-677-1116 or you can search the web by using the Eldercare. gov web link or by calling 2-1-1 to find the Area Agency on Aging that serves your loved one's region.)
Arthritis Foundation	Offers expert advice on arthritis and possible treatments, and the main website offers practical tips on a wide variety of arthritic conditions and has a link to locate an office and support groups for a wide variety of populations within your loved one's region. (References: 800-283-7800. The Arthritis Foundation's website offers a wealth of information including an A-Z resource guide you may find useful.)
Autism	Autism spectrum disorder (ASD) is a developmental disability caused by differences in the brain. Some people with ASD have a known difference, such as a genetic condition. People with ASD may behave, communicate, interact, and learn in ways that are different from most other people. There is often nothing about how they look that sets them apart from other people. The abilities of people with ASD can vary significantly. For example, some people with ASD may have advanced conversation skills, whereas others may be nonverbal. Some people with ASD need a lot of help in their daily lives; others can work and live with little to no support. Look through the following for references. For your research on autism, you merely need to type in your web browser "autism resources," and you will find a wide variety of web links you can explore for information on what might be available to help you in your role.

Caregiver Action Network	Caregiver Action Network (CAN) is the nation's leading family caregiver organization working to improve the quality of life for the more than 90 million Americans who care for loved ones with chronic conditions, disabilities, disease, or the frailties of old age. Caregiver help desk: (855) 227-3640 Office phone: (202) 454-3970
cardiac rehabilitation	Cardiac rehab is a medically supervised program designed to improve your cardiovascular health if you have experienced heart attack, heart failure, angioplasty, or heart surgery. Cardiac rehab has three equally important parts: exercise, education, and counseling. Your loved one may benefit if they have or have experienced the following: • heart attack (myocardial infarction) • heart condition, such as coronary artery disease (CAD), angina, or heart failure • heart procedure or surgery, including coronary artery bypass graft (CABG) surgery, percutaneous coronary intervention (PCI, including coronary or balloon angioplasty and stenting), valve replacement, or a pacemaker or implantable cardioverter defibrillator (ICD)
Centers for Disease (CDC) Control and Prevention	The Centers for Disease Control and Prevention (CDC) is the national public health agency of the United States. It is a United States federal agency under the Department of Health and Human Services and is headquartered in Atlanta, Georgia. The agency's main goal is the protection of public health and safety through the control and prevention of disease, injury, and disability in the US and worldwide. The CDC focuses national attention on developing and applying disease control and prevention. It especially focuses its attention on infectious disease, foodborne pathogens, environmental health, occupational safety and health, health promotion, injury prevention, and educational activities designed to improve the health of United States citizens.

	The CDC also conducts research and provides information on noninfectious diseases, such as obesity and diabetes, and is a founding member of the International Association of National Public Health Institutes. Under the tab labeled Health Topics A–Z, you will be able to research any health topic.
Centers for Independent Living	Designed and operated by individuals with disabilities, Centers for Independent Living (CILs) provide independent living services for people with disabilities. CILs are at the core of the Administration for Community Living's (ACL's) independent living programs, which work to support community living and independence for people with disabilities across the nation based on the belief that all people can live with dignity, make their own choices, and participate fully in society. These programs provide tools, resources, and supports for integrating people with disabilities fully into their communities to promote equal opportunities, self-determination, and respect. At a minimum, centers funded by the program are required to provide the following IL (Independent Living) core services: • Information and referral • IL skills training • Peer counseling • Individual and systems advocacy • Services that facilitate transition from nursing homes and other institutions to the community, provide assistance to those at risk of entering institutions, and facilitate transition of youth to postsecondary life Centers also may provide, among other services, psychological counseling, assistance in securing housing or shelter, personal assistance services, transportation referral and assistance, physical therapy, mobility training, rehabilitation technology, recreation, and other services necessary to improve the ability of individuals with significant disabilities to function independently in the family or community or to continue in employment.

	The Independent Living Resources and Utilization (ILRU) is a national center to provide information and services for the disabled and independent living. For example, under the tab Contact Us, there is a wealth of information of the disabled and services you may wish to explore, and the website also contains information on many of the key legislation and national acts, such as the Developmental Disabilities Act, Rehabilitation Act of 1973, Assistive Technology Act, Public Health Services Act, and more. (References: 202-401-4634. You may also find information by calling the Eldercare Locator at 800-677-1116.)
Centers for Medicare and Medicaid Services website for Medicare information	The Centers for Medicare and Medicaid Services (CMS) is the agency within the US Department of Health and Human Services (HHS) that administers the nation's major healthcare programs. CMS oversees programs including Medicare, Medicaid, the Children's Health Insurance Program (CHIP), and the state and federal health insurance marketplaces. CMS collects and analyzes data, produces research reports, and works to eliminate instances of fraud and abuse within the health care system. The Centers for Medicare and Medicaid Services (CMS) is a part of Health and Human Services (HHS) and is not the same as Medicare. Medicare is a federally run government health insurance program, which is administered by CMS. CMS is headquartered in Maryland and has ten regional offices throughout the US—located in Boston, New York, Philadelphia, Atlanta, Dallas, Kansas City, Chicago, Denver, San Francisco, and Seattle.
child care	Find local resources on child care, health and social services, financial assistance, support for children with disabilities, and more. This website allows you to enter your zip code to find resources in your local community. (references: 202-290-6782, or you can do research on child care and find a state resource guide by using the Childcare.gov resource web link.)

Child Protective Services (CPS)	Child protective services (CPS) is the name of a government agency in many states of the United States responsible for providing child protection, which includes responding to reports of child abuse or neglect. Some states use other names, often attempting to reflect more family-centered (as opposed to child-centered) practices, such as Department of Children and Family Services (DCFS). CPS is also sometimes known by the name of Department of Social Services (DSS or simply Social Services for short), though these terms more often have a broader meaning. Here is a list of other names and acronyms for CPS. • Children, youth, and family (CYF) • Department of children and families (DCF) • Department of children and family services (DCFS) • Department of social services (DSS) • Department of human services (DHS) • Department of child safety (DCS) • Department of child services (DCS) • Department of human resources (DHR) CPS/DCF is a department under a state's health and human services organization. See also abuse of a person mentioned earlier in this section (reference: 202-690-6782).
Children's Health Insurance Program (CHIP)	The Children's Health Insurance Program (CHIP) provides health coverage to eligible children, through both Medicaid and separate CHIP programs. CHIP is administered by states, according to federal requirements. The program is funded jointly by states and the federal government. The beneficiary resources website allows you to search for your state and local office to work with. You can do your own research on the Medicaid.gov CHIP weblink and search for information that may be of help to you.

| Children and Youth with Special Health Care Needs | CYSHCN are children who have or are at increased risk for chronic physical, developmental, behavioral, or emotional conditions. They also require health and related services of a type or amount or complexity beyond that required by children generally.

This is a program that has been modified over the many years but was originally created by Title V of the Social Security Act of 1935. This act created programs for maternal and child health and at one point was known primarily by the name Crippled Children's Services, or CCS.

While no longer is the term "crippled children" used, it is a program whereby all states provide a range of services for children with crippling or special medical needs; this includes locating these children; diagnosing their medical condition; providing or locating skilled care for them in hospitals, in convalescent and foster homes, and in their own homes; and cooperating with agencies and professional groups concerned with the care and treatment of children with special care and medical needs. Because no state has funds sufficient to do this comprehensive job for all handicapped boys and girls, all states necessarily have to restrict some services to certain parts of the state or to certain groups of children—most commonly children with handicapping conditions that require orthopedic or plastic treatment.

For example, in California, the eligibility criterion are, the child must be the following:

• Under age twenty-one
• Have a chronic, disabling, or life-threatening medical condition that meets the state's eligibly diagnosis listing
• Meet income requirements and be eligible for full scope Medicaid or Share-Of-Cost Medicaid or family's adjusted gross income (AGI) is under $40,000 or, if the family's AGI is over $40,000, may be eligible if their out-of-pocket costs for the eligible condition are expected to exceed 20 percent of AGI |

	This is not an income program but provides medical care if your loved one meets eligibility requirements.
Chron's disease and other digestive diseases	You can find information on Crohn's disease and other digestive disease on the National Institute of Diabetes, Digestive, and Kidney Diseases website. Under the tab labeled Digestive Diseases, you will find a variety disease listed, and should your loved one have such a disease, you can start your research here. Each will define, at a minimum, what the disease is and will give you information on symptoms and causes, diagnosis, treatment, possible clinical trials, and related diseases and disorders (reference: 800-860-8747).
COBRA continuation coverage questions and answers	COBRA stands for the Consolidated Omnibus Budget Reconciliation Act of 1985. The Centers for Medicare and Medicaid (CMS) has advisory jurisdiction over the continuation coverage requirements of COBRA as they apply to group health plans, which are sponsored by state, county, municipal, or public school districts (Public Sector COBRA). If you or your loved one has to termination employment and you or they are covered by an employer health plan, you are given the opportunity to elect to continue any health plan benefits by signing up for COBRA. (References: 877-696-6775. As COBRA is expensive, and you may be on a limited income, before you sign up, do your own research so you can make the right choice if COBRA is right for you or should you explore other options for health care insurance.)
community transportation	Finding transportation when your loved one doesn't qualify for nonemergent transport via gurney or wheelchair van can pose problems and is one of the biggest reasons patients are often not compliant with follow-up medical appointments. Your best way to see what is available in your loved one's region is to use the United Way 2-1-1 phone system. Dependent upon the urgency of need to see a provider, if transportation is an issue, work with your loved one's physician to see if a video or facetime visit can be arranged.

If your loved one's community does offer transportation these services are financed through federal, state, and local governments; and they will be public transportation systems that fixed routes and set schedules. Dependent upon the system, some may offer discounted fares for older adults and people with disabilities. Vouchers may be available as well. Unfortunately, this type of transportation is not suitable for persons who have issues with stairs, waiting, or walking to and from bus stops.

Thus, if this is the case for your loved one, you will want to consider what public transit services are available in his or her area. This service will be termed Paratransit and public transit agencies are required by law to provide complementary paratransit service for people who are unable to use regular lines. Paratransit operates during the same hours as normal service and covers comparable routes.

Riders must meet eligibility criteria set out in the federal Americans with Disabilities Act (ADA). Vehicles typically are vans outfitted for accessibility. Trips should be scheduled at least a day in advance and generally are shared with other passengers who have booked similar times. Paratransit providers typically have a thirty-minute pickup window, from fifteen minutes before to fifteen minutes after the scheduled time, so riders need to be ready and waiting at least fifteen minutes early.

Another type of public transport is called demand response. This type of transportation is referred to as dial-a-ride and is a service that is another shared ride service, carrying multiple passengers who book individually with different pickup points and destinations. Reservations usually must be made at least twenty-four hours in advance, online or by phone. Other sources of transportation will be to use a taxi or ride-hailing.

Taxis

Some communities require locally licensed taxi fleets to include accessible vehicles, but this will be community- and city-specific and possibly one of your best sources for information on this might be from your loved one's Area on Aging. Dependent upon the company, some will have vouchers that may allow a discount for an older or and disabled rider.

Ride-Hailing

Ride-hailing companies such as Lyft and Uber connect passengers with drivers who provide point-to-point transportation in their own vehicles. Booking and payment are typically done via mobile apps. In some cities, riders can request wheelchair assistance as part of their booking, and the companies have expanded accessibility efforts in recent years. The Uber Assist program trains drivers to accommodate passengers who have mobility issues and use wheelchairs, walkers, or scooters. Lyft is teaming with United Way to provide free rides through the 2-1-1 phone service for people who have difficulty using public transit.

Volunteer Programs

Some nonprofit and faith-based organizations offer transportation for medical appointments or other destinations. This might include door-to-door or door-through-door service for passengers who need someone to help them get in and out of cars and buildings or stay with them throughout the trip.

Volunteer drivers provide rides in their own cars or agency-owned vehicles. The drawback with ride-hailing or volunteer drivers is your loved one must be able to get in and out of the car without the assistance of the driver. In most cases, such trips are free.

	Some websites to use to locate transportation might be the following: • The Eldercare Locator • The National Center for Mobility Management The National Aging and Disability Transportation Center (NADTC) can also provide technical assistance on transportation for older persons and those with disabilities. (Reference: 2-1-1)
craniofacial	Craniofacial is a medical term that relates to the bones of the skull and face. Craniofacial abnormalities are birth defects of the face or head. Some, like cleft lip and palate, are among the most common of all birth defects. Others are very rare. Most of them affect how a person's face or head looks. These conditions may also affect other parts of the body. The National Craniofacial website has a wealth of information on craniofacial topics, including potential financial assistance allowed under its FACES program (Reference: 800-332-2373).
deaf and blind-ness services	There are many causes of deaf-blindness. Those that are present or occur around the time a child is born include prematurity, childbirth complications, and numerous congenital syndromes, many of which are quite rare. Deaf-blindness may also occur later in childhood or during adulthood due to causes such as meningitis, brain injury, or inherited conditions. It is not uncommon for the same conditions that cause deaf-blindness to also lead to additional cognitive, physical, or other disabilities and health care needs. Each state has a federally-funded deaf-blind project that provides information and assistance, and as your child's IEP is developed you, you should be directed to the services available to assist your child with the special education they will require. Regardless if your loved one is a child, adolescent or adult, your best resources to explore will be any of the websites devoted to *deaf-blindness*.

DEERS	You or your loved one must be registered in the Defense Enrollment Eligibility Reporting System (DEERS). DEERS is a database of information on uniformed services members (sponsors), US-sponsored foreign military, DoD and uniformed services civilians, other personnel as directed by the DoD, and their family members. You need to register in DEERS to get TRICARE and get your TRICARE benefits. Sponsors are automatically registered in DEERS, but they must register eligible family members. If both parents are service members, choose one to be listed as the child's sponsor in DEERS.
Department of Developmental and Intellectual Services	Developmental disability (DD) involves severe cognitive or physical impairments and might be Down syndrome but more commonly referred to in the past as mentally retarded. Federal law states a developmental disability is a substantially handicapping disability that originated prior to the person attaining the state's designated age for eligibility and the disability is expected to last a lifetime. Developmental disabilities (DD) are a group of conditions due to an impairment in physical, learning, language, or behavior areas. These conditions begin during the developmental period, may impact day-to-day functioning, and usually last throughout a person's lifetime. Intellectual disability (ID) is characterized by significant limitation in intellectual functioning (such as reasoning, learning, and problem solving) and adaptive behavior (such as social functioning and practical skills). This is often caused by a brain injury at birth or one that occurs before the age of eighteen. If your child is identified before the age of three with an ID or DD diagnosis, and while all states will have their own requirement and programs for early intervention services, an individualized family service plan (IFSP) must be created to meet the individual needs, concerns, and priorities of individual children, from birth to age three, and their families. The plan states the family's desired outcomes for their child and themselves and lists the early intervention services and supports that will help meet those outcomes. It also describes when, where, and how the services will be delivered.

	If your loved one is over the age of three and deemed eligible for services an individualized program plan (IPP) must be developed. The IPP is completed initially and updated at a three-year interval, but some require it to be updated annually or more frequently if other issues arise. The IPP describes what the person's issues are that require help and the services that will be provided to the individual. This document is produced in cooperation with the parents and the DDS agency. In all cases, the individual is placed in the least restrictive environment (LRE) that can meet and provide the care and services the individual requires. Each state varies in the services they provide for the ID and DD population, and each state's name for the agency that offers ID and DD services varies vastly. To find your loved one's state and the agency that serves the Intellectual and Developmentally Disabled, type in your web browser the state name and then the words services for the intellectually and developmentally disabled. This should bring up the information you might need. The National Association of State Directors of Developmental Disability Services (NASDDDS) represents the nation's agencies in fifty states, Puerto Rico, and the District of Columbia providing services to persons with intellectual and developmental disabilities (ID and DD) and their families. You can locate your loved one's agency on the NASDDDS website. Here you can click on the link for state agencies.
Department of Motor Vehicles lDMV) Placards, Licenses for Handicapped and Removal of license	The DMV or state motor vehicle agency gives disabled license plates to disabled drivers for their personal use while a disabled placard can be moved from one vehicle to another. Usually, a placard or handicapped license plate is the best option for a caregiver who transports the disabled person. Unfortunately, the medical requirements vary state by state. You will need to speak to your doctor or physician first to determine if you qualify for a disabled driver license plate or placard.

	While qualifications vary by state, some of the medical conditions that could cause you to receive one of these special license plates are: • The loss of use of your legs or hands. • The inability to walk two blocks without resting. • Heart, lung, or circulatory disease. • Strokes or epilepsy. • Mental health problems. • Age and other forms of serious illness. To apply for a placard, go to your loved one's local DMV office. While the website listed below is a private website, it does allow you to click on your loved one's state to read about where and how that state's placard can be used. Reference: Disability Plates & Placards | DMV. ORG If your loved one will be a danger to themselves or others when they drive, you can make an anonymous report to the local DMV office or your loved one's physician or nurse practitioner or physician assistant can request the DMV to remove your loved one's license by completing the state specific form.
Disabilities per the Americans with Disabilities Act (ADA)	A person with a disability is someone • who has a physical or mental impairment that substantially limits one or more major life activities, • has a history or record of such an impairment (such as cancer that is in remission), • and is perceived by others as having such an impairment (such as a person who has scars from a severe burn).

	If a person falls into any of these categories, the ADA protects them. Because the ADA is a law and not a benefit program, you do not need to apply for coverage. The rights of an individual with a disability are protected under this law. You can do your own research on the ADA by merely typing in your web browser ADA and disability rights.
dual eligible	Dual eligible means you have both Medicare and Medicaid, or often referred to as Medi-Medi. Medicare pays covered dually eligible beneficiaries' medical services first, because Medicaid is generally the payer of last resort. Medicaid may cover medical costs. Medicare may not cover or partially covers (such as nursing home care, personal care, and home- and community-based services). Coverage for dually eligible beneficiaries varies by state. Some states offer Medicaid through Medicaid managed care plans while others provide fee-for-service Medicaid coverage. Some states contract with health plans that include all Medicare and Medicaid benefits. Federal law defines Medicaid and MSP (Medicare Savings Program) income and resource standards, but states can effectively raise those limits above the federal floor (except for QDWIs—Qualified Disabled Working Individual). Annually, the Centers for Medicare and Medicaid Services (CMS) releases eligibility standards for dually eligible beneficiaries.
early and periodic screening and diagnostic treatment (EPSDT)	States are required to provide comprehensive services and furnish all Medicaid coverable, appropriate, and medically necessary services needed to correct and ameliorate health conditions based on certain federal guidelines. • Early—assessing and identifying problems early • Periodic—checking children's health at periodic, age-appropriate intervals

- Screening—providing physical, mental, developmental, dental, hearing, vision, and other screening tests to detect potential problems
- Diagnostic—performing diagnostic tests to follow up when a risk is identified
- Treatment—control, correct, or reduce health problems found

Screening may include any other necessary health care services, which include any medically necessary diagnostic services to further evaluate the individual's health and make the necessary referrals without delay. State Medicaid agencies are required to inform all Medicaid-eligible individuals under age 21 that EPSDT services are available and of the need for age-appropriate immunizations.

States must also develop periodicity schedules for periodic screening, vision, and hearing services must be provided at intervals that meet reasonable standards of medical practice. States must consult with recognized medical organizations involved in child health care in developing their schedules.

Alternatively, states may elect to use a nationally recognized pediatric periodicity schedule (i.e., Bright Futures). A separate dental periodicity schedule is also required. Periodic developmental and behavioral screening during early childhood is essential to identify possible delays in growth and development when steps to address deficits can be most effective. These screenings are required for children enrolled in Medicaid and are also covered for children enrolled in CHIP. As it is critical you know your rights and what is available under the Medicaid EPSDT program, you can type in your web browser "Medicaid and EPSDT," and here you will find a wealth of information on the topic.

Easterseals	Easterseals provides a variety of services at four hundred sites nationwide for children and adults with disabilities, including adult day care, in-home care, camps for special needs children, and more. Services vary by site. Under Services and Support and Education, you will find a wealth of information Easterseals provides. Easterseals also provides for camping and other recreational activities for the disabled.
end-of-life planning	Advance care planning involves discussing and preparing for future decisions about your medical care if you become seriously ill or unable to communicate your wishes. It also often means having those hard conversations with your loved one; it is key and one of the most important parts of end-of-life planning. Even though you have such a discussion, make sure it is put in writing what you want and complete and documents referred to as advance directives. Having an end-of-life plan in place has several advantages. For instance, an end-of-life plan ensures your wishes are followed if you're longer able to make them known. An end-of-life plan allows you to decide in advance which medical steps and medical care you want to receive. (references: 800-222-2225. To help you plan for your loved one's end of life, the National Institute on Health and their National Institute on Aging end-of-life website offers some valuable information you may wish to use.)
Epilepsy Foundation	The epilepsy website contains a link where you can enter your zip code to find a support group in your area. It also offers a wealth of information on epilepsy. Here you will find links to information on such topics as lifestyle toolkit, medication resources, or information for anyone that is new to epilepsy, seizure first aid resource, and much more.

Ethnic Social Services	Ethnic social services agencies are community based and provide a variety of services to a specific ethnic population in a region, offering a variety of services such as facilitate the social adjustment and cultural transition of refugees by providing a broad range of services, including case management, translation and interpretation services, information and referral, employment assistance, English language training, health promotion education, emergency assistance, and a variety of other services specific to that population served. Services are delivered in a linguistically and culturally appropriate manner. Your best resources to find such an agency if you are new to the region will be to use the United Way 2-1-1 phone services. You can also use the Health and Human Services website for the Office of Minority Health to locate minority agencies within your loved one's community. References: 800-444-6472 or 2-1-1
Family Caregiver alliance	Supports and assists families and caregivers of adults with debilitating health conditions. Offers programs and consultation on caregiving issues at local, state, and national levels. (References: 415-434-3388 or 800-445-8106.)
Federal Communications Commission and Free Phones and Lifeline Services	Recognizing the importance of having access to a phone and concerned that low-income households may not be able to afford phone service on their own, the federal government created the Lifeline Assistance Program in 1985. Consumers who qualify based on federal or state-specific eligibility criteria can obtain free phone service through the Lifeline Assistance Program (references: 888-225-5322). For Lifeline eligibility criteria and applicable terms and conditions, visit www.lifewireless.com/tac or call 1-888-543-3620. Life Wireless is a service of Telrite (Free Government Cell Phone Lifeline Program - Life Wireless).

Genetically Handicapped Persons Program (GHPP)	The mission of GHPP is to promote high quality, coordinated medical care through case management services that assure partnership among the special care center team and the client's community health care providers. At this point, there are only two states, California and Nebraska, that offer a specific program designed to assist any person with a genetic handicap. This program is designed to serve those over age twenty-one who have a specific genetic disorder. California has five that are legislatively mandated for coverage, and there are three in Nebraska.
Guide Dogs for the Blind and Service Dogs for the Disabled	Both types of dogs are specifically trained to help a person who is blind to navigate successfully around while a service dog actually performs specific duties for a disabled person. (Reference: 800-295-4050)
Health and Human Services	This is a government program and using the website and the tab named programs and services, you will find a wealth of information on a variety of topics you may want to explore to see if they are right for your situation. HHS programs protect the health of all Americans and provide essential human services, especially for those who are least able to help themselves. HHS administers more than one hundred programs across its operating divisions.
Health Insurance Marketplace	The Health Insurance Marketplace is a service run by the federal government that helps people, families, and small businesses if they want to do the following: • Compare health insurance plans for coverage and affordability • Enroll in or change a health insurance plan • Find out about tax credits for private insurance or health programs like Medicaid or the Children's Health Insurance Program (CHIP) • Get answers to questions about health care insurance.

	Some states, including Washington DC have their own Market Place and these are: California, Colorado, Connecticut, Idaho, Kentucky, Maine, Maryland, Massachusetts, Minnesota, Nevada, New Jersey, New Mexico, New York, Pennsylvania, Rhode Island, Vermont, Washington. If you are denied coverage by the state, you have 90 days to file an appeal. References: 1-800-318-2596 (TTY: 1-855-889-4325)
Help with Utility Bills	This website lists a variety of ways to lower utility bill costs. The first way of course is to contact the utility company directly to see what programs they offer and to see if you or your loved one qualifies. If you type in your web browser "help with utility bills" you will find a variety of ways to lower utility bill costs.
hospice services	A medical team with a 24-7 approach of care for people with an anticipated life expectancy of six months or less when cure isn't an option, and the focus shifts to comfort, symptom management, and quality of life. To find a hospice provider in your loved one's region, you can use the Hospice Foundation of America directory. Online consumer database that lists hospices in North America and the US. All hospices are listed at no cost. It is a free service that assists families and individuals in locating a hospice within their community quickly. It also provides reliable information about hospice and end-of-life care and dealing with grieve to consumers.
incontinence supplies and diapers	While catheters and ostomy products are covered, other incontinence supplies and diapers for children and adults fall under the optional, personal care category as a type of medical supply. Thus, Medicare and many health plans do not cover them, and while some states may cover them under their Medicaid program, this is an optional benefit and incontinence supplies and diapers may not be covered. This includes youth and adult diapers and pull-ones from sizes youth to bariatric.

Individuals with Disabilities Education Act (IDEA)	The Individuals with Disabilities Education Act (IDEA) or better known as special education is a law that makes available a free appropriate public education to eligible children with disabilities throughout the nation and ensures special education and related services to those children. Infants and toddlers, birth through age two, with disabilities and their families receive early intervention services under IDEA Part C. Children and youth ages three through twenty-one receive special education and related services under IDEA Part B. Referrals for special education should be made in writing to the local school district or county office of education in which your loved one resides. The school district must complete the needed assessments and tests and develop what is called an individual education plan (IEP) within a specific period of time, usually fifty to ninety days after intake. The IEP is a written statement that serves as the database for the designed education and services your loved one needs to allow them to get a free and public education. To ensure the IEP is tailored to the individual needs, it must cover the following areas: relevant health issues visual abilities; hearing abilities; motor, self-help, and mobility abilities; emotional and psychological status; language spoken or understood; and vocational abilities and interests. The IEP, individualized education program, is a written document that's developed for each public school child who is eligible for special education. The IEP is created through a team effort and reviewed at least once a year. Before an IEP can be written, your child must be eligible for special education. By federal law, a multidisciplinary team must determine that the child has a disability, and they will require special education and related services to benefit from the general education program.

	The IEP is a document that is designed to meet your child's unique educational needs. It is not a contract, but it does guarantee the necessary supports and services that are agreed upon and written for your child. Unfortunately, specific devices or equipment identified in the IEP to assist the child with their learning will be devices or equipment that will remain at school. Thus, you may need to work with your loved one's health plan to see if the same will be available at home. Because states and local school systems may include additional information, forms and services differ from state to state and may even vary between school systems within a state. Thus, you will want to learn as much as you can on IDEA. So do your research on the IDEA law within your loved one's state as this will help you advocate for your loved one's educational needs.
insure kids now	Medicaid and CHIP offer free or low-cost health insurance for kids and teens. Find information on health insurance programs and dental providers in your state by clicking on your state in the map shown on the website or selecting it from the drop-down menu (Reference: 877-543-7669).
Lifeline	Lifeline is an assistance program providing government cell phone service for free to eligible customers in low-income households. This program helps ease the burden of monthly phone bills for qualified individuals and their families by covering monthly data, texting, and monthly minutes. If you receive assistance from Medicaid/Medi-Cal, SNAP/CalFresh, or other government assistance programs. Or if you are considered low income, you may be approved for free Lifeline phone service.

Lupus Foundation of America	Lupus is a chronic (long-term) disease that can cause inflammation and pain in any part of your body. It's an autoimmune disease, which means that your immune system—the body system that usually fights infections—attacks healthy tissue instead. When people talk about lupus, they're usually talking about systemic lupus. But there are four kinds of lupus: • Systemic lupus erythematosus (SLE), the most common form of lupus • Cutaneous lupus, a form of lupus that is limited to the skin • Drug-induced lupus, a lupus-like disease caused by certain prescription drugs • Neonatal lupus, a rare condition that affects infants of women who have lupus The main lupus website has a link you can click that will allow you to search for your loved one's local area for a support group.
Make a Wish	Make a Wish is a nonprofit organization that grants critically ill children a wish they may have with the hope the wish when granted will serve as a turning point, and it will give them the strength to fight harder against their disease.
Medicare Compare	The Centers for Medicare and Medicaid (CMS) has developed and maintain this website which allows you to search by zip code for health care providers in your loved one's area. The highest star rating will be a five and when possible, you should strive to find a 5-star provider in your loved one's immediate area.
Medicare Publications	Medicare maintains a website that offers a wealth of information on various topics and while written for persons with Medicare, many of the topics might help you navigate and learn about specific health care topics your loved one has. All the brochures are downloadable and this site has hyperlinks you can use to find and compare providers, durable medical equipment, and suppliers, as well as information on what Medicare covers.

Medicare Rights Center	This is an independent source of health care information and assistance for older and disabled Americans, their caregivers, and the professionals who serve them. Medicare Interactive (MI) is the one-stop source for information about health care rights, options, and benefits; and it is designed to help people find answers to all their Medicare questions.
Medicaid	Medicaid is a joint federal and state program that provides free or low-cost health coverage to millions of Americans, including some low-income people, families and children, pregnant women, the elderly, and people with disabilities. This program was implemented under the Social Security Act of 1965 and is titled Title XIX of the SS Act. The federal government provides a portion of the funding for Medicaid and sets guidelines for the program. Medicaid programs vary from state to state. They may also have different names, like medical assistance. The joint program, funded by the federal government and administered at the state level, varies. In California, the program is called Medi-Cal; in Arizona, their program is called Arizona Health Care Cost Containment System (AHCCCS). Under federal law states must include the following as what are called core benefits, and they also have the opportunity to include what are called optional benefits. States establish and administer their own Medicaid programs and determine the type, amount, duration, and scope of services within broad federal guidelines. The mandatory/core benefits include the following: • Inpatient hospital services • Outpatient hospital services • EPSDT: Early and Periodic Screening, Diagnostic, and Treatment Services • Nursing facility services • Home health services • Physician services • Rural health clinic services

	<ul><li>Federally qualified health center services</li><li>Laboratory and X-ray services</li><li>Family planning services</li><li>Nurse midwife services</li><li>Certified Pediatric and Family Nurse Practitioner Services</li><li>Freestanding Birth Center services (when licensed or otherwise recognized by the state)</li><li>Transportation to medical care</li><li>Tobacco cessation counseling for pregnant women</li></ul>The optional benefits are the following:<ul><li>Prescription drugs</li><li>Clinic services</li><li>Physical therapy</li><li>Occupational therapy</li><li>Speech, hearing, and language disorder services</li><li>Respiratory care services</li><li>Other diagnostic, screening, preventive and rehabilitative services</li><li>Podiatry services</li><li>Optometry services</li><li>Dental services</li><li>Dentures</li><li>Prosthetics</li><li>Eyeglasses</li><li>Chiropractic services</li><li>Other practitioner services</li><li>Private duty nursing services</li><li>Personal care</li><li>Hospice</li><li>Case management</li><li>Services for individuals age sixty-five or older in an Institution for Mental Disease (IMD)</li><li>Services in an intermediate care facility for individuals with intellectual disability</li></ul>

	• State plan home and community-based services—1915(i) • Self-directed personal assistance services—1915(j) • TB-related services • Inpatient psychiatric services for individuals under age twenty-one
Medicare	Medicare is a federal government program established under Title XVIII of the Social Security Act of 1965 to provide hospital expense and medical expense insurance to elderly and disabled persons. Benefits allowed are consistent nationwide. Medicare is a taxpayer-funded program for seniors aged sixty-five and older. Eligibility requires the senior to have worked and paid into the system through the payroll tax, either by Social Security or Railroad Retirement System. Medicare also provides health coverage for people with recognized disabilities and specific end-stage diseases as confirmed by the Social Security Administration (SSA). Medicare consists of four parts, titled A, B, C, and D. Parts of Medicare are the following: • Part A covers inpatient hospital stays, skilled nursing facility (SNF) stays, some home health visits, and hospice care. Part A benefits are subject to a deductible ($1,600 per benefit period in 2023). Part A also requires coinsurance for extended inpatient hospital and SNF stays—for example, the Part A coinsurance ($400 a day for days 61–90, $800 a day for days 91–150 [lifetime reserve days], $200 a day for days 21–100 [SNF]). • Part B covers physician visits, outpatient services, preventive services, and some home health visits. Many Part B benefits are subject to a deductible Part B Standard Premium ($164.90 a month Part B deductible—$226 a year) and typically coinsurance of 20 percent. No coinsurance or deductible is charged for an annual wellness visit or for preventive services that are rated A or B by the US Preventive Services Task Force, such as mammography or prostate cancer screenings.

	• Part C refers to the Medicare Advantage program, through which beneficiaries can enroll in a private health plan, such as a health maintenance organization (HMO) or preferred provider organization (PPO), and receive all Medicare-covered Part A and Part B benefits and typically also Part D benefits. • Part D covers outpatient prescription drugs through private plans that contract with Medicare, including standalone prescription drug plans (PDPs) and Medicare Advantage plans with prescription drug coverage (MA-PDs). The Part D benefit helps pay for enrollees' drug costs and provides coverage for extremely high drug costs. Additional financial assistance is available for beneficiaries with low incomes and modest assets. Enrollees pay monthly premiums and cost sharing for prescriptions, with costs varying by plan. Enrollment in Part D is voluntary. Deductibles vary between Medicare drug plans. No Medicare drug plan may have a deductible more than $505 in 2023. Some Medicare drug plans don't have a deductible. In some plans that do have a deductible, drugs on some tiers are covered before the deductible.
Medicare hospice benefit	The Medicare hospice benefit, as are other benefits allowed, serves as a plan for how health plans design and allow a benefit or as health care providers provide care. You can find full information on hospice on the Medicare Hospice Care website.
Mental Health America (MHA)	Mental Health America is the nation's leading community-based nonprofit dedicated to addressing the needs of those living with mental illness and promoting the overall mental health of all.

mental health equity	Mental health care is important for mental well-being, yet many people from racial and ethnic minority groups face obstacles in accessing needed care. These obstacles may include lack of or insufficient health insurance, lack of racial and ethnic diversity among mental healthcare providers, lack of culturally competent providers, financial strain, and stigma.
MentalHealth. gov	MentalHealth.gov provides one-stop access to US government mental health and mental health problems information. MentalHealth.gov aims to educate and guide • the general public, • health and emergency preparedness professionals, • policymakers, • government and business leaders, • school systems, and • local communities.

modified vehicles for the disabled	Modifying a vehicle to accommodate a disabled person is costly, and private health plans do not cover this expense. They may pay for a rehabilitation therapist to evaluate you for what might be needed, as well as what you might need, but payment for any vehicle modifications is not a benefit. The only health coverage that may pay for the actual modifications will be the VA, workers' compensation, your loved one's state Department of Developmental Services, or your loved one's state Department of Vocational Rehabilitation, if your loved one can possibly return to some form of employment. According to the Department of Veterans Affairs official site, veterans and currently serving troops may be eligible for VA disability benefits related to the AUTO Act if one of the following is true for you: • You have loss, or permanent loss of use, of one or both feet; • You have loss, or permanent loss of use, of one or both hands; • You have decreased vision in both eyes: 20/200 vision or less "in your better eye with glasses" or greater than 20/200 vision "but with a visual field defect that has reduced your peripheral vision to 20 degrees or less" in your better eye according to VA.gov. • You have a severe burn. • You have amyotrophic lateral sclerosis (ALS). • You have ankylosis in one or both knees or hips (restrictions may apply). Some websites you may wish to explore to see what is available and what might be covered will be.

	References:
	• National Highway Traffic and Safety Administration Association (NHTSA)—this site offers a brochure on vehicle modification that contains a wealth of information.https://specialkidsfund.org/about-us/https://www.utires.com/articles/vehicle-modifications-for-drivers-with-disabilities/#lc-6
Mothers Against Drunk Drivers (MADD)	If your loved one's injury was caused by a drunk driver, you may want to research the MADD site for a support group or join the group as they advocate against drunk or impaired substance driving (877-MADD-HELP Home-MADD).
National Adult Day Services Association	This association provides information about locating adult day care and day health centers in your local area. Adult Day Services (ADS) centers are a key provider of long-term care services in the United States. They provide a program of activities, health monitoring, socialization, and assistance with daily activities which allows individuals to continue to lives in their homes and receive needed care in a supportive, professionally staffed, community-based setting.
National Alliance of Caregiving (NAC)	NAC plays a pivotal role in shaping public policy for family caregivers and those in their care. When it originally started its focus was on the elderly, but this has evolved over the years to address at a minimum such issues as those related to the caregiver role and supporting family responsibilities in the workplace and children as caregivers.
National Alliance of Mental Health (NAMI)	By using their website, you can find your local NAMI resources, as well as both local and online support groups. NAMI has partnered with the National Alliance of Caregiving (NAC) and has a handbook, and you can download both the handbook, as well as some fact sheets on different topics. The handbook is called *Circle of Care: A Guidebook for Mental Health Caregivers*. (References: 800-950-6264; 62640)

National Amputation Foundation	The National Amputation Foundation Inc. (NAF) is a nonprofit organization comprised of amputee volunteers who offer their support to amputees and their families. People with amputations that were present at birth (congenital) are also served by the foundation. NAF's objective is to aid a new amputee in returning too as normal a life as possible within the sphere of his or her potential. Established in 1919, the foundation provides affected individuals with appropriate referrals to support groups, and promotes education of amputees, family members, healthcare professionals, and the general public.
	The amputee coalition website offers a wealth of information for amputees such as: support groups, resources for mental health and wellness; coping with limb loss, emergency preparedness, employment, and job training resources, pain management, medical issues, recreation and sports activities (references: 888-267-5669).
Amputee Coalition	Amputee Coalition—using the Amputee website, you can learn about amputation and prosthetic care, and you can request information on support groups for people living with limb loss, their families, caregivers, and clinicians who care for amputees.
National Council on Aging	The National Council on Aging, a private group, has a free service called BenefitsCheckUp. This website can be invaluable for seniors who need help in finding federal and state benefit programs. After providing some general information about the person who needs care, you can see a list of possible benefit programs to explore. These programs can help pay for prescription drugs, heating bills, housing, meal programs, assistive technology and legal services. You don't have to give a name, address, or Social Security number to use this.
National Council on Independent Living (NCIL)	The National Council on Independent Living is the longest-running national cross-disability, grassroots organization run by and for people with disabilities.

National Kidney Foundation and Renal Disease	This website has a wealth of information, including dialysis and treatment options, sexual help, financial information, nutrition, and the right diet for persons with kidney disease and support groups. To find a dialysis center, you can use the US renal care site at https://www.usrenalcare.com/.
National Library Services (NLS) for the blind or print disabled in the Library of Congress	Here you can order talking books or books in Braille. Books can be downloaded or mailed free of charge directly to your home. Once used, the book(s) can be put in a mailbox and sent back, free of charge. NLS offers books for children and adults, and they also offer Bible and other sacred writings, calendars, and music. You can also sign up for the e-version and download books or music without the hassle of mailing any material back. (References: 888-NLS-READ [888-657-7323]).
National Multiple Sclerosis Society	The National Multiple Sclerosis Society website offers information and resources for you to explore and also information on support groups and educational material.
National Resource Center for Traumatic Brain injury (NRCTBI)	While this is a site for persons dealing with a loved one with a brain injury, it has information that might be useful for others as this site has some great information on such topics as: • Caregiver Basics • Family Relationships • Caregiver Emotions • Staying Positive • Health and Self Care • Legal and Finances • military caregiving • caregiver personal blog Under the tab People with TBI, you will find links to various resources you may want to explore. There is a link in this tab where you can type in your zip code, and it will bring up local resources you may want to explore.

National Scleroderma Foundation	Scleroderma (sklair-oh-dur-muh), also known as systemic sclerosis, is a group of rare diseases that involve the hardening and tightening of the skin. It may also cause problems in the blood vessels, internal organs and digestive tract. Scleroderma is often categorized as limited or diffuse, which refers only to the degree of skin involvement. Both types can involve any of the other vascular or organ problems. Localized scleroderma, also known as morphea, affects only the skin. While there is no cure for scleroderma, treatments can ease symptoms, slow progression and improve quality of life. The National Scleroderma Foundation website contains links to local resources and support.
Office of Disability and US Department of Labor	This website has helpful information to assist people with disabilities in seeking meaningful work and succeeding once on the job. DOL also advises employers on effective strategies for recruiting and retaining qualified people with disabilities, as well as educating both federal agencies and federal contractors and private subcontractors about their obligations related to affirmative action and nondiscrimination in hiring. To locate potential transportation services for the disabled in your loved one's area, you can use the 2-1-1 phone system.
Pediatric Day Health Care Centers (PDHC)	The names of such centers vary across the US but these are day health centers for very medically fragile children, providing a full range of skilled nursing and rehabilitation services to very medically fragile children. (Reference: 2-1-1 to locate a pediatric day health center in your loved one's region.)

Permanent Residence Under Color of Law (PRUCOL)	PRUCOL is a term used to describe certain noncitizens living in the United States. It stands for persons residing under color of law or permanent residence under color of law. The official definition of PRUCOL is any noncitizen living in the United States with the knowledge and consent of the DHS (Department of Homeland Security) and whose departure the DHS does not contemplate enforcing. This category of residents has the ability to apply for SSI and any benefits allowed under the program.
poison control	To access poison control, the main number is 800-222-1222, and you can find a poison control center in your area by using the website to your state's site(s).
pulmonary rehabilitation	Pulmonary rehabilitation is a program of education and exercise to increase awareness about your lungs and your disease and is a program offered as an outpatient either in a clinic or hospital. The program is designed to teach your loved one how to exercise with less shortness of breath. The classes are offered in a group setting so your loved one will get a chance to meet others with their same condition while also providing an opportunity to give and receive peer support. The skills and knowledge learned in the program will help your loved one feel better and be able to manage their chronic lung disease. Pulmonary rehabilitation may even decrease the need for hospital visits.

presumptive eligibility for Medicaid, VA benefits, and SSI	According to the Affordable Care Act, all states can now allow hospitals, the Veterans Administration, and Supplemental Security Income the opportunity to make presumptive eligibility determinations regardless of whether the state had previously adopted the presumptive eligibility option. Every state now has the ability to enroll individuals who are likely eligible under a state's Medicaid eligibility guidelines, including children, pregnant women, parents and caretaker relatives, and former foster children. Hospitals may also make PE determinations for other groups that are covered by their state Medicaid programs, including individuals with income above 133 percent of the federal poverty level and under age sixty-five; individuals eligible for family planning services; and individuals needing treatment for breast and cervical cancer. At the discretion of each state, hospitals may also be allowed to make hospital PE determinations for other groups such as aged, blind, and disabled persons, as well as groups whose eligibility is established by section 1115 waivers. Hospital PE determinations are not limited to patients but can also be made for patients' families and eligible individuals from the broader community. At the initial visit of an individual who is not already enrolled in Medicaid, a hospital employee who is trained in doing the PE application. The only program that does not allow PE is when you or your loved one applies for Social Security Disability Insurance (SSDI).
printable medication records	This site offers to you as a caregiver fifty-eight different forms you can download for free. Thus, this allows you to record the daily medications you give to your loved one.

prescription assistance	You might be thinking about buying your medicines online to save some money. These websites may be of help. Family caregivers can do the following: 1. Contact the pharmaceutical company directly that manufactures the drug to see what services they offer for discounting their drug. If eligible, you will be required to complete and application, as well as possibly show proof of the fact paying for the drug presents a financial hardship. 2. Contact you loved one's county or state Department of Health and Human Services for financial programs, which may provide assistance for acquiring health insurance and prescription medications. 3. Other possible financial resources may include social service agencies, such as Catholic Charities, the Association of Jewish Families, and Children's Agencies. Local chapters of voluntary health agencies may also offer financial support programs or information on how to apply for such programs. 4. The National Council on the Aging, Benefits Check-Up, and Benefits Check-UP RX are designed to help people over the age of fifty-five find federal, state, and local public and private programs that may pay for some of their medical care or prescription costs. 5. Another resource will be to use your loved one's health plan and use their mail-order pharmacy benefit, as this will allow you to get a three months' supply and only pay three co-payments instead.

PTSD for veterans and non-veterans	Post-traumatic stress disorder (PTSD) is a psychiatric disorder that can occur following a traumatic experience. Many people think about PTSD in the context of military combat and war veterans. However, PTSD symptoms can develop from experiences involving natural disasters, serious accidents, life-threatening illnesses, physical abuse, and sexual assault during childhood or adulthood. A traumatic event that precedes the onset of PTSD can be experienced either directly or indirectly by an individual. For Veterans, the VA is the national center for PTSD and offers a wealth of information on the treatment and support for families and a veteran with PTSD. All VA medical centers offer PTSD treatment even if there is no specific PTSD program. Contact your local VA medical center and ask for the mental health clinic.
Rare Diseases	The National Organization for Rare Disease (NORD) is committed to the identification, treatment, and cure of rare diseases through education, advocacy, research, and service programs. The website lists in alphabetical order the various rare disease one might have. NORD also provides patient assistance programs to help individuals living with rare diseases. • Obtain medication • Receive financial help with insurance premiums and co-pays • Get diagnostic testing assistance • Receive travel assistance for clinical trials or consultation with disease specialists • Provide caregiver respite • Offer support during emergencies • Gain knowledge about rare diseases • Connect with other patient assistance programs

Religious Social Service Agencies and Goodwill Industries	Religious organizations have become a central component of the safety net of providers in any given community, and they assist low-income families in America, and they fill in the gap where it is most needed. This often is providing shelter, food, clothing, or other essential goods or offering critical services, such as counseling, rehabilitation, job placement, foster-care placement, and adoption. Examples of the most common religious organizations include (a) Catholic Social Services, (b) Church of Jesus Christ of Latter-day Saints (LDS Church), (c) Lutheran Social Services, (d) Jewish Social Services, (e) Salvation Army, and (f) Volunteers of America While the Goodwill Industries stated out as a religious organization, it is not now, as it is a nonprofit, nondenomenational organization that offers a myriad of services in any community, including employment and job training for the disabled.
respite resources	This site links you not only to respite providers and programs but also to state-by-state fact sheets on funding and program eligibility with state contacts for the state's respite programs. To assist with finding respite for a caregiver who is tending to a loved one with Alzheimer's' disease, the Alzheimer's Association website has a link to use.
Ronald McDonald House	These are free housing / apartment units near major tertiary hospitals where children are getting their medical treatments. The goal is to help reduce the stress and financial burden families face when their loved one is getting the medical care they need.
Senior Living Directory	This website allows you to search for a wide variety of senior living options and also allows you to drill down so you can conduct your search by city or zip code. To find resources for senior living options in your loved one's area, another resource will be to use the 2-1-1 phone directory. You can find similar resources for a veteran if you use the VA.gov website.

sickle cell disease	Sickle cell disease is a lifelong illness. A blood and bone marrow transplant is currently the only cure for sickle cell disease, but there are effective treatments that can reduce symptoms and prolong life. Your health care team will work with you on a treatment plan to reduce your symptoms and manage the condition. The NHLBI is leading and supporting research and clinical trials to find a cure for sickle cell disease. You can find a fact sheet on the National Institute of Health Heart Lung Blood Institute website, and this same site offers tips on pain control and tips for healthy living. The Mayo Clinic website lists many symptoms and complications and has a link where you can connect with others.
Shriners Hospitals for Children	The mission of Shriners Hospitals for Children is to provide the highest quality care to children with neuro-musculoskeletal conditions, burn injuries, and other special health care needs within a compassionate, family-centered, and collaborative care environment regardless of the family's ability to pay. (References: 813-281-0300).
American Sign Language	The National Association of the Deaf (NAD) website has a wealth of information not only on sign language but also on other resources you may wish to explore. The NAD recognizes that American Sign Language (ASL) is the backbone of the American deaf culture. The NAD values the acquisition, usage, and preservation of ASL and is a recognized leader in promoting the acquisition, learning, teaching, and interpreting of ASL. The NAD was created in part to promote and preserve ASL as a legitimate language and an optimal educational tool for deaf children and adults.
Social Security Administration (SSA)	By all means, explore any of the programs offered by the Social Security Administration for your loved if they are disabled. This includes any child under the age of eighteen, and they are eligible for SSI. The SSA website on disability benefits listed below contains all the information, including a link to access the application and any documents you might need to complete the application process. (References: 800-772-1213).

Social Security Disability Insurance (SSDI)	Social Security Disability Insurance (SSDI) programs provide assistance to people who meet the requirements for disability. The SSDI program pays benefits to you if you have worked long enough (forty quarters) and paid Social Security taxes on your earnings. The SSDI program pays benefits to adults who meet the requirements for a qualifying disability. If you meet the medical requirements, monthly benefits are paid if you have a medical condition expected to last at least one year or result in death. As the approval timeline from application to the final approval can be at least five months, it is important as soon as the health care team has issued a determination your loved one's disability will not allow gainful employment; it is key to start the application. Once your loved one has been on SSDI for twenty-four months, they will be eligible for Medicare Part A, and they must sign up for Part B at the same time.

| State Health Insurance Counseling Programs (SHIPS) | State Health Insurance Counseling Programs (SHIPS) offer no-cost, unbiased health benefit counseling, education, and advocacy services to help empower people to make informed benefit decisions. To find a SHIP that serves your area, enter your ZIP code or city and state in the orange search bar at the top of the page. SHIP services are available to Medicare-eligible individuals, their family members, and their caregivers. SHIPs provide personalized counseling and education to help someone make informed choices about their health care benefits. This service is free and not affiliated with insurance companies, which means that counselors will not try to sell any products or services. Not all states term their program as SHIPS, some call it HICAP or a variety of other names. SHIPs help people with the following topics:

• Original Medicare (Part A and Part B)
• Medicare Advantage plans (Part C)
• Medicare prescription drug coverage (Part D)
• Medicare Supplement Insurance (Medigap)

SHIP services are available to Medicare-eligible individuals, their family members, and their caregivers. People in the US are typically eligible for Medicare when they reach sixty-five years of age, although younger people with certain disabilities may also qualify.

• People who will soon be eligible for Medicare may also get SHIP services.
• SHIPs provide their services free of charge. |
| St. Jude Children's Research Hospital | The mission of St. Jude Children's Research Hospital is to advance cures and means of prevention for pediatric catastrophic diseases through research and treatment. Consistent with the vision of our founder, Danny Thomas, no child is denied treatment based on race, religion, or a family's ability to pay. |

	Free housing is available close to campus for up to four family members. They have three different housing options: Ronald McDonald House, housing for eight days to three months; Tri Delta, short-term housing for one to seven days; and Target house for families needing to stay greater than ninety days. St. Jude has eight affiliate clinics across the United States. <ul><li>Baton Rouge, Louisiana</li><li>Charlotte, North Carolina</li><li>Huntsville, Alabama</li><li>Johnson City, Tennessee</li><li>Peoria, Illinois</li><li>Shreveport, Louisiana</li><li>Springfield, Missouri</li><li>Tulsa, Oklahoma</li></ul> (References: 888-226-4343).
Substance Abuse and Mental Health Services Administration (SAMHSA)	The Substance Abuse and Mental Health Services Administration (SAMHSA) is the agency within the US Department of Health and Human Services (HHS) that leads public health efforts to advance the behavioral health of the nation and to improve the lives of individuals living with mental and substance use disorders and their families. The SAMHSA website allows you to find mental health and substance abuse treatment programs in your loved one's local area. SAMHSA also has a helpline that offers free and confidential 24-7 365-day-a-year treatment referral and information service (in English and Spanish) for individuals and families facing mental or substance use disorders. FindSupport.gov is an online guide that helps people navigate through common questions when they are at the start of their journey to better behavioral health.

	The SAMHSA website offers a wealth of information and has links where you can find information on such topics as: • Finding health care or support • How to set up an appointment • Types of treatment and providers • How to help someone • Finding help for someone with early serious mental
Supplemental Security Income (SSI)	Supplemental Security Income (SSI) is a federal program in the United States that provides additional monthly income for older adults and people with disabilities that have little to no income. SSI is a federal program that pays monthly checks to people in need who are blind or otherwise disabled. The purpose of the program is to provide sufficient resources so that qualified individuals can have a basic monthly income. Eligibility is based on income and assets. The field office locator helps you find the nearest SSA office. This website gives you information on who is eligible (both adults and children). This site also explains who is eligible and defines a disabled adult or child, as well as other terms.
Supplemental Nutrition Assistance Program (SNAP)	Under the tab Programs, you will find listed the many programs they offer. The goal is reducing hunger for children and low-income people so they have access to food, a healthy diet, and education. This site also allows you to find the programs in your or your loved one's area.
telephone support or reassurance program	A program operated within a community where someone will volunteer to call your loved one to check in on them. Which agency that provides this service is dependent upon each local community. Your best resource to find a telephone reassurance program in your loved one's region will be to use the telephone 2-1-1 directory system.

Temporary Assistance for Needy Families (TANF)	Temporary Assistance for Needy Families (TANF), enacted in 1996, replaced Aid to Families with Dependent Children (AFDC), which provided cash assistance to families with children experiencing poverty. TANF cash assistance can play a critical role in supporting families during times of need. Under TANF, the federal government provides a fixed block grant to states, which use these funds to operate their own programs.

The programs go by different names in states—for example, CalWORKs in California. In order to receive federal funds and avoid a fiscal penalty, states must also spend some of their own dollars, known as maintenance of effort (MOE) spending.

TANF's funding structure differs greatly from AFDC, where the federal government contributed at least one dollar in matching funds for every dollar that states spent. States can use federal TANF and state MOE dollars to meet any of the four purposes set out in the 1996 law.

- Assisting families in need so children can be cared for in their own homes or the homes of relatives
- Reducing the dependency of parents in need by promoting job preparation, work, and marriage
- Preventing pregnancies among unmarried persons
- Encouraging the formation and maintenance of two-parent families.

States define what constitutes a needy family for the first and second purposes and do not have to limit assistance to needy families for the third and fourth purposes.

transplants	If your loved one requires an organ transplant, the process is not as simple of your loved one's doctor making a referral. Your loved one will undergo a multitude of medical and psychological testing to help determine if they are a right candidate for a transplant. If it is determined they are a candidate, they are placed on a registry waiting list. • The organs that have successfully transplanted include the heart, kidneys, liver, lungs, pancreas, intestine, thymus, and uterus. • Tissues include bones, tendons (both referred to as musculoskeletal grafts), cornea, skin, heart valves, nerves, and veins. The government site Health Resources and Service Administration (HRSA) and its website—organdonor.gov—offers a wealth of information on a wide variety of transplant-related topics.
TRICARE	TRICARE is a health care program of the Military Health System. TRICARE provides civilian health benefits for US Armed Forces military personnel, military retirees, and their dependents, including some members of the Reserve Component. TRICARE is the civilian care component of the Military Health System, although historically it also included health care delivered in military medical treatment facilities. TRICARE functions similar to a single-payer health care system.

TRICARE for Life (TFL)	The following are the TRICARE regions:
	<table><tr><td>West Health Net 844-866-9378 (www. tricare-west.com)</td><td>East Humana Military 800-444-5445 (www. tricare-east.com)</td></tr><tr><td>Alaska, Arizona, California, Colorado, Hawaii, Idaho, Iowa (excludes Rock Island arsenal area), Kansas, Minnesota, Missouri (except St. Louis area), Montana, Nebraska, Nevada, New Mexico, North Dakota, Oregon, South Dakota, Texas (southwestern corner, including El Paso), Utah, Washington, and Wyoming</td><td>Alabama, Arkansas, Connecticut, Delaware, the District of Columbia, Florida, Georgia, Illinois, Indiana, Iowa (Rock Island area), Kentucky, Louisiana, Maine, Maryland, Massachusetts, Michigan, Mississippi, Missouri (St. Louis area), New Hampshire, New Jersey, New York, North Carolina, Ohio, Oklahoma, Pennsylvania, Rhode Island, South Carolina, Tennessee, Texas (excluding El Paso area), Vermont, Virginia, West Virginia, and Wisconsin</td></tr></table> TRICARE for Life (TFL) is Medicare-wraparound coverage for TRICARE-eligible beneficiaries who have Medicare Parts A and B. TFL is not insurance. It is a benefit program that pays medical expenses, and the member is not required to pay a premium (https://tricare.mil/tfl; https://tricare.mil/Publications/Handbooks/tricare_for_life).TRICARE For Life Handbook | TRICARE

United Cerebral Palsy	This site offers a wealth of information under its Resource tab and has a link where you can find the nearest agency you may be able to utilize. Once you locate your local office, you can work with them on transportation options and other services they provide in your area.
United Network for Organ Sharing (UNOS)	United Network for Organ Sharing (UNOS) is the private, nonprofit organization that serves as the nation's organ transplant system—the Organ Procurement and Transplantation Network (OPTN)—under contract with and oversight by the federal government. References: 800-292-9548 Organ Transplant | US Organ Donation System | UNOS
United Ostomy Association (UOAA)	This is a nonprofit organization that supports, empowers, and advocates for people who have had or who will have an ostomy or continent diversion surgery.
USA.gov	Under the tab All Topics and Services, you can click on a variety of topics, any one of which may be helpful to your situation.
US Department of Health and Human Services (HHS)	The US Department of Health and Human Services protects the health of all Americans and provides essential human services. On this site, they offer an A–Z weblink to all US government offices, as well as information on Indian tribes and resources for Native Americans. You can click on any of the agencies under HHS, and you can find added information that may be of help. The agencies are below. • CDC (Centers for Disease Control and Prevention) • FDA (Federal Drug Administration) • NIH (National Institute of Health) • CMS (Centers for Medicare and Medicaid Services) • SAMHSA (Substance Abuse and Mental Health Services Administration)

	<ul><li>IHS (Indian Health Service)</li><li>HRSA (Health Resources and Services Administration)</li><li>AHRQ (Agency for Healthcare Research and Quality)</li><li>ACL (Administration for Community Living)</li><li>ACF (Administration for Children and Families)</li><li>US Public Health Services</li></ul>
Veterans Affairs and VA benefits	If your loved one served in the military, they may be entitled to receive benefits because of their status as a veteran. The VA offers a wealth of benefits for our country's veterans by providing health care, housing, and long-term care options. Unfortunately, like so many programs, many veterans do not use them well, because navigating these benefits can be confusing, especially for the elderly retired veterans. The main criterion for being eligible for VA benefits is being a veteran, but the actual eligibility rules are a bit more complex than this. Each program has its own eligibility requirements. Universally, however, veterans must have something other than an honorable discharge to qualify. Veterans also must complete a minimum time in the service to qualify for If you were dishonorably discharged, you lose your right to claim veterans' benefits. Veterans also must complete a minimum time in the service to qualify for health benefits. The rules the VA indicates apply include the following: <ul><li>For those who enlisted after September 7, 1980, or who entered active duty after October 16, 1981, they must serve twenty-four continuous months or their full active duty period to qualify.</li><li>For those who enlisted or served before September 7, 1980, no minimum duty requirement is required.</li></ul>

<table>
<tr><td></td><td>

- For veterans discharged for a service-related disability or who took an early out for a hardship, the minimum duty requirement does not apply.
- These are the requirements for general health care eligibility. Elderly veterans who need help paying for long-term care or care in their homes have additional requirements to qualify for A&A or housebound veterans services.

For A&A, veterans must

- need help with the activities of daily living, like bathing or dressing;
- need to stay in bed for a large part of the day due to their illness;
- be a patient in a nursing home because of their physical or mental health need; or
- have eyesight that is 5/200 or less in both eyes, even with corrective lenses.

For housebound benefits, veterans must have a health need or permanent disability that requires them to spend most of their time at home.

The VA health care program assigns priority groups to ensure that those who need care the most can get it quickly. This is often due to low income or a serious disability level. For example, someone who has a service-related disability that is 50 percent or more disabling or that makes the veteran unable to work will get priority over someone who can work and has a high income.

The VA currently has eight priority groups. Some factors that can impact your loved one's priority group assignment as a veteran include these:

- *Honors received for your service.* Those with Purple Heart medals or Medal of Honor recipients are placed higher than those without.

</td></tr>
</table>

- *Disabilities connected to service.* Service-related disabilities increase the priority level for a veteran, and disabilities that led to discharge also impact eligibility.
- *Disability and housebound status.* Veterans who are unable to leave the house receive priority over those who can.
- *Medicaid and VA pension benefits status.* If your loved one qualifies for Medicaid or VA pension benefits, it will impact their priority group.

CHAMPVA Benefits

In addition to the benefits paid directly to a veteran, the VA offers the Civilian Health and Medical Program of the Department of Veterans Affairs.

What Is CHAMPVA?

CHAMPVA covers services and supplies that are medically necessary for the individual, such as durable medical equipment, inpatient care, outpatient care and skilled nursing care. It's a program for the spouses and qualifying children of some veterans who can no longer rely on their veteran family members to provide income.

Who Is Eligible for CHAMPVA?

CHAMPVA allows the surviving spouse or child of a veteran who has died or one with disabilities to get health insurance for themselves. This program is offered to those who do not qualify for TRICARE.

To qualify for CHAMPVA, you must be the spouse or child of a veteran who has suffered a permanent, total disability for a service-related issue or who has died because of a service-related disability. You may also be able to receive CHAMPVA if you're the child or spouse of a veteran who was permanently and totally disabled at the time of his death. Finally, the children and spouses of soldiers who died in the line of duty but who do not qualify for TRICARE may also receive CHAMPVA.

Caregiver Support Program

The Department of Veteran Affairs Caregiver Support Program (CSP) offers clinical services to caregivers of eligible and covered veterans enrolled in the VA health care system. There is a CSP team locator located at every VA facility. The VA also offers the Program of General Caregiver Support Services (PGCSS), one of two programs within the Caregiver Support Program. PGCSS provides peer support mentoring, skills training, coaching, telephone support, online programs, and referrals to available resources to caregivers of veterans.

The veteran must be enrolled in Veterans Affairs (VA) health care and be receiving care from a caregiver in order for the caregiver to participate. Caregivers who participate in PGCSS are called general caregivers. General caregivers do not need to be a relative or live with the veteran.

The VA also offers another program known as aid and attendant care. Your loved one may be eligible for this benefit if he gets a VA pension, and they spend most of their time in their home because of a permanent disability, one that doesn't go away.

victims of violent crimes (VOCA)	All states receive federal Victims of Crime Act (VOCA) funds from the Office of Violent Crimes (OVC) to help support crime victim assistance and compensation programs. There are resources in your immediate area that offer services to victims of crime. You may be eligible for crime victim compensation benefits, including reimbursement for medical services, mental health counseling, lost wages, and other costs incurred as a result of the crime. You can find more information on victims of violent crimes by visiting the Department of Justice website and their link to Office of Violent Crimes.
vocational rehabilitation	If your loved one has recovered enough from his injury of illness and desires to possibly return to work and they cannot return to their previous employment, he can work with the Social Security Administration or their state's Division of Vocational Rehabilitation to see if they can be retrained for another type of work.
warmline	The National Alliance for Mental Illness (nami.org) maintains a national directory of services called warmline to help offer telephonic support for persons who are living with a mental illness or the families or caregiver of a person with a mental illness. This is a service that is volunteer peer hotline that offers callers emotional support and is staffed by trained volunteers who are in recovery themselves. References: (520) 770-9909; (877) 770-9912.

waivers	Medicaid and the Children's Health Insurance Program (CHIP) allow states the ability to expand services to specific populations via Section 1915 demonstrations and waiver authorities. Section 1915 of the Social Security Act are vehicles states can use to test new or existing ways to deliver and pay for health care services in Medicaid and the Children's Health Insurance Program (CHIP). All current and concluded state programs authorized under these authorities may be accessed using the below dynamic list to find what waivers are allowed in your loved one's state (see the Medicaid website and the state waiver listing). Many states have elected to receive an exemption to the Title XIX of the Social Security Act from the Centers for Medicare and Medicaid Services (CMS) that allows them to offer in specific regions added services for specific groups or individuals to provide medical coverage. Medicaid waivers are programs that provide additional services to specific groups of individuals, limit services to specific geographic areas of the state, and provide medical coverage to individuals who may not otherwise be eligible under traditional Medicaid rules. There are Section 1915 demonstrations in place for substance abuse disorders, serious mental health illnesses, or serious emotional disturbances. You can find your state using the website in the reference area of this chapter. Unlike nearly all other Medicaid-covered services, states use optional waivers to provide most home- and community-based services (HCBS). Seniors, people with disabilities, and those with chronic conditions rely on Medicaid HCBS to live independently outside nursing homes and other institutions. HCBS waivers enable states to expand Medicaid financial eligibility and offer benefits targeted to a particular population; these waivers also allow states to choose and limit how many people are served. States' ability to cap HCBS waiver enrollment can result in waiting lists when the number of people seeking services exceeds the number of waiver slots available.

Medicare and Medicaid Waiver

Medicare also has a waiver called PACE (Program of All-Inclusive for the Elderly).

PACE provides comprehensive medical and social services to certain frail, elderly people (participants) still living in the community. Most of the participants who are in PACE are dually eligible for both Medicare and Medicaid. PACE-enabling legislation is active in thirty-eight states and DC, and PACE programs are now active (launched and operating) in thirty states and DC residential. PACE is currently offered in California, Florida, and Missouri. The Program of All-Inclusive Care for the Elderly (PACE) benefits include but are not limited to all Medicaid and Medicare covered services.

- Adult day care
- Dentistry
- Emergency services
- Home care
- Hospital care
- Laboratory/X-ray services
- Meals
- Medical specialty services
- Nursing home care
- Nutritional counseling
- Occupational therapy
- Physical therapy
- Prescription drugs
- Primary care (including doctor and nursing services)
- Recreational therapy
- Social services
- Social work counseling
- Transportation

	PACE also includes all other services determined necessary by the health professionals' team to improve and maintain an individual's health. PACE programs provide services primarily in an adult day health center and are supplemented by in-home and referral services in accordance with the enrollee's needs. Since comprehensive care is provided to PACE participants, individuals who need end-of-life care will receive the appropriate medical, pharmaceutical, and psychosocial services. If the individual wants to elect the hospice benefit, they must voluntarily disenroll from the PACE program. Enrollment in the PACE program is voluntary. If an individual meets the eligibility requirements and elects PACE, then an enrollment agreement is signed. Enrollment continues as long as desired by the individual, regardless of change in health status, until voluntary or involuntary disenrollment.
white cane training	A white cane is a mobility aid that can be used by people of all ages who have low vision or blindness. This is a tool that will help your loved one move independently while providing safety and balance. There are different types of canes available depending on your level of vision loss. It's used around the world so that people everywhere can recognize it and its purpose. To see what is available, as well as possibly any white cane training in your loved one's local area, contact the local area's Society for the Blind. One of the best resources to locate this will be the 2-1-1 phone directory.
women, infant, and children (WIC)	The Special Supplemental Nutrition Program for Women, Infants, and Children (WIC) provides federal grants to states for supplemental food, health care referrals, and nutrition education for low-income pregnant, breastfeeding, and non-breastfeeding postpartum women and to infants and children up to age five who are found to be at nutritional risk. You can find your loved one's state by using the US Department of Agriculture website. Reference: WIC Program Contacts | Food and Nutrition Service (usda.gov)

Health Care and Insurance Terms and Abbreviations

LIKE MANY WORK-RELATED entities, the language and lingo used can be very confusing. Definitely, health care is not exempt, and it has a language of its own. It is full of complex terms and acronyms that can be very confusing. Thus, we live in a world of what I call alphabet soup, funny words, or gobbledygook. Believe it or not, some of us working in the health industry even struggle if the word is not familiar to us.

Over the course of writing so many proposals and policies and other related medical documents, I want to share with you some common acronyms (those funny letters that may be written on any note or document) and their definitions. To assist you, I have included many websites you can search on your own if you desire more information on the term. I am also giving you some of the health care terms I identified in my first nursing test book: *Case Management in Health Care: A Practical Guide* (1999).

This section will not include any traditional bibliography, as I feel that too confusing. So if I have used a medical term I have found in a specific website, I have included the website after the term used. I did that, as often, that same website may have other hyperlinks to other sites you may wish to explore.

Remember, you, as the caregiver, may end up being the eyes, ears, and voice of your loved one. So by all means, practice the following:

1. Keep a pad handy or use your cell phone, where you can either write down or record notes on anything you want further information on or if you want to ask a question to the health care team on the next visit.
2. Ask questions when present during a physician's hospital rounds, an office visit, or to any other provider who is helping your loved one.
3. If you do not understand what is said, request they tell you in simple terms and how to spell it so then you can further your research once you are home. As there as so many funny or confusing big words in health care, you can then look them up if you feel more information is needed.
4. If you or your loved one does not understand mental health and how important it is to take care of yourselves, educate yourselves and know the facts; and as you learn, educate others. According to the American Psychiatric Association, approximately half of those with a mental illness do not receive the help they need. Many find it difficult to seek help because they fear stigmatization. Experts say that although talking about mental health may not be easy, it is essential. Open dialogues support those who live with a condition while also helping dispel false ideas and prejudices.

   In everyday terms, mental health is about living a balanced life and coping with its ups and downs while keeping a positive attitude and frame of mind and functioning to the best of your ability emotionally, cognitively, and socially. It's more than just the absence of mental illness, but it doesn't mean that a person is happy all the time. In fact, mental health problems, issues, or concerns can be experienced temporarily and as a reaction to the stresses of life by anyone, particularly when going through some major event or significant change, even the good ones, like a new job or the birth of a child. These problems, issues, or concerns should be addressed and dealt with adequately, as they do interfere with how you think, feel, and behave on a daily basis even if to a much lesser extent than a mental illness.

5. If you do not speak English, no matter if in the hospital or during an office visit or a telehealth visit, request they use a phone interpreter service. While you may have a friend or family member who can translate, they often may not give the full information as a professionally trained health care interpreter will do. Interpreter services are not a luxury but a requirement of at least three federal laws.

- The first law to require this service was Title VI of the Civil Rights Act of 1964, outlawing discrimination based on race, color, religion, sex, or national origin. Then in 2000, President Clinton did an executive order to the act. The act now requires any health care agency or institution that receives federal money to provide interpreters.

- Under Section 1557 of the Affordable Care Act, any health care provider or health insurance company that receives federal money must provide limited English proficiency (LEP) patients with a qualified interpreter.

- The Americans with Disabilities Act (ADA) requires that Title II entities (state and local governments) and Title III entities (businesses and nonprofit organizations that serve the public) communicate effectively with people who have communication disabilities. The goal is to ensure that communication with people with these disabilities is equally effective as communication with people without disabilities.

  However, your best device is, if you have an iPhone or an Android phone, purchase a translator app. This will allow you to have translation services immediately available, especially when key information will be important and help you in your role.

If you need more information on any of the terms listed below, you can type in your web browser the Medical Term listed in column one.

Medical Term	Acronym	Meaning
abuse and fraud by a health care provider		Abuse is defined as practices that are inconsistent with accepted, sound fiscal, business, or medical practices and result in an unnecessary cost or in reimbursement for services that are not medically necessary or that fail to meet professionally recognized standards for health care. • Misusing codes on a claim • Charging excessively for services or supplies • Billing for services that are not medically necessary or billing for services not rendered If you suspect provider abuse, you can report it by calling your health plan's Member Services. The number is on the back of the member's insurance card. If a person believes they may have noticed Medicare abuse or fraud, they can report it in three ways: calling Medicare at 1-800-633-4227, or 1-877-486-2048 for TTY users; contacting the Senior Medicare Patrol (SMP) resource center at 877-808-2468; and contacting the Office of Inspector General fraud hotline at 1-800-447-8477.

abuse of a person		Abuse is cruelty, violence, or demeaning or invasive behavior from one person to another person, causing physical, sexual, psychological, or emotional harm. It also can include financial or material exploitation, as well as neglect or negligence. Abuse can affect a child, an adult, or an elder whether they are residing either at home or in an institution. If you suspect abuse of a person, call your local CPS or APS office, and the best number to use to find the one in your local area will be 2-1-1.
access to health care		Access to health care means having "the timely use of personal health services to achieve the best health outcomes." Access to health care consists of four components. • *Coverage.* This facilitates entry into the health care system. • *Services.* Having a usual source of care is associated with adults receiving recommended screening and prevention services. • *Timeliness.* This refers to the ability to provide health care when the need is recognized. • *Workforce.* This consists of capable, qualified, culturally competent providers.

accredita-tion		Accreditation is the process of quality assurance through an external agency conducting review of an institution of a specialized program. When an institution or specialized program is accredited, it has demonstrated that it meets standards set by organizations representing the academic community, professionals, and other stakeholders. To become accredited, an institution or program voluntarily undergoes an investigation of its services, management, and other practices by a professional organization that specializes in accreditation. For hospitals, this may include the Joint Commission (JC). For a comprehensive rehabilitation program, there's the Commission on Accreditation of Rehabilitation Facilities (CARF). Accreditation tells patients the provider is committed to providing high-quality care.
activities of daily living	ADLs	ADLs are activities that are oriented toward taking care of your own body on a daily basis. The activities are broken down into nine areas. • Bathing/showering • Toileting and toilet hygiene • Dressing • Eating/swallowing • Feeding (setting up, arranging, and bringing food to the mouth) • Functional mobility (the ability to get from place to place while performing ADLs either under one's own power or with the assistance of a walker, wheelchair, or other assistive device) • Personal device care (utilizing essential personal care items, such as hearing aids, contact lenses, glasses, orthotics, a walker, etc.) • Personal hygiene and grooming • Sexual activity

| acute care in a hospital | | This is defined as a level of care in a hospital where a person receives active and short-term treatment for a severe new injury or a new onset of an episode of illness (health plans often say within the last seven days), an emergent or urgent medical condition, or care during recovery from surgery that requires an overnight hospital stay and one that cannot be performed in an outpatient setting.

Acute care is a diverse group of medical specialties, but it can be organized into a few different types.

• *Emergency care.* Emergency care is any acute treatment that is administered for a life- or limb-threatening illness or injury. It may also be used to treat illnesses or injuries that are causing severe pain or may lead to serious consequences if not addressed immediately.
• *Urgent care.* This is a type of outpatient or ambulatory care that is administered from a clinic rather than an emergency room and that typically does not require an appointment. Urgent care is used for pressing but not emergency health care needs.
• *Trauma and acute surgery.* Acute surgery is used to treat patients with immediate needs, such as the removal of the appendix before it bursts. It may also be used for treating traumatic injuries, like internal bleeding after a car accident. |

		• *Prehospital care.* This is care provided for a patient before they arrive at the hospital. It may be emergency care administered by paramedics or emergency medical technicians (EMTs), or it may be evaluation by an urgent care or other doctor, who then decides to transfer the patient to the hospital. • *Critical and intensive care.* Intensive or critical care units are typically found in hospitals and are used to treat and monitor patients who have life-threatening conditions but do not require emergency treatment. Patients are often transitioned from emergency to critical care after emergency treatment. • *Short-term stabilization.* This is a type of care that is used to stabilize a patient ahead of the actual treatment. For example, a patient may need to be stabilized and hydrated.
acute onset versus sub-acute or chronic		Acute onset in reference to a disease happens suddenly, and acute often also connotes an illness that is of short duration, rapidly progressive, and in need of urgent care. *Acute* is a measure of the time scale of a disease and is in contrast to *subacute* and *chronic. Subacute* indicates longer duration or less rapid change. *Chronic* indicates indefinite duration or virtually no change.

Adaptive clothing		This is clothing that is easy for you to put on your loved one, as it has concealed snaps or hooks on key donning sites, such as arm holes, pant openings for legs, or openings in the crotch area for ease of toileting or changing soiled diapers. Many large chain stores, such as JCPenney and Target, and other clothing providers have a variety of clothing not only for adult women and men but also for children, many of which allow the consumer to purchase such online.
adaptive equipment		Assistive and adaptive equipment is any kind of tool or device that can simplify caregiving or make the environment safer for a person who is ill, disabled, or elderly. Medical and assistive devices make navigating the home and performing daily tasks easier for those with mobility, vision, or hearing impairment. They can include but are not limited to mobility aids, grab bars, alarm systems, adaptive phones, and shower seats. For eating, there are such devices as plate guards or special handles for silverware; and for dressing, sock pullers, zipper pulls, and so forth.
administrative law judge	ALJ	One is used as the final and fifth level of appeal when either Medicare or a Medicare Advantage health plan denies an item or service, and the party filing the appeal appeals the decision by requesting an administrative law judge (ALJ) hearing. In order to request a hearing by an ALJ, the amount remaining in controversy must meet the threshold requirement. This amount may change each year. For example, for 2023, the amount in controversy is $180 (reference: Medicare).

admission date		This is the day on which a person is formally admitted to a hospital as an inpatient, and the physician has not only written the order, but it is also signed and dated. It is the first inpatient day the patient is receiving services.
admission status		Your hospital status, whether you're an inpatient or an outpatient, affects how much you pay for hospital services, like X-rays, drugs, and lab tests. Your hospital status may also affect whether Medicare or your health plan will cover care you get in a skilled nursing facility (SNF) following your hospital stay. • You are an inpatient starting when you are formally admitted to the hospital with a doctor's order. • The day before you are discharged is your last inpatient day. • You are an outpatient if you're getting emergency department services, observation services, outpatient surgery, lab tests, X-rays, or any other hospital services; and the doctor hasn't written an order to admit you to a hospital as an inpatient. In these cases, you are an outpatient even if you spend the night in the hospital.

		If you or your loved one has their health care paid by Medicare or a Medicare plan, it is especially important you ask your or their status to see if it is an inpatient or observation. If observation, this means Medicare considers this to be outpatient care. Thus, if you do not have a secondary health plan, you will be financially responsible for 20 percent of the bill. To assist you to further understand, you may want to visit the Medicare.gov publication site and type in the "Are You a Hospital Inpatient or Outpatient—If You Have Medicare—Ask" and download the brochure.
admitting physician or doctor		An admitting physician is a doctor on staff at the hospital and one who has privileges to practice within the hospital. While one physician may be the admitting doctor, they often are not the one who may be considered the attending physician.
advance beneficiary notice	ABN	An advance beneficiary notice (ABN), also known as a waiver of liability, is a notice a provider should give you before you receive a service if, based on Medicare coverage rules, your provider has reason to believe Medicare will not pay for the service. The ABN allows you to decide whether to get the care in question and to accept financial responsibility for the service (pay for the service out of pocket) if Medicare denies payment. The notice must list the reason why the provider believes Medicare will deny payment.
advance directives	AD	Advance directives are legal documents that provide instructions for medical care and only go into effect if you cannot communicate your own wishes. Advance care planning is not just for people who are very old or ill. At any age, a medical crisis could leave you unable to communicate your own health care decisions.

<table>
<tr><td></td><td></td><td>

The two most common advance directives for health care are the living will and the durable power of attorney for health care.

- *Living will.* A living will is a legal document that tells doctors how you want to be treated if you cannot make your own decisions about emergency treatment. In a living will, you can say which common medical treatments or care you would want, which ones you would want to avoid, and under which conditions each of your choices applies.
- *Durable power of attorney for health care.* A durable power of attorney for health care is a legal document that names your health care proxy, a person who can make health care decisions for you if you are unable to communicate these yourself. Your proxy, also known as a representative, surrogate, or agent, should be familiar with your values and wishes. A proxy can be chosen in addition to or instead of a living will. Having a health care proxy helps you plan for situations that cannot be foreseen, such as a serious car accident or stroke.

</td></tr>
</table>

<table>
<tr><td></td><td></td><td>

Other types of advance directives may include the following:

- *Do not resuscitate (DNR) order.* A DNR becomes part of your medical chart to inform medical staff in a hospital or nursing facility that you do not want CPR or other life support measures to be attempted if your heartbeat and breathing stop. Sometimes, this document is referred to as a do not attempt resuscitation order or an allow natural death (AND) order. Even though a living will may state that CPR is not wanted, it is helpful to have a DNR order as part of your medical file if you go to a hospital. Posting a DNR next to your hospital bed may avoid confusion in an emergency. Without a DNR order, medical staff will attempt every effort to restore your breathing and the normal rhythm of your heart.
- *Do not intubate (DNI) order.* A similar document, a DNI informs medical staff in a hospital or nursing facility that you do not want to be on a ventilator.
- *Do not hospitalize (DNH) order.* A DNH indicates to long-term care providers, such as nursing home staff, that you prefer not to be sent to a hospital for treatment at the end of life.
- *Out-of-hospital DNR order.* An out-of-hospital DNR alerts emergency medical personnel to your wishes regarding measures to restore your heartbeat or breathing if you are not in a hospital.

</td></tr>
</table>

		• *Physician Orders for Life Sustaining Treatment (POLST) and Medical Orders for Life Sustaining Treatment (MOLST) forms.* These forms provide guidance about your medical care that health care professionals can act on immediately in an emergency. They serve as a medical order in addition to your advance directive. Typically, you create a POLST or MOLST when you are near the end of life or critically ill and understand the specific decisions that may need to be made on your behalf. These forms may also be called portable medical orders or physician orders for scope of treatment (POST). Check with your state department of health to find out if these forms are available where you live.
advocacy		In health care, advocacy means promoting the desired goal of a person or group. A health care advocate can help you express your wishes, concerns, and needs to your health care providers. Your family, guardians, care partners, and friends may serve as your health care advocates. An advocate can also be a professional you hire to partner with you to understand and promote either your own or your loved one's health care goals. Thus, in the role of a caregiver, you will often have to assume an advocacy role, especially if your loved one is a child or is an adult who has impaired thought processes.
Affordable Care Act	ACA	The Patient Protection and Affordable Care Act (commonly called the ACA) was a federal act signed into law in 2010. This act addresses access, quality, and cost in the health care industry (https://www.healthcare.gov/glossary/affordable-care-act/).

against medical advice	AMA	This is when a patient leaves the hospital before the health care team makes the discharge official.
allowed amount		This term refers to the maximum reimbursement the member's health plan policy allows for a specific service. It is the maximum dollar amount assigned for a procedure based on various pricing mechanisms. Allowed amounts are generally based on the rate specified by the insurance company. This amount may be (a) a fee negotiated with participating providers, (b) an allowance established by law, and (c) an amount set on a fee schedule of allowance.
ambulatory care facility	ACF	This is a medical care center that provides a wide range of health care services, including acute care, surgery, and outpatient services, such as infusion therapy and rehabilitation therapies—all in a centralized facility.
Americans with Disabilities Act	ADA	The Americans with Disabilities Act (ADA) protects people with disabilities from discrimination. Disability rights are civil rights. From voting to parking, the ADA is a law that protects people with disabilities in many areas of public life and describes what a health care disability means.

American Medical Association	AMA	"The American Medical Association (AMA) is the largest and only national association that convenes 190+ state and specialty medical societies and other critical stakeholders. Throughout history, the AMA has always followed its mission: to promote the art and science of medicine and the betterment of public health. As the physicians' powerful ally in patient care, the AMA delivers on this mission by representing physicians with a unified voice in courts and legislative bodies across the nation, removing obstacles that interfere with patient care, leading the charge to prevent chronic disease and confront public health crises, and driving the future of medicine to tackle the biggest challenges in health care and training the leaders of tomorrow."
ambulatory surgery center	ASC	A center that specializes in performing various types of surgeries, the Centers for Medicare and Medicaid has designed not to be on its Inpatient Only listing, and it is anticipated the patient can be discharged without an overnight hospital stay. While the Inpatient Only listing is a document developed for Medicare, it is a list used by many health plans to help determine the right place for surgery to be performed.
American Sign Language	ASL	American Sign Language (ASL) is the primary language of the deaf community in North America. It uses a combination of hand movements, facial expressions, and body posture.

ancillary services		Ancillary services are supportive or diagnostic measures that supplement and support a primary physician, nurse, or other health care provider in treating a patient. Some examples of ancillary services include imaging tests (e.g., X-rays, MRI, CT scan, and ultrasound), lab tests, pharmacies, and physical therapy. Ancillary services are typically found in medical offices, hospitals, or free-standing diagnostic testing facilities. Additionally, a patient may have to go to a separate facility to receive ancillary services. For example, a primary care physician may refer a patient to an imaging center for an X-ray.
ankle-foot orthosis	AFO	This is any of a class of external orthopedic appliances, braces, or splints devised to control, limit, or assist foot and ankle motion and provide leg support. Typically, orthotics are made of lightweight materials, such as thermoplastics.
appeal process		This is the reconsideration of a denial issued by your health plan. If your health insurer refuses to pay a claim or ends your coverage, you have the right to appeal the decision and have it reviewed by a third party. The health plan may deny a claim for many reasons, including the following: • The treatment or service is not deemed medically necessary or appropriate. • The plan does not cover the treatment, service, medication, or goods. • The health care provider is not in your loved one's provider network, and there is no letter of agreement between the health plan and the provider submitting the claim.

| | | <ul><li>Your loved one's health plan requires preauthorization or a referral from their primary care physician.</li><li>The treatment is considered investigational or experimental.</li><li>Your loved one's health plan coverage has lapsed, or they are not enrolled with the insurer any longer.</li><li>A paperwork or data entry error (often a diagnosis or procedure code) is missing and prevents the claim from being processed correctly.</li><li>The claim was not filed on time.</li></ul>All health plan insurers have an appeal process you can follow, so one of the first things to do is contact them and request a reconsideration of its decision. Insurers must tell you why they have denied your claim or ended your coverage, and they must let you know how you can dispute their decisions. Challenging a coverage denial by a health insurance plan is a legal right guaranteed to all insured individuals. Every plan, including private policies, employer-sponsored health plans, Medicare, Medicare medication plans, and Medicaid, must provide a process for reconsideration of any adverse determination of coverage by the plan. There are two ways to appeal a health plan decision.<ul><li>*Internal appeal.* If your claim is denied or your health insurance coverage is canceled, you have the right to an internal appeal. You may ask your insurance company to conduct a full and fair review of its decision. If the case is urgent, your insurance company must speed up this process.</li></ul> |

<table>
<tr><td></td><td></td><td>

• *External review.* You have the right to take your appeal to an independent third party for review. This is called external review. External review means that the insurance company no longer gets the final say over whether to pay a claim.

Most health plans only offer two (2) internal levels of appeal; Medicare allows five (5) levels of appeal. If you or your loved one has Kaiser Permanente, Kaiser only allows for arbitration. The five levels of appeal for either the original Medicare or for a Medicare Advantage plan are as follows:

Level 1: Reconsideration by the health plan
Level 2: Review by an independent review entity (IRE) level
Level 3: Decision by the Office of Medicare Hearings and Appeals (OMHA)
Level 4: Review by the Medicare Appeals Council
Level 5: Judicial review by a federal district court

</td></tr>
</table>

appeal process timelines		Your internal appeal must be completed within thirty days if the appeal is for a service your loved one has not received yet. If your appeal is for a service your loved one has already received, the appeal must be completed within sixty days. You can file an expedited appeal if the timeline for the standard appeal process would seriously jeopardize your loved one's life or their ability to regain maximum function. An expedited appeal is used when you need urgent medical care. In this case, the decision must be made within seventy-two hours. The expedited appeal process can be used if you are hospitalized, and if your health plan is a Medicare plan, you will be given a letter called the Important Message from Medicare that you are to be discharged. Yet if you feel you or your loved one is not ready, you can appeal and be allowed to stay in the hospital while awaiting a decision. At the end of the internal appeals process, your health plan must provide you with a written decision. If your insurance company still denies you the service or payment for a service, you can ask for an external review. The insurance company's final determination must tell you how to ask for an external review.
assisted living		Basically, assisted living is for people who can live independently but need assistance with some of the tasks of daily living, such as cooking and cleaning.
assisted living facility	ALF	An assisted living facility can provide a wide array of services and services, and these might include the following: • Resident dining serving three meals daily • Medication management

		• Weekly housekeeping, laundry, and linen services • Emergency 24-7 call system with on-site staff response • Social, spiritual, recreational, and educational programs • Transportation Assisted living facilities do not provide medical care or skilled nursing care. Each state has its own requirements for regulating this type of facility. The cost of assisted living is not covered by medical insurance or Medicaid and is either paid by private individuals and their family or a long-term care insurance policy, if premiums are current.
assisted living technology		Assisted living (or assistive) technologies include telehealth (remote monitoring for clinical biomarkers) and telecare (for example, alarms, sensors, or voice-activated reminders), designed to deliver health and social care services to the home.
augmentative or alternative communication devices	ACC	An AAC might be either augmentative when it is used to supplement existing speech or alternative when it is used in place of speech that is absent or not functional. AAC means all the ways someone communicates besides talking. People of all ages can use AAC if they have trouble with speech or language skills. Augmentative means to add to someone's speech. Alternative means to be used instead of speech.

autism spectrum disorder	ASD	Autism spectrum disorder (ASD) is a developmental disability that can cause significant social, communication, and behavioral challenges. A diagnosis of ASD now includes several conditions that used to be diagnosed separately: autistic disorder, pervasive developmental disorder not otherwise specified, and Asperger's syndrome.
autoimmune diseases		Autoimmune disease happens when the body's natural defense system can't tell the difference between your own cells and foreign cells, causing the body to mistakenly attack normal cells. There are more than eighty types of autoimmune diseases that affect a wide range of body parts.
auxiliary aids and services		Auxiliary aids and services are terms identified under the Americans with Disabilities Act (ADA), and they refer to the ways to communicate with people who have communication disabilities. • For people who are blind, who have vision loss, or who are deaf-blind, this includes providing a qualified reader, information in large print, braille, electronically for use with a computer screen reading program, or an audio recording of printed information. A qualified reader means someone who is able to read effectively, accurately, and impartially using any necessary specialized vocabulary.

		<ul><li>For people who are deaf, who have hearing loss, or who are deaf-blind, this includes providing a qualified notetaker, a qualified sign language interpreter, an oral interpreter, a cued-speech interpreter, a tactile interpreter, real-time captioning, written materials, or a printed script of a stock speech, such as what is given on a museum or historic house tour. A qualified interpreter means someone who is able to interpret effectively, accurately, and impartially both receptively (i.e., understanding what the person with the disability is saying) and expressively (i.e., having the skill needed to convey information back to that person) using any necessary specialized vocabulary.</li><li>For people who have speech disabilities, this may include providing a qualified speech-to-speech translator (a person trained to recognize unclear speech and repeat it clearly), especially if the person will be speaking at length, such as giving testimony in court, or just taking more time to communicate with someone who uses a communication board. In some situations, keeping paper and pencil on hand so the person can write out words that staff cannot understand or simply allowing more time to communicate with someone who uses a communication board or device may provide effective communication. Staff should always listen attentively and not be afraid or embarrassed to ask the person to repeat a word or phrase they do not understand.</li></ul>

aversion		This means a strong dislike or opposition.
balance billing		Balance billing is when a health care provider bills you the difference between their charge and what the health plan paid. If you visit a preferred provider, that provider isn't allowed to balance bill because in-network providers have an agreement with the insurance company to provide services for the agreed-upon amount.
basic life support (BLS) ambulance versus advanced life support (ALS) ambulance		Basic life support (BLS) is transportation by ground ambulance vehicle and the provision of medically necessary supplies and services. For BLS, the ambulance must be staffed by an individual who is qualified in accordance with state and local laws as an emergency medical technician-basic (EMT-B). These laws may vary from state to state or within a state. For example, only in some jurisdictions is an EMT-B permitted to operate limited equipment onboard the vehicle, assist more qualified personnel in performing assessments and interventions, and establish a peripheral intravenous (IV) line. Advanced life support level 1 (ALS-1) is the transportation by ground ambulance vehicle and the provision of medically necessary supplies and services, including the provision of an ALS assessment or at least one ALS intervention. Advanced life support level 2 (ALS-2) is the transportation by ground ambulance vehicle and the provision of medically necessary supplies and services, including (1) at least three separate administrations of one or more medications by intravenous push/bolus or by continuous infusion (excluding crystalloid fluids) or (2) ground ambulance transport, medically necessary supplies and services, and the provision of at least one of the ALS-2 procedures listed below. a) Manual defibrillation/cardioversion b) Endotracheal intubation

		c) Central venous line d) Cardiac pacing e) Chest decompression f) Surgical airway.
bedbound		*Bedbound* is a synonym of *bedridden*. It is when a person is bedridden or confined to bed because of infirmity or illness and is unable to leave one's bed for some reason.
behavioral health	BH	This is the provision of mental health services.
beneficiary		This is a term used by CMS and means the same as a health plan may term a person who is insured by them. The term health plans use will be *member*.
beneficiary notice imitative	BNI	Both Medicare beneficiaries and providers have certain rights and protections related to financial liability and appeals under the fee-for-service (FFS) Medicare and the Medicare Advantage (MA) programs. These financial liability and appeal rights and protections are communicated to beneficiaries through notices (written letters) given by providers. The various beneficiary notices can be found on the Centers for Medicare and Medicaid Services BNI website. The site lists the various letters you or your loved one may receive and its purpose. It also allows you to view a sample of the notice.
best prac-tice		A best practice is a method or technique that has been generally accepted as superior to other known alternatives because it often produces results that are superior to those achieved by other means or because it has become a standard way of doing things (e.g., a standard way to perform nursing care or other health care procedures).

birthday rule		Created by the National Association of Insurance Commissioners (NAIC), the birthday rule is a method many insurance companies use to determine when a plan is primary or secondary for a dependent child covered by both parents' insurance plans. States and insurers can use different approaches, but most have adopted the birthday rule as a uniform, unbiased means of determining primary and secondary coverage in situations where a child has coverage under both parents' plans. This means whichever parent has the first birthday date or year.
board and care	B&C	Board and care homes, also known as residential care homes, group homes, or foster care homes, are a type of assisted living facility that offers personal assistance with basic daily tasks. They often tend to be set up in a homelike setting in a single-family home with around six beds and public areas for everyone to share, each offering services dependent on how licensed. Most will have available semiprivate or private rooms, and they will provide meals and laundry services, 24-7 supervision of residents, assistance with medications, and transportation to and from medical appointments. If they are licensed, they can provide services for mental health conditions, psychiatric assistance or monitoring, and dispensation of medications to residents. Licensure for nonmental health conditions can include non-bedbound and bedbound, and some also have a hospice waiver. States vary as to what agency licenses such facilities.
board certified		Health care professionals seeking board certification in a given area of specialty must successfully complete and pass an examination process designed to test their mastery of the minimum knowledge and skills contained in the core competency document for their licensure.

body mechanics		Body mechanics are the way you move during daily activities. Proper body mechanics can help you avoid injury and muscle fatigue, and if you are a caregiver, it is critical you have someone (preferably a physical therapist) show you proper body mechanics for moving your loved one about.
bowel and bladder	B&B	These are body organs for elimination of feces (poop) and urine (pee).
Braden Scale		This is a tool for assessing pressure ulcer risk.
Bright Future		Bright Future is a national health promotion and prevention initiative led by the American Academy of Pediatrics (AAP) and supported in part by the US Department of Health and Human Services, Health Resources and Services Administration (HRSA), and Maternal and Child Health Bureau. Bright Futures guidelines provide theory and evidence-driven guidance for all preventative care screenings and health supervision visits.
caregiver		A caregiver is a person who tends to the needs or concerns of a person with short- or long-term limitations due to illness, injury, or disability. The term "family caregiver" describes individuals who care for members of their family of origin but also refers to those who care for their family of choice. This could be members of their congregation, neighbors, or close friends. Family caregivers play a significant role in health care, as they are often the main source of valuable information about the patient.

care plan		A care plan is a legal document that contains an assessment of a patient's needs and details the level of care and services that he should receive. It is used to coordinate the care given to the patient by different members of the health care team. It is also important that the services to be provided include short- and long-term goals. This plan will be one any one of your loved one's case managers will develop.
cardiac rehabilitation		Cardiac rehab is a medically supervised program designed to improve your cardiovascular health if you or your loved one has experienced a heart attack, heart failure, angioplasty, or heart surgery. Cardiac rehab has three equally important parts: (a) exercise counseling and training, (b) education for heart-healthy living, and (c) counseling to reduce stress. The Department of Health and Human Services (hhs.gov) has a great tip sheet on their site millionhearts.hhs.gov website you may want to review as it contains a wealth of information. Million Hearts is a national initiative led by the Centers for Disease Control and Prevention and the Centers for Medicare and Medicaid Services (CMS).

case man-agement	CM	The definition of case management is the planning, processing, and monitoring of the health care services given to a patient; and it is to provide for a patient's needs while controlling costs. Case management is an area of specialty practice within the health and human services professions. Its underlying premise is that everyone benefits when clients reach their optimum level of wellness, self-management, and functional capability. The case manager helps identify appropriate providers and facilities throughout the continuum of services while ensuring that available resources are being used in a timely and cost-effective manner in order to obtain optimum value for both the client and the reimbursement source.
catatonia		Catatonia is a neuropsychiatric condition that affects both behavior and motor function and results in unresponsiveness in someone who otherwise appears to be awake. For the purpose of diagnosis, there are three types of catatonia, including catatonia associated with another mental disorder, catatonia disorder due to another medical condition, and unspecified catatonia. Although often associated with schizophrenia and other affective disorders, catatonia may be a result of or due to any number of psychotic disorders, mood disorders, or general medical conditions. This website contains a wealth of information on types of catatonia, causes, symptoms, and treatments.

Centers for Medicare and Medicaid Services and the Food and Drug Administration	CMS and FDA	CMS and FDA are both regulatory agencies that focus on evidence-driven delivery of health care products and services. However, the FDA ensures proper regulation of the marketing and use of pharmaceutical products and medical products while CMS regulates the reimbursement practices for health care products and services through Medicare and Medicaid.
Certificate of medical necessity	CMN	A certificate of medical necessity (CMN) or a DME information form (DIF) is a form required to help document the medical necessity and other coverage criteria for selected durable medical equipment, prosthetics, orthotics, and supplies (DMEPOS). CMNs must be completed by both the provider and by the ordering physician. In most cases, it does not require a narrative description of equipment or a physician's signature.
certification for health care professionals		Certification demonstrates that the health care professional possesses the education, skills, knowledge, and experience required to render appropriate services delivered according to sound principles of practice.
chronic		A lasting or prolonged illness or symptom.

chronic disease		Chronic diseases are defined broadly as conditions that last one year or more and require ongoing medical attention or limit activities of daily living or both. Chronic diseases, such as heart disease, cancer, and diabetes, are the leading causes of death and disability in the United States. To read more on how to prevent chronic disease, the CDC offers some tips on the topic. If you or your loved one has one or more chronic diseases, one of your best resources will be to talk with your physician about a referral to the palliative care team in your area. The palliative care approach is to teach you how to live and manage the symptoms of a chronic disease.
claim		This is an itemized statement of health care services and their costs provided by a hospital, physician's office, or other provider facility. Claims are submitted to the health plan or managed care plan by either the plan member or the provider for payment of the costs incurred.
claim denial versus rejected claim		A health insurance company may deny a claim for many reasons, including the following: • The treatment or service is not deemed medically necessary or appropriate. • The plan does not cover the treatment, service, medication, or goods. • The health care provider is not in your plan's network. • Your insurer requires preauthorization or a referral from your primary care physician. • The treatment is considered investigational or experimental. • Your coverage has lapsed, or you aren't enrolled with the insurer any longer.

<table>
<tr><td></td><td></td><td>

- A paperwork or data entry error prevented the claim from being processed correctly.
- The claim was not filed on time.

A denied claim is different from a rejected claim. Here are the differences.

- A denied claim is one that the insurer finds is not payable. These claims may be unpayable because of vital errors, or they violate the provider's contract.
- A rejected claim has one or more errors discovered before the claim is processed, often because there is missing or incomplete information on the claim form.

Patients or providers are typically informed about a denied claim through a mailed or emailed explanation of benefits (EOB) or electronic remittance advice. Insurers will usually explain why they deny a claim when they send the denied claim back to the submitting party. Most denied claims can be appealed. Rejected claims must be corrected and resubmitted by you or your health care provider. If they are eventually denied, rejected claims most likely can be appealed.

</td></tr>
</table>

clinical practice guidelines		Clinical practice guidelines are collated by the National Guideline Clearinghouse. This allows access by health care providers to stay current on what the standard of care is for their area. A standard of care in one community will not necessarily be the same standard in another. Further, one health care provider's standard can vary from another health care provider's standard. If you want to research the clinical practice guidelines for a disease, condition, treatment, or intervention or for health services administration, you can browse them on a website that is maintained by the Agency for Healthcare Research and Quality, which is part of the US Department of Health and Human Services.
clinical trial		Clinical trials are designed for research studies performed in people who are aimed at evaluating a medical, surgical, or behavioral intervention. They are not a source of income for any caregiving needs, nor will your loved one's health plan cover any costs related to the trial. All costs related to the trial are the financial responsibility of the sponsor of the trial. Clinical trials are the primary way that researchers find out if a new treatment, like a new drug or diet or medical device (for example, a pacemaker), is safe and effective on people. Often, a clinical trial is used to learn if a new treatment is more effective or has less harmful side effects than the standard treatment. Clinical trials of drugs are usually described based on their phase. The FDA typically requires phase I, II, and III trials to be conducted to determine if the drug can be approved for use. • A phase I trial tests an experimental treatment on a small group of often healthy people (twenty to eighty) to judge its safety and side effects and to find the correct drug dosage.

		• A phase II trial uses more people (one hundred to three hundred). While the emphasis in Phase I is on safety, the emphasis in Phase II is on effectiveness. This phase aims to obtain preliminary data on whether the drug works in people who have a certain disease or condition. These trials also continue to study safety, including short-term side effects. This phase can last several years. • A phase III trial gathers more information about safety and effectiveness, studying different populations and different dosages, using the drug in combination with other drugs. The number of subjects usually ranges from several hundred to about three thousand people. If the FDA agrees that the trial results are positive, it will approve the experimental drug or device. • A phase IV trial for drugs or devices takes place after the FDA approves their use. A device or drug's effectiveness and safety are monitored in large, diverse populations. Sometimes, the side effects of a drug may not become clear until more people have taken it over a longer period of time.

Code of Federal Regulations	CFR	The Code of Federal Regulations (CFR) is the codification of the general and permanent rules published in the *Federal Register* by the executive departments and agencies of the federal government. It is divided into fifty titles that represent broad areas subject to federal regulation. Each volume of the CFR is updated once each calendar year and is issued on a quarterly basis. The Code of Federal Regulations (CFR) are created to carry out regulations (rules) under the authority of Congress to help the government carry out public policy.
cognition		Cognition is a term referring to the mental processes involved in gaining knowledge and comprehension. These cognitive processes include thinking, knowing, remembering, judging, and problem-solving.
coinsurance		The percentage of coinsurance is about the maximum out-of-pocket amount that you can spend in a year, after which the company will bear the full expenses. Coinsurance refers to the percentage of a treatment cost you'll have to pay once you've paid the deductibles—the amount of money that you, as a member, pay out of pocket each year for allowed amounts for covered medical care before your health plan begins to pay. This is usually a fixed percentage and is like co-payment. Features of coinsurance are the following: a. Policyholders will have to pay the deductible before claiming coinsurance b. The percentage is fixed.

comfort care		The National Hospice and Palliative Care Organization defines comfort care as care that is focused on symptom control, pain relief, and quality of life. Confusingly, the term is often used interchangeably with palliative care and hospice care. It may be part of either one but doesn't accurately describe the entire offering of either. Their website offers a wealth of information on hospice, palliative care, curative or therapeutic care, comfort care, and bereavement care.
Commission on Accreditation of Rehabilitation	CARF	An independent, nonprofit organization founded in 1966 as the Commission on Accreditation of Rehabilitation Facilities, CARF International is an independent, nonprofit accreditor of health and human services in the following areas: • Aging Services • Behavioral Health • Child and Youth Services • Employment and Community Services • Visio Rehabilitation Services • Medical Rehabilitation • Opioid Treatment Program CARF provides accreditation services worldwide at the request of health and human service providers, whether one is seeking rehabilitation for a disability, treatment for addiction and substance abuse, home and community services, retirement living, or other health and human services. Providers that meet CARF standards have demonstrated that facilities have commitment to being among the best available.

common assessment scales used to measure pain		A pain scale measures a patient's pain intensity or other features. Pain scales are a necessity to assist with better assessment of pain and patient screening. Pain measurements help determine the severity, type, and duration of the pain and are used to make an accurate diagnosis, determine a treatment plan, and evaluate the effectiveness of treatment. The most common pain scales are the numeric system, where one describes pain on a scale of 1–10, and the Wong-Baker Faces Pain Rating Scale. There are other scales one may use, which are found on the Verywell website.
complaint		A grievance is a complaint you make about a health plan or one of its network providers or pharmacies. This includes a complaint about the quality of your care. Health plans have special procedures in place to help members who file grievances. Filing a complaint will not change your health care services or your benefits coverage. You may want to file a grievance if • your provider or an employee did not respect your rights; • you had trouble getting an appointment with your provider in a reasonable amount of time; • you were unhappy with the care or treatment you received; • your provider or an employee was rude to you; • your provider or an employee did not respect your cultural needs or other special needs you may have; • your provider does not give you the service in a timely manner; and • your provider or the health plan does not answer your appeal in a timely manner.

com-pounded drugs		Drug compounding is often regarded as the process of combining, mixing, or altering ingredients to create a medication tailored to the needs of an individual patient. Compounding includes the combining of two or more drugs. Compounded drugs are not FDA-approved. A drug may be compounded for a patient who cannot be treated with an FDA-approved medication, such as a patient who has an allergy to a certain dye and needs a medication to be made without it or an elderly patient or a child who cannot swallow a tablet or capsule and needs a medicine in a liquid dosage form.
comprehensive inpatient rehabilitation		Comprehensive inpatient rehabilitation is the most intensive therapy program available. Provided by an interdisciplinary team that works under the direction of a physiatrist, a physician who specializes in physical medicine and rehabilitation medicine, treatment includes physical therapy, occupational therapy, rehabilitation nursing, case management, and often, speech and language therapy.
comprehensive perinatal care		To ensure Title V of the Social Security Act of 1935 is followed, all fifty states offer a comprehensive perinatal program for low-income pregnant women. Most programs are provided by a regional public health clinic.
Comprehensive Outpatient Rehabilitation Facility	CORF	CORFs must provide coordinated outpatient diagnostic, therapeutic, and restorative services at a single fixed location to outpatients for the rehabilitation of injured, disabled, or sick individuals.

concurrent review		Concurrent review is a process used by a health plan whereby the patient's chart or medical record is reviewed during the care a patient is receiving during a patient's stay or course of treatment in a facility, the office of a health care professional, or other inpatient or outpatient health care setting.
Conditions of Participation and Conditions for Coverage	CoPs and CfCs	"CMS develops Conditions of Participation (CoPs) and Conditions for Coverage (CfCs) that health care organizations must meet in order to begin and continue participating in the Medicare and Medicaid programs. These health and safety standards are the foundation for improving quality and protecting the health and safety of beneficiaries. CMS also ensures that the standards of accrediting organizations recognized by CMS (through a process called 'deeming') meet or exceed the Medicare standards set forth in the CoPs. The CoPs are the "minimum health and safety standards that providers and suppliers must meet in order to be Medicare and Medicaid certified." In addition, the CoPs provide a foundation for healthcare organizations to improve and protect the quality of care administered to beneficiaries.
conservatorship		Under US law, conservatorship is the appointment of a guardian or a protector by a judge to manage the financial affairs or daily life of another person due to old age or physical or mental limitations. A person under conservatorship is a conservatee, a term that can refer to an adult. A person under guardianship is a ward, a term that can also refer to a minor child. A conservator of the person is more typically called a legal guardian. Conservatorship is established either by court order (with regard to individuals) or via a statutory or regulatory

authority (with regard to organizations, such as business entities). In other legal terms, a conservatorship may refer to the legal responsibilities over a person who has a mental illness, including individuals who are psychotic, suicidal, demented, incapacitated, or in some other way unable to make legal, medical, or financial decisions on behalf of themselves.

Conservatorship is a legal term referring to the legal responsibilities of a conservator over the affairs of a person who has been deemed gravely disabled by the court and unable to meet their basic needs of food, clothing, and shelter. They are governed by the state's individual laws. Terminology varies, and some states or jurisdictions may refer to a conservator as a guardian of the estate or as a trustee.

Conservatorships are generally put in place for people who are significantly disabled by mental illness, elderly individuals who lack mental capacity due to medical conditions, such as dementia, or individuals with developmental disabilities who lack the capacity to manage their own affairs. In typical conservatorship proceedings, an allegedly mentally incapacitated person must be evaluated by a qualified physician or psychiatrist, who prepares a report documenting the person's mental capacity that is provided to the court and may be used as evidence.

A limited conservatorship usually refers to the limited legal responsibilities of a conservator over the affairs of an individual who is developmentally disabled but still capable of making important decisions for themselves. In these cases, the conservatee to whom the limited conservatorship applies can retain more control over their personal affairs than other conservatees can; for example, they may retain their right to decide where they may live.

| contin-uum of care | | The continuum of care matches ongoing needs of the individuals with the appropriate level and type of health, medical, financial, legal, and psychosocial care for services within a setting or across multiple settings.

1. For the general acute care patient who requires ongoing care, this consists of a variety of health care service providers, such as inpatient acute rehabilitation unit, long-term acute care hospitals, subacute hospitals (adult and children), skilled nursing facilities, and home health agencies.
2. For mental health, it may include residential/community integration, home care, partial/day hospital, and intensive outpatient and traditional outpatient therapy; and many may reside in a residential care facility.

For the developmentally disabled, the goal is to keep them at the lowest level of care as possible. So many may live at home with a caregiver, or they may reside in one of four (4) levels assigned to residential care facilities, with the fourth level subdivided into levels 4A through 4I, in which staffing levels are increased to correspond to the escalating severity of disability levels. Or they may be admitted to an intermediate care facility (ICF), which includes such as an ICF-DDH (habilitation), ICF-DDN (nursing), and ICF-DDCN (complex nursing). California offers another level of care: an Adult Residential Facility for Persons with Special Health Care Needs (ARFPSHN). These are specialized homes that provide very complex care for the medically fragile, many of whom are on life-sustaining equipment. |

contrac- ture		A muscle contracture, also known as a contracture deformity, is a permanent shortening and tightening of muscle fibers that reduces flexibility and makes movement difficult. It is caused when a muscle loses elasticity. If a muscle cannot move and be stretched, the nearby joints also lose mobility and become painful. While being inactive for any length of time is one of the biggest risks and causes for contracture, this inactivity is often the result of such medical conditions and the severity of the condition, such as scarring from burns or injuries, cerebral palsy, muscular dystrophy, nerve damage, stroke, central nervous system diseases, rheumatoid arthritis, and traumatic injury.
coordi- nation of benefits	COB	Coordination of benefits (COB) applies to a person who is covered by more than one health plan. The COB regulations, as well as the HIPAA Privacy Rule, permit Medicare to coordinate benefits with other health plans and payers to reduce administrative burden and enable patients to obtain payment of the maximum benefit they are allowed. The same applies in situations where Medicare is the secondary payer, and a provider must file a COB claim to Medicare. COB claims are those sent to secondary payers with claims adjudication information included from a prior or primary payer (the health plan or payer obligated to pay a claim first). These claims can be sent (1) from provider to payer to payer or (2) from provider to payer.

co-pay-ment of co-pay		This is a specified or fixed dollar amount the health plan requires to be paid out of pocket each time a specified service at the time the service is rendered. Co-pay ranges from five dollars to twenty-five dollars, and the amount you need to pay will be specified in the health plan's Evidence of Coverage (EOC) and also on the insurance card they issue that you can carry with you.
cranial prosthesis		Wig.
Current Procedural Terminol-ogy		Current Procedural Terminology, more commonly known as CPT, refers to a medical code set created and maintained by the American Medical Association. This code is used on the claims submitted for payment to the insurer. It is used by physicians, allied health professionals, nonphysician practitioners, hospitals, outpatient facilities, and laboratories to represent the services and procedures they perform.
custodial care		This is care provided primarily to assist a patient in meeting the activities of daily living but not requiring skilled nursing or rehabilitation services or care.
deci-sion-mak-ing capacity		A person's capacity to make a specific decision is their ability to • understand information and facts relevant to the decision, • retain that information long enough to make a voluntary choice, • use or weigh up that information as part of the process of making the decision, and • communicate the decision by any means, including by assistive technology.

deductible		This is a flat amount the member or beneficiary must pay before the insurer will make any benefit payments. The deductible is usually a set amount or percentage determined by the member's or beneficiary's health plan and is set for a given period of time.
dementia		This is a progressive mental disorder that affects memory, judgment and cognitive powers. One type of dementia is Alzheimer's disease.
denial		A health plan decision to not allow prior authorization if services have not occurred or to not pay a claim (called a claims denial) for services already rendered. In either case, you can file an appeal, and your physician can submit information that supports the reason services should be covered. See also appeals process and appeals process timeline.
Detailed Explanation of Non-Coverage	DENC	A notice given to a Medicare beneficiary that requests an expedited determination and explains the specific reasons for the end of covered services.
Detailed Notice of Discharge	DND	Notice given only if a beneficiary requests expedited review of a discharge decision and explains the specific reasons for the discharge.
determination or organization determination		An organization determination is any decision made by a health plan regarding 1. authorization or payment or denial of a health care item or service, 2. the amount a health plan requires a beneficiary to pay for an item or service, and 3. a limit on the quantity of items or services.

diagno-sis-related group	DRG	Medicare's DRG system is called the Medicare Severity Diagnosis Related Group, or MS-DRG, which is used to determine hospital payments under the inpatient prospective payment system (IPPS). It's the system used to classify various diagnoses for inpatient hospital stays into groups and subgroups so that Medicare can accurately pay the hospital bill.
Diagnostic and Statistical Manual of Mental Disorders	DSM-5	The DSM-5 (the last revision of the codes) is the authoritative guide for diagnosing mental health disorders in the US. It is also used internationally as a research standard. This text describes and lists the symptoms of hundreds of mental health diagnoses, conditions, and social problems. It promotes consistency and a common language among health care professionals and researchers. Each mental health diagnosis has a corresponding International Classification of Diseases (ICD) code developed by the World Health Organization (WHO). These codes are used for billing and data collection purposes.
dialysis		Dialysis is a type of treatment that helps your body remove extra fluid and waste products from your blood when the kidneys are not able to, as your loved one has been diagnosed with end-stage renal disease (ESRD). There are two type of dialysis: (1) peritoneal and (2) hemodialysis that both perform normal kidney functions, filtering waste and excess fluid from the blood. One of your best resources to explore to help you decide which method might be the best for you will be to explore the National Kidney Foundation website. Here you will find a wealth of information that will allow you to make an informed decision.

difference between coinsurance and deductible		Coinsurance refers to the percentage of treatment cost you will have to pay once you've paid the deductibles. This is usually a fixed percentage and is similar to co-payment. The deductible is the amount that you need to pay as a share toward your medical bill, upon which your policy comes into effect.
disability		It is important to remember that in the context of the ADA, *disability* is a legal term rather than a medical one. Because it has a legal definition, the ADA's definition of *disability* is different from how *disability* is defined under some other laws, such as for Social Security disability-related benefits. The ADA defines a person with a disability as a person who has a physical or mental impairment that substantially limits one or more major life activity. This includes people who have a record of such an impairment even if they do not currently have a disability. It also includes individuals who do not have a disability but are regarded as having a disability. The ADA also makes it unlawful to discriminate against a person based on that person's association with a person with a disability.
discharge planning	DCP	Discharge planning is the process of assessing the patient's needs of care after discharge from a health care facility and ensuring that the necessary services are in place before discharge. This process ensures a patient's timely, appropriate, and safe discharge to the next level of care or setting, including appropriate use of resources necessary for ongoing care.
disease management		A coordinated system of preventive, diagnostic, and therapeutic measures intended to provide cost-effective, quality health care for a patient population who have or are at risk for a specific chronic illness or medical condition. Also known as disease state management.

domestic partner-ship		Two people of the same or opposite sex who live together and share a domestic life but are not married or joined by a civil union. In some states, domestic partners are guaranteed some legal rights, like hospital visitation.
drug for-mulary		A formulary is a list of generic and brand-name prescription drugs covered by your health plan. Each health plan, including Medicare and an individual's state Medicaid plan, lists the drugs they cover, and the listing includes if the drug will require prior authorization. Medications not on the list are considered non-formulary. In most health plans, the formulary is developed by a pharmacy and therapeutics committee composed of pharmacists and physicians from various medical specialties. Each health plan, Medicare and Medicaid, has their own pharmacy review committee, and this committee reviews new and existing medications and selects drugs to be included in the health plan's formulary based on safety and how well they work. The committee then selects the most cost-effective drugs in each therapeutic class. A therapeutic class is a group of medications that treats a specific health condition or work in a certain way. Most health plan formularies have procedures to limit or restrict certain medications. This does not mean your drug may not be covered, but it may require you and your physician to submit a letter of medical necessity to your health plan on why the specific drug is the one necessary for your medical condition. Any information that would support the patient's need for the treatment should be added. This would be including any other publications supporting the letter of medical necessity, as well as any lab or test results. Providing lab results gives hard evidence of the severity of the medical condition.

| drug tiers | | Drug tiers or levels are organized as follows:

• Level or tier 1: preferred and low-cost generic drugs
• Level or tier 2: non-preferred and low-cost generic drugs
• Level or tier 3: preferred brand-name and some higher-cost generic drugs
• Level or tier 4: non-preferred brand-name drugs and some non-preferred, highest-cost generic drugs
• Level or tier 5: highest-cost drugs, including most specialty medications

Both prescription medicine and over-the-counter medicine can have brand-name and generic versions. Brand-name and generic drugs use the same active ingredients, and they have the same dosage, strength, instructions, and use. The Food and Drug Administration (FDA) requires generic drugs to be as effective as brand-name drugs. The main differences between generic and brand-name drugs are their appearance and cost. Trademark laws require generic drugs to look different from brand-name versions. Generic drugs also usually cost less than the brand-name versions. Specialty drugs tend to be high-cost drugs, often used to treat complex or rare conditions. |
| Drug Utilization Review | DUR | A health plan's pharmacy or drug utilization review program evaluates whether drugs are being used safely, effectively, and appropriately and if a drug should be added or removed from the health plan's drug formulary. |

dual eligible		The term "dual eligible" is most often used when the patient is insured by both Medicare and Medicaid, but it can also apply when the patient is • covered by their own private insurance or health maintenance organization (HMO) or managed care plan and that of their spouse, • covered by their own private insurance, which their spouse has also (i.e., the primary payer will be determined by what is called the birthday rule, meaning whichever parent has the first birthday in the year will be deemed the primary payer), • eligible for both Medicare and Medicaid, • eligible for both a private insurance and also Medicaid, • eligible for both Medicare and also a secondary insurer or third-party payer, and • eligible for public entitlement programs, such as the Title V Children with Special Health Care Needs program.
durable medical equipment	DME	Equipment and supplies ordered by a health care provider for everyday or extended use. Coverage for DME may include oxygen equipment, wheelchairs, crutches, or blood testing strips for diabetics. One of your best resources to use to educate yourself on durable medical equipment and supplies that will be covered under Medicare and even private health insurance will be to search the Medicare.gov/publications site and in the search bar type in "durable medical equipment."

efficacy		Refers to the ability of a product or treatment to provide a beneficial effect. Efficacy can refer to drugs, medical devices, surgical or medical procedures, and even public health interventions.
electronic medical record	EMR	A computerized record of a patient's clinical, demographic, and administrative data, also known as a computer-based patient record.
Emergency Medical Treatment and Labor Act	EMTALA	The Emergency Medical Treatment and Labor Act (EMTALA) was enacted in 1986 to ensure public access to emergency services regardless of ability to pay and prevent hospital dumping in the event the patient is uninsured or without the ability to pay. The act imposes specific obligations on Medicare-participating hospitals that offer emergency services to provide a medical screening examination (MSE) when a request is made for examination or treatment for an emergency medical condition (EMC), including active labor. Hospitals must then provide stabilizing treatment for patients with EMCs. If a hospital is unable to stabilize a patient within its capability or if the patient requests, an appropriate transfer should be attempted and implemented if a hospital is found that can meet the medical needs of the patient.
emergent care		This means you need immediate care or surgery when life or limb loss is possibly imminent, or you are in a mental health crisis and are in danger of self-harm.

emergency medical technician versus paramedic	EMT	Emergency medical technicians provide out-of-hospital emergency medical care and transportation for critical and emergent patients who access the emergency medical services (EMS) system. EMTs have the basic knowledge and skills necessary to stabilize and safely transport patients ranging from nonemergency and routine medical transports to life-threatening emergencies. Emergency medical technicians function as part of a comprehensive EMS response system under medical oversight. Emergency medical technicians perform interventions with the basic equipment typically found on an ambulance. Emergency medical technicians are a critical link between the scene of an emergency and the health care system. The paramedic is an allied health professional whose primary focus is to provide advanced emergency medical care for critical and emergent patients who access the emergency medical system. This individual possesses the complex knowledge and skills necessary to provide patient care and transportation. Paramedics function as part of a comprehensive EMS response under medical oversight. Paramedics perform interventions with the basic and advanced equipment typically found on an ambulance.
Employee Retirement Income Security Act	ERISA	The Employee Retirement Income Security Act of 1974 (ERISA) is a federal law that sets minimum standards for most voluntarily established retirement and health plans in private industry to provide protection for individuals in these plans. ERISA requires plans to provide participants with plan information, including important information about plan features and funding and providing fiduciary duties. (The primary duty or responsibilities

		of fiduciaries is to run the plan solely in the interest of participants and beneficiaries and for the exclusive purpose of providing benefits and paying plan expenses.) The duties also extend to those who manage and control plan assets and requires plans to establish a grievance and appeals process for participants to get benefits from their plans and gives participants the right to sue for benefits and breaches of fiduciary duty.
end-stage renal disease	ESRD	ESRD is partial or complete failure of the kidneys. Individuals with ESRD typically are on dialysis or have had a kidney transplant.
enteral therapy		Enteral therapy, commonly referred to as tube feeding, is the administration of food (formula) through a tube directly into your stomach or intestines. Enteral feeding allows a person, who is unable to eat or maintain weight, to receive optimized nutrition. To be a covered benefit of a health plan, most health plans require the formula to be your loved one's sole source of nutrition.
essential health benefits		A set of ten categories of services health insurance plans must cover under the Affordable Care Act (ACA). These include doctors' services, inpatient and outpatient hospital care, prescription drug coverage, pregnancy and childbirth, mental health services, and more. Some plans cover more services. Plans must offer dental coverage for children. Dental benefits for adults are optional.

evidence-based medicine		Evidence-based medicine is the conscientious, explicit, and reasonable use of best evidence and making decisions about the case of individual patients—a way of providing health care that is guided by a thoughtful integration of the best available scientific knowledge with clinical expertise. This approach allows the practitioner to critically assess research data, clinical guidelines, and other information resources in order to correctly identify the clinical problem, apply the most high-quality intervention, and reevaluate the outcome for future improvement.
evidence of benefits	EOB	EOB gives you information about how an insurance claim from a medical provider, such as a doctor, hospital, or lab, is paid on your behalf. The EOB will indicate that the insurer has paid some or all of the bill and how much you are responsible for paying yourself.
Evidence of Coverage	EOC	The Evidence of Coverage is a comprehensive resource guide issued by your health plan to explain your health care coverage. It explains your benefits, premiums, and cost-sharing; conditions and exclusions and any limitations of coverage; and plan rules.
Exclusive Provider Organization	EPO	An EPO typically offers a local network of providers and hospitals for enrollees to choose from and usually costs less than a PPO plan. Out-of-network care is generally not covered except in cases of emergencies. While premiums for EPOs can be lower, the restrictions around seeking in-network care are important for enrollees to consider.

expedited appeal		An expedited appeal occurs when a participant believes that his life, health, or ability to regain maximum function would be seriously jeopardized absent provision of the service in dispute. The organization will respond to the appeal as expeditiously as the participant's health condition requires but no later than seventy-two hours after it receives the appeal. The seventy-two-hour time frame may be extended by up to fourteen calendar days for either of the following reasons: 1. The participant requests the extension 2. The organization justifies the need for additional information and how the delay is in the interest of the participant
experimental or investigational		Experimental or investigational means any treatment, therapy, procedure, drug or drug usage, facility or facility usage, equipment or equipment usage, device or device usage, or supplies that are not recognized as being in accord with generally accepted professional medical standards or as being safe and effective for use in the treatment of an illness, injury, or condition at issue.
extra-contractual		Extra-contractual benefits are benefits that are given to the insured, which are not covered under the health plan. This is almost always done as a cost-saving to the health plan and is done on a case-by-case basis. Extra-contractual benefits may be offered when analysis of all relevant information, including the opinion of the member's provider(s) and cost benefit projections, indicates that such benefits will enhance member health outcomes and maximize member benefits through cost-effective, efficient use of resources. All such cases

		are reviewed on an individual basis, and the decision to offer extra-contractual benefits is at the sole discretion of the health plan. Once approved, a letter of agreement is sent to the patient and provider outlining the details of the individualized plan.
face-to-face	F2F or FTF	The Affordable Care Act (ACA) established a face-to-face (F2F) encounter requirement for certification of eligibility for Medicare home health services and some other services, such as specific durable medical equipment, by requiring the certifying physician to document that he or a nonphysician practitioner working with the physician has seen the patient. The encounter must occur within ninety days prior to the start of care or within thirty days after the start of care.
Family and Medical Leave Act	FMLA	A federal law that was enacted in 1993 to grant family and temporary medical leave under certain circumstances. The FMLA entitles eligible employees of covered employers to take unpaid, job-protected leave for specified family and medical reasons with continuation of group health insurance coverage under the same terms and conditions as if the employee had not taken leave. Eligible employees are entitled to twelve workweeks of leave in a twelve-month period for the following: • the birth of a child and to care for the newborn child within one year of birth • the placement with the employee of a child for adoption or foster care and to care for the newly placed child within one year of placement • to care for the employee's spouse, child, or parent who has a serious health condition

		<ul><li>a serious health condition that makes the employee unable to perform the essential functions of his job</li><li>any qualifying exigency arising out of the fact that the employee's spouse, son, daughter, or parent is a covered military member on covered active duty</li><li>to care for a covered service member with a serious injury or illness if the eligible employee is the service member's spouse, son, daughter, parent, or next of kin (military caregiver leave)</li></ul>
family practice physician		Family practice physicians are primary care providers who see patients of all ages and provide basic care for a variety of common ailments. They are usually the first to recognize major health problems, order diagnostic tests, and refer patients to specialists when needed.
fiscal intermediary		A fiscal intermediary is a business contracted by the federal government to administer a program and process its payments in a specific geographic location, such as a metro area or a state. These businesses are usually private companies that work in the insurance industry. For Medicare beneficiaries, a fiscal intermediary may make determinations on how local providers may cover a specific service or piece of medical equipment for local beneficiaries, or they may help process and resolve your Medicare appeals.
Federal Employee Health Benefit Program	FEHBP	A voluntary health insurance program for federal employees, retirees, and their dependents and survivors.

Federal Drug Administration	FDA	The Food and Drug Administration (FDA) is an agency within the US Department of Health and Human Services. It consists of the Office of the Commissioner and four directorates overseeing the core functions of the agency: Medical Products and Tobacco, Foods and Veterinary Medicine, Global Regulatory Operations and Policy, and Operations. The FDA is responsible for protecting the public health by assuring the safety, efficacy, and security of human and veterinary drugs, biological products, medical devices, our nation's food supply, cosmetics, and products that emit radiation. The FDA also provides accurate, science-based health information to the public.
federal fraud and abuse laws		The five most important federal fraud and abuse laws that apply to physicians are the following: 1. False Claims Act (FCA) 2. Anti-Kickback Statute (AKS) 3. Physician Self-Referral Law (Stark law) 4. Exclusion Authorities 5. Civil Monetary Penalties Law (CMPL) Government agencies, including the Department of Justice, the Department of Health and Human Services, the Office of Inspector General (OIG), and the Centers for Medicare and Medicaid Services (CMS), are charged with enforcing these laws.
Federal Poverty Guidelines		The Federal Poverty Guidelines are federally set poverty lines that indicate the minimum amount of annual income that an individual/family needs to pay for essentials, such as housing, utilities, clothing, food, and transportation. These guidelines, also called Federal Poverty Levels (FPLs), are based on the size of a household and the state in which one resides.

federally qualified health center	FQHC	FQHCs include community health centers, migrant health centers, health care for the homeless health centers, public housing primary care centers, and health center programs. FQHC services include physician services; services and supplies incident to the services of physicians; nurse practitioner (NP), physician assistant (PA), certified nurse-midwife (CNM), clinical psychologist (CP), and clinical social worker (CSW) services; services and supplies incident to the services of NPs, PAs, CNMs, CPs, and CSWs; Medicare Part B–covered drugs furnished by and incident to services of a FQHC practitioner; visiting nurse services to the homebound in an area where CMS determined there is a shortage of home health agencies; and outpatient diabetes self-management training (DSMT) and medical nutrition therapy (MNT) for patients with diabetes or renal disease furnished by qualified practitioners of DSMT and MNT. Some also provide dental and podiatry services. They also provide comprehensive services, either on-site or by arrangement with another provider, and they provide preventive health services, mental health and substance abuse services, and transportation services necessary for adequate patient care.
Federally Recognized Indian Tribe		Any Indian or Alaska Native tribe, Alaska Native Claims Settlement Act corporation (regional or village), band, nation, pueblo, village, rancheria, or community that the Department of the Interior acknowledges to exist as an Indian tribe. If you explore this website, you will find a wealth of information that will assist you in finding health care and services for a loved one if they are an American Indian, Alaskan native and what is available in their area.

fee-for-service	FFS	A benefit payment system in which an insurer reimburses the group member or pays the provider directly for each covered medical expense after the expense has been incurred. The original Medicare program is an example of a fee-for-service plan.
five-star rating for nursing homes		If your loved one requires placement in a nursing home, this is the rating you can use as you make your selection for care. The five-star rating was developed by the US government through the Centers for Medicare and Medicaid Services (CMS), and it offers citizens the five-star rating on over 15,000 nursing homes across the country. The system includes data on all these nursing homes, as well as a rating of between one and five stars for each so that you can get a quick view of the best facilities. A five-star rating is given when a nursing home is found to provide care that is well above average quality. A one-star rating means that the facility's care is below average in quality. In addition to the overall star rating, CMS gives each facility a separate rating for three important areas. 1. *Staffing.* The rating for staffing describes how many hours of care per day residents receive from staff on average. It takes into account the fact that some patients need more care than others. 2. *Health inspections.* Nursing homes undergo regular inspections and the health inspections score collects the resulting information from the previous three years. The rating also includes information from surveys and complaints.

		3. *Quality measures.* There are eleven separate clinical and physical measures that are used to come up with the quality measures score for a nursing home. It gives a measurement of the quality of care that residents receive in a facility.
Flexible Spending Account	FSA	Allows members to use pre-tax dollars for certain eligible medical and dependent care expenses. Members fund their FSAs with contributions that come out of their paycheck.
formulary		A listing of drugs, classified by therapeutic category or disease class, that are considered preferred therapy for a given managed population and that are to be used by an MCO's (managed care organization) providers in prescribing medications.
foot drop		Foot drop isn't a disease. Rather, it is a sign of an underlying neurological, muscular, or anatomical problem. While it can be caused by an injury to the ankle or knee or the result of a neurogenic disorder, the risk of peroneal nerve damage and foot drop increases if a person (a) sits for a prolonged period of time with their legs crossed at the knee, (b) has a cast on their leg, and (c) is on bed rest or has prolonged periods of time in bed with the weight of blankets or a bedspread resting on their toes for a prolonged period of time. Possible treatments include physical and occupational therapy to help stretch and strengthen your muscles and help you walk better braces, splints, or shoe inserts (orthotics) to help support your ankle and foot and keep it in a more natural position. In some cases, people need surgery to relieve pressure on their peroneal nerve or to try to repair it.

fraud by a health care provider		Fraud is the intentional deception to secure unfair or unlawful gain or to deprive a victim of a legal right. It is estimated that nearly $60 billion are lost annually due to health care fraud and abuse. The following are examples of health care fraud, which you may encounter and should report: • Misrepresentation of the type or level of service provided • Misrepresentation of the individual rendering service • Billing for items and services that have not been rendered • Billing for services that have not been properly documented • Billing for items and services that are not medically necessary • Seeking payment or reimbursement for services rendered for procedures that are integral to other procedures performed on the same date of service (unbundling) • Seeking increased payment or reimbursement for services that would be correctly billed at a lower rate (upcoding)
Functional Independence Measure	FIM	The Functional Independence Measure (FIM) is an instrument that was developed as a measure of disability for a variety of populations and is not specific to any diagnosis. The FIM instrument includes measures of independence for self-care, including sphincter control, transfers, locomotion, communication, and social cognition. It is an eighteen-item, seven-level ordinal scale intended to be sensitive to changes over the course of a comprehensive inpatient medical rehabilitation program, and

		it uses the level of assistance an individual needs to grade functional status from total independence to total assistance. The tool is used to assess a patient's level of disability and a change in patient status in response to rehabilitation or medical intervention.
gainfully employed		To be eligible for Social Security Disability Insurance (SSDI), a person must be unable to engage in substantial gainful activity (SGA). A person who is earning more than a certain monthly amount (net of impairment-related work expenses) is ordinarily considered to be engaging in SGA. The amount of monthly earnings considered as SGA depends on the nature of a person's disability. The Social Security Act specifies a higher SGA amount for statutorily blind individuals. Federal regulations specify a lower SGA amount for non-blind individuals. Both SGA amounts generally change with changes in the national average wage index.
generally accepted standards of medical practice		Generally accepted standards of medical practice means standards that are based upon credible scientific evidence published in peer-reviewed medical literature and generally recognized by the relevant medical community; physician and health care provider specialty society recommendations; the views of physicians and health care providers practicing in relevant clinical areas; and any other relevant factor, as determined by statute(s) and regulation(s). For these purposes, generally accepted standards of medical practice means the following: 1. Standards that are based on credible scientific evidence published in peer-reviewed medical literature generally recognized by the relevant medical community

<table>
<tr><td></td><td></td><td>

2. Physician Specialty Society recommendations
3. The views of physicians practicing in the relevant clinical area

Generally accepted standards of care are those standards that are based on credible scientific evidence and generally recognized by behavioral health experts. Some sources of generally accepted standards of care are the following:

1. American Society of Addiction Medicine (ASAM) Criteria
2. Level of Care Utilization System (LOCUS)/Child and Adolescent LOCUS (CALOCUS)
3. Child and Adolescent Service Intensity Instrument (CASII)
4. Medicare Benefit Policy Manual
5. Practice Guidelines for the Treatment of Patients with Substance Abuse Disorders
6. Practice Guidelines for the Treatment of Patients with Major Depressive Disorder
7. Principles of Care for Treatment of Children and Adolescents with Mental Illnesses in Residential Treatment Centers

A standard of care can also refer to informal or formal guidelines that are generally accepted in the medical community for the treatment of a disease or condition. It may be developed by a specialist society or organization and the title of standard of care awarded at their own discretion. It can be a clinical practice guideline or a formal diagnostic and

</td></tr>
</table>

		treatment process a healthcare provider will follow for a patient with a certain set of symptoms or a specific illness. That standard will follow guidelines and protocols that experts would agree as most appropriate, also called best, practice. Standards of care are developed in a number of ways. Sometimes, they are simply developed over time; and in other cases, they are the result of clinical trial findings.
generic drug		Generic drugs are required to have the same active ingredient, strength, dosage form, and route of administration as the brand name.
geriatrician		An expert in the branch of medicine or social science dealing with the health and care of old people.
Glasgow Coma Scale		The Glasgow Coma Scale provides a practical method for assessment of impairment of conscious level in response to defined stimuli after a head injury or trauma to the head and brain.
grievance		A complaint that you communicate to your or your loved one's health insurer or plan.
group home		Residents of group homes are typically children or adults with chronic disabilities requiring continual assistance to complete ADLs/IADLs or behavioral problems that may make them dangerous to themselves or others. These homes usually have less than eight residents who share common areas, such as kitchen, living room, and laundry facilities. And depending on the facility, some may be required to do chores, if they can.

habili-tative or habili-tation services		These are health care services that help you keep, learn, or improve skills and functioning for daily living. Examples include therapy for a child who isn't walking or talking at the expected age. These services may include physical and occupational therapy, speech-language pathology, and other services for people with disabilities in a variety of inpatient or outpatient settings.
Healthcare Common Procedural Coding System	HCPCS	HCPCS is an acronym for Healthcare Common Procedural Coding System (HCPCS). HCPCS codes is the national procedure code set for health care practitioners, providers, and medical equipment suppliers when filing health plan claims for medical devices, supplies, medications, transportation services, and other items and services.
health care proxy		A health care proxy is a document that gives someone the power to make health care decisions for a person who is unable to do so. Its purpose is to nominate someone to make one's health care decisions in the event of an illness or injury. Other names for the person nominated include proxy, agent, surrogate, or representative. On a proxy, a person names someone they trust to act on their behalf in the event of a serious injury or illness. It may work together with a living will, but it can also stand on its own. Most states give people the flexibility to decide which medical decisions they want to delegate to their representative on the proxy. While state requirements vary greatly, the American Bar Association generally recommends not choosing the following: • Your health care provider or their spouse, employee, or spouse of an employee

		• The owner or operator of your health or residential care facility or someone working for a government agency financially responsible for your loved one's care • A professional evaluating your loved one's ability to make decisions • Your loved one's court-appointed guardian or conservator • Someone who serves as a health care proxy for ten or more other people Contact your state legal aid office or state bar association to confirm your state's rules and find out if there are any other limitations on who can be your proxy. You may also pick an alternate proxy, a backup, if your primary proxy is unavailable for any reason.
Health Insurance Portability and Accountability Act	HIPAA	The Health Insurance Portability and Accountability Act of 1996 (HIPAA) is a federal law that required the creation of national standards to protect sensitive patient health information from being disclosed without the patient's consent or knowledge.
health literacy		Personal health literacy is the degree to which individuals have the ability to find, understand, and use information and services to inform health-related decisions and actions for themselves and others. Health literacy incorporates a range of abilities: reading, comprehending, and analyzing information; decoding instructions, symbols, charts, and diagrams; weighing risks and benefits; and ultimately, making decisions and taking an action.

health maintenance organization	HMO	This is a health care system that assumes or shares both the financial risks and the delivery risks associated with providing comprehensive medical services to a voluntarily enrolled population in a particular geographic area, usually in return for a fixed, prepaid fee. HMOs often have lower monthly premiums and manage care by placing restrictions around which providers enrollees can see. HMOs typically require enrollees to see in-network providers— those providers for whom the plan is directly contracted (providers not included in the plan's network are referred to as out-of-network providers). Frequently, HMOs also require enrollees to see their primary care provider and obtain a referral before seeing a specialist. Preventive care appointments, such as annual wellness visits, are fully covered. HMOs often cost less but offer fewer choices than other options.
health savings		Allows members to save money into tax-advantaged accounts. Qualified contributions made to HSAs are tax-deductible, and funds withdrawn to pay for qualified medical expenses are tax-free.
homebound		The Centers for Medicare and Medicaid Services (CMS) released a clearer definition of *homebound* to be used when deciding if patients are eligible for home health services under Medicare. Patients are considered confined to the home, or homebound, if they meet these two criteria: 1. Patients either need supportive devices, such as crutches, canes, wheelchairs, and walkers, special transportation, or help from someone else in order to leave their home because of illness or injury or a condition that makes leaving the home medically inadvisable.

		2. "There must exist a normal inability to leave home; and leaving home must require a considerable and taxing effort." Documentation from the certifying physician's medical records or the acute / post-acute care facility's medical records is used to support the certification of home health eligibility. This documentation must support the patient's need for skilled services and homebound status, and the physician must make the recommendation for home care only after having a face-to-face (F2F or FTF) visit with your loved one. The home health agencies documentation, such as the initial or comprehensive assessment of the patient, can be incorporated into the certifying physician's medical record and used to support the patient's homebound status and need for skilled care. As a rule, the home health agency should document the homebound status frequently enough to reflect the beneficiary's current functional status and at a minimum at least once per episode. It is recommended that homebound status be documented in clear, specific, and measurable terms. Documentation of the homebound status needs to be clear throughout care. Whether stated or implied, the homebound status must be obvious from a reviewer's standpoint.
home health agency care	HHA	Home health agency care is a wide range of health care services that can be given in your home for an illness or injury. Home health care is usually less expensive, more convenient, and just as effective as care you get in a hospital or skilled nursing facility (SNF). A home health agency is staffed and licensed to provide health services to individuals in their own homes.

		Home health care provides intermittent skilled care to patients in their home. Skilled nursing, physical therapy, occupational therapy, speech therapy, and medical social worker visits are services that home health agencies provide. For a patient to qualify for home health, they must be deemed homebound. To qualify as homebound, the patient must be unable to leave their home, or it would require great effort to leave.
Home Health Change of Care Notice	HHCCN	A letter or notice issued to beneficiaries receiving home health care benefits for notification of plan of care changes.
hospice care		A set of specialized health care services that provide support to terminally ill patients and their families. A system of inpatient and outpatient care, which is supportive and palliative family-centered care, designed to assist the individual with terminal illness to be comfortable and maintain satisfactory lifestyle through the end of life.
hospital readmission		A situation where you were discharged from the hospital and wind up going back in for the same or related care within thirty, sixty, or ninety days. The number of hospital readmissions is often used in part to measure the quality of hospital care since it can mean that your follow-up care wasn't properly organized or that you weren't fully treated before discharge.
hospitalist		A hospitalist is a physician who only treats or attends to patients who are in a hospital, and he does not have a practice outside the hospital either in an outpatient setting or general practice office.

hospital-ization		Care in a hospital that requires admission as an inpatient and usually requires an overnight stay with your head in a bed. An overnight stay for observation is not hospitalization but is basically outpatient care until the treating physician determines you need admission or can be discharged.
hospi-tal-issued notice of non-cover-age	HINN	Is a formal written letter issued in order to transfer financial liability to beneficiaries (your loved one) if the hospital determines that the care he receiving or is about to receive is not covered in a specific case. There are currently four different HINNs which you can review on the CMS BNI website. The four HINNs are as follows: • HINN 10, also known as the Notice of Hospital Requested Review (HRR), should be issued by hospitals to beneficiaries whenever a hospital requests Beneficiary and Family Centered Care Quality Improvement Organization (BFCC-QIO) review of a discharge decision without physician concurrence. HIINN 10 may be used for original Medicare beneficiaries or Medicare Advantage enrollees. • HINN 11 is used for noncovered items or services provided during an otherwise covered stay. • HINN 12 should be used in association with the hospital discharge appeal notices to inform beneficiaries of their potential financial liability for a noncovered continued stay. • The Preadmission/Admission HINN, used prior to an entirely noncovered stay, is also known as HINN 1

Important Message from Medicare and Detailed Letter of Discharge	IM and DND	The Important Message from Medicare is a notice your loved one will receive from the hospital to sign within two days of being admitted as an inpatient. This notice explains his rights as a patient. They will also receive another copy up to two days and no later than four hours before the discharge. Hospitals are required to deliver the Important Message from Medicare to all Medicare beneficiaries (Original Medicare beneficiaries and Medicare Advantage plan enrollees) who are hospital inpatients and have Medicare Part A. The IM informs hospitalized inpatients of their hospital discharge appeal rights. If you or your loved one files an appeal, as you do not agree with the discharge plan, the hospital must issue a Detailed Letter of Discharge (DND). The DND explains the specific reasons for the discharge. To educate yourself on the IM letter and the Detailed Letter of Discharge, you can view samples of the letters on the Beneficiary Notices Initiative (BNI) | CMS website.
immunization program		Preventive care programs designed to monitor and promote the administration of vaccines to guard against childhood illnesses, such as chicken pox, mumps, and measles, as well as adult illnesses, such as pneumonia and influenza.
in area		The geographic area in which your health plan that limit which doctors and hospitals you may use. It is generally the area where you can get routine (nonemergency) services, as the health plan has contracts in place with a wide range of providers—physician, hospitals, laboratories, and other health care providers.

inconti-nence		Loss of the ability to control when or where one eliminates waste (urine or pee or feces or poop). Incontinence can come in a variety of forms. Those that affect a person's ability to empty his bladder are classified as urinary incontinence (UI) while those that disrupt the person's ability to pass gas or stool are classified as bowel incontinence (BI).
indemnity or fee-for-service	FFS	Traditional insurance, also known as indemnity or fee-for-service, allows members to select any health care provider for services. Traditional insurance offers the most freedom of choice.
Inde-pendent Medical Review	IMR	IMRs are a right provided to health plan members as part of the Affordable Care Act (ACA) and are used to determine coverage of medical necessity, experimental or investigational treatments, preexisting conditions, and other similar issues. An independent medical review (IMR) or external review is the process where a physician not affiliated with the health care entity that denied the care or services reviews a medical case in order to provide a claims determination for health insurance payers, workers' compensation insurance payers, or disability insurance payers. To request such a review, contact your health plan's Member Services department, or you can contact your state's Department of Insurance. To find your state's Department of Insurance, it can be located on the National Association of Insurance Commissioners web link.
Indian Health Service	IHS	The Indian Health Service (IHS) is an operating division within the US Department of Health and Human Services (HHS). IHS is responsible for providing direct medical and public health services to members of federally recognized Native American tribes and

		Alaska Natives. IHS is the principal federal health care provider and health advocate for Indian people. The IHS provides health care in thirty-seven states to approximately 2.2 million out of 3.7 million American Indians and Alaska Natives. As of April 2017, the IHS consisted of twenty-six hospitals, fifty-nine health centers, and thirty-two health stations. Thirty-three urban Indian health projects supplement these facilities with a variety of health and referral services. Several tribes are actively involved in IHS program implementation. Many tribes also operate their own health systems independent of HIS. It also provides support to students pursuing medical education in order to staff Indian health programs.
informed consent		Informed consent is the process in which a health care provider educates a patient about the risks, benefits, and alternatives of a given procedure or intervention. The patient must be competent to make a voluntary decision about whether to undergo the procedure or intervention. Informed consent is both an ethical and legal obligation of medical practitioners in the US and originates from the patient's right to direct what happens to their body. Implicit in providing informed consent is an assessment of the patient's understanding, rendering an actual recommendation and documentation of the process.
in lieu of		A term used when the extra contractual process may be used to medically support the need for a requested service. Often, it is used to replace a level of care. For example, if the plan is home, the case manager may use the term "in lieu of continued stay at an acute hospital."

in network		Providers that are contracted with a health plan and offer services within a specific geographic area. Same as in area.
Inpatient Only list		Few people are aware that the Centers for Medicare and Medicaid Services (CMS) has established a list of surgeries that will be covered by Medicare Part A. Every year, CMS releases an updated Inpatient Only (IPO) surgery list. The surgeries on this list are not arbitrarily selected. The surgeries on this list are more complex and pose a higher risk for complications, and they require postoperative monitoring even if it is overnight or for a longer period of time. Other surgeries, as long as there are no complications and the person undergoing surgery does not have significant chronic conditions that put them at high risk for complications, default to Medicare Part B, and the surgery is performed in an outpatient surgery center. Thus, this affects not only how much you will pay but also where your surgery can be performed.
inpatient psychiatric services for under the age of twenty-one		"This benefit referred to as 'Psych under 21' is an optional benefit that most states have chosen to provide. Services are provided in psychiatric hospitals or psychiatric units in a hospital, or psychiatric facilities for which states may define accreditation requirements, subject to requirements at 42 CFR 441 Subpart D [a specific section in the Code of Federal Regulations]. Among the requirements for this service are certification of need for inpatient care, and a plan of care for active treatment, developed by an interdisciplinary team.

			"This benefit is significant as a means for Medicaid to cover the cost of inpatient mental health services. The federal Medicaid program does not reimburse states for the cost of institutions for mental diseases (IMDs) except for young people who receive this service, and individuals age 65 or older served in an IMD. No later than age 22, individuals are transitioned to community services, or non-Medicaid inpatient services. "Many states provide psych under 21 services through psychiatric residential treatment facilities (PRTFs). A PRTF provides comprehensive mental health treatment to children and adolescents (youth) who, due to mental illness, substance abuse, or severe emotional disturbance, need treatment that can most effectively be provided in a residential treatment facility. All other ambulatory care resources available in the community must have been identified, and if not accessed, determined to not meet the immediate treatment needs of the youth.
inpatient rehabilitation facility	IRF		An IRF is a hospital or part of a hospital that provides an intensive rehabilitation program to inpatients. Patients who are admitted must be able to tolerate an intensive level of rehabilitation services and benefit from a team approach. The IRF benefit is not to be used as a substitute to complete the full course of treatment in the referring hospital. A patient who has not yet completed the full course of treatment in the referring hospital is expected to remain there, with appropriate rehabilitative treatment provided until the full course of treatment has been completed. The medical records must sufficiently demonstrate that the admission to an IRF was reasonable and necessary.

insurance methods of pay- ment		The most common reimbursement methodologies can be described as follows: • *Indemnity.* This method pays a specific amount for services regardless of the provider or vendor. Any balance between what was billed and paid is the responsibility of the patient. • *Per diem.* This method pays for various types of care but is commonly used for hospital care or services. The incentive is to maximize days in the hospital and minimize the use of services and resources. • *DRGs or per hospital stay.* This method pays a predetermined amount for hospital or aftercare. The incentive is to do only what is appropriate or necessary. Length of stay and use of resources or other services are minimized, and if the stay is over the geometric mean length of stay (GMLOS), payment will be via an outlier methodology. • *Capitation.* This method pays a predetermined amount for all care related to resolving the problem. The incentive is on coordination of care reducing resource use and offering only necessary services in the least number of days. • *Discounted fee-for-services.* This method pays services after a negotiated rate is agreed upon between the insurer or third-party payer and a hospital or provider.

| instru-mental activities of daily living | IADLS | Instrumental activities of daily living (IADLS) refer to activities that support daily life and are oriented toward interacting with your environment. IADLs are typically more complex than ADLs. They are important components of home and community life but can be easily delegated to another person.

• Care of others
• Care of pets
• Child-rearing
• Communication management
• Driving and community mobility
• Financial management
• Health management and maintenance
• Home establishment and management
• Meal preparation and cleanup
• Religious and spiritual activities and expressions
• Safety procedure and emergency responses
• Shopping |
| Interna-tional Classifi-cation of Diseases | ICD | The International Classification of Diseases (ICD) is the classification used to code and classify mortality data from death certificates. The International Classification of Diseases, Clinical Modification is used to code and classify morbidity data from the inpatient and outpatient records, physician offices, and most National Center for Health Statistics (NCHS) surveys. The International Classification of Diseases (ICD) codes are a set of designations used by health care staff to communicate diseases, symptoms, abnormal findings, and other elements of a patient's diagnosis in a way that is universally accepted by those in the medical and insurance fields. The tenth and most recent edition is known as ICD-10. ICD-10 |

		codes are passed to insurance companies to establish the medical necessity of the services a provider is asking to be paid for. There are more than 70,000 of them, and their highly specific definitions are understood by all who use them. The 10 after ICD indicates the latest edition, which occurred in 2014.
intermediate care facility / developmentally dis-abled-habilitative intermediate care facility	ICF/DDH	"ICF/DD-H (Habilitative): 'Intermediate care facility/developmentally disabled-habilitative' is a facility with a capacity of 4 to 15 beds that provides 24-hour personal care, habilitation, developmental, and supportive health services to 15 or fewer developmentally disabled persons who have intermittent recurring needs for nursing services but have been certified by a physician and surgeon as not requiring availability of continuous skilled nursing care."
intermediate care facilities	ICF	The ICF benefit is an optional Medicaid benefit. The Social Security Act created this benefit to fund institutions (four or more beds) for individuals with intellectual disabilities and specifies that these institutions must provide active treatment, as defined by the secretary. Currently, all fifty states have at least one ICF/IID facility. This program serves over one hundred thousand individuals with intellectual disabilities and other related conditions. Most have other disabilities as well as intellectual disabilities. Many of the individuals are nonambulatory and have seizure disorders, behavior problems, mental illness, visual or hearing impairments, or a combination of the above. All must qualify for Medicaid assistance financially. Intermediate care is a level of care for patients who require more assistance than custodial care and may require nursing supervision but do not have a true skilled

		need. Most insurance companies do not cover intermediate care. Intermediate care facilities are institutions that provide health related long-term care and services to individuals who require custodial care and not the degree of care that hospitals or skilled nursing facilities provide but because of their physical or mental condition require care and services above the level of room and board.
Integrated Denial Notice	IDN	This is a letter that is issued when a Medicare health plan issues a denial, whether the denial is for all the services or only a portion of the services you receive.
Integrated Behavioral Health	IBH	Behavioral health is an umbrella term that includes mental health and substance abuse conditions, life stressors and crises, stress-related physical symptoms, and health behaviors. Behavioral health conditions often affect medical illnesses. Integrated behavioral health care blends care in one setting for medical conditions and related behavioral health factors that affect health and well-being. Integrated behavioral health care, a part of whole-person care, is a rapidly emerging shift in the practice of high-quality health care. It is a core function of the advanced patient-centered medical home. Providers practicing integrated behavioral health care recognize that both medical and behavioral health factors are important parts of a person's overall health. Medical and behavioral health clinicians work together as a team to address a patient's concerns. Care is delivered by these integrated teams in the primary care setting unless patients request or require specialty services. The advantage is better coordination and communication while working toward one set of overall health goals.

Kaiser Family Foundation	KFF	KFF (Kaiser Family Foundation) is a nonprofit organization focusing on national health issues, as well as the US role in global health policy. KFF develops and runs its own policy analysis, journalism, and communications programs, sometimes in partnership with major news organizations. KFF serves as a nonpartisan source of facts, analysis, and journalism for policymakers, the media, the health policy community, and the public. Our product is information, always provided free of charge, from the most sophisticated policy research to basic facts and numbers, in-depth health policy news coverage provided by our news service, KHN, and information young people can use to improve their health or the general public can use to understand health insurance.
letter of agreement	LOA	A letter of agreement is a formal contractual agreement between a health plan and a specific provider when the health plan does not have the health care provider needed to deliver the medically necessary services a patient requires in the health plan's provider network. The LOA will include all the terms and conditions, including the payment amount and timelines for claims submission agreed upon between the two parties.
letter of medical necessity	LMN	This is a document you and your physician can submit to your loved one's health plan when a treatment, drug, or service is either (a) medically necessary and your physician is requesting a prior authorization or (b) denied and you wish to appeal the health plan's denial of coverage. CMS has their own forms that can be completed by your physician for requesting Medicare coverage of an item or service. It is

| | | important to note here that unrelated medical history should be avoided. The last thing you want is information that has nothing to do with your medical condition and the treatment that is needed. |
| | | As your physician writes your letter, it is critical to include at least the following three sections: |

- *Medical history.* This section is for the history of symptoms related to the diagnosis; any hospitalizations or procedures related to the diagnosis should be stated in this section. If you have tried past treatment options and they failed, add a brief description of any adverse effects—whatever key information that can help support the need for the requested or denied treatment, medical equipment, surgery, or drug.
- *Medical necessity.* This section is crucial. This is where your physician should state why the new treatment is medical necessary. Include here how the medication or treatment being prescribed will cure or prevent any decline in your health. It will also be beneficial to explain why other treatment options did not or are not ones you can use, whether this may be due to costs or no other medications you have tried (make sure you list them and the dose you were on) provided the effectiveness you or your physician anticipated. If you found you had an allergic or adverse reaction, include all the signs, symptoms, and issues you encountered.

		• *Supporting literature.* Any information that would support your need for the treatment or requested item or service should be added. This would be including any other publications supporting the letter of medical necessity, as well as any lab or test results. Providing lab or imaging or other test results gives hard evidence of the severity of the medical condition.
levels of care by physicians or specialists or specialty centers	LOC	Levels of care refer to the complexity of medical cases, the types of conditions a physician treats, and their specialties. Primary care involves your primary health care provider. You see them for things like acute illnesses, injuries, or screenings or to coordinate care among specialists. Secondary care is the care of a specialist. These specialists may include oncologists, cardiologists, and endocrinologists. Tertiary care is a higher level of specialized care within a hospital. Similarly, quaternary care is an extension of tertiary care, but it is more specialized and unusual.
levels of care for a newborn or premature baby		A well baby nursery provides care to healthy babies born close to their due dates. Well baby nurseries provide routine medical care, including assessment and state-mandated newborn screening. Regular well baby nurseries can typically care for premature babies born at thirty-five weeks (called late preterm babies) and those with minor medical problems. A special care nursery, sometimes called a level 2 NICU, can care for babies born at thirty-two weeks gestational age or greater (often referred to as moderately preterm babies) or babies who are full-term but require close monitoring or intravenous antibiotics after birth.

Special care nurseries can treat babies with some health problems of prematurity, such as jaundice and trouble eating or staying warm. Feeding is one of the tasks that often determines when a baby can be sent home from a special care nursery.

Special care (level 2) nurseries may be further divided into the following:

- Level 2A nurseries, which do not provide respiratory assistance.
- Level 2B nurseries, which provide some respiratory assistance, such as continuous positive airway pressure (CPAP).
- A level 3 NICU can provide intensive care for babies born at almost all gestational ages—from very premature babies, babies born at twenty-seven to thirty weeks, and above.

The definition of a level 3 NICU may vary in different states or hospitals, but all level 3 NICUs can care for babies born at more than twenty-eight weeks, are able to provide respiratory support for babies who are having trouble breathing, and can deliver intravenous fluids to babies who cannot take milk feedings.

According to some classification systems, a level 3 NICU is the highest level of neonatal care. Under these classifications, a level 3 NICU can provide the same level of care as a level 4 NICU below.

For states and hospitals who use this classification, a level 4 NICU is an intensive care unit that can care for babies as young as twenty-two to twenty-four weeks gestational age. The term *micro-preemies* is used to describe babies born between twenty-two and twenty-six weeks of gestation or smaller than one pound, thirteen ounces.

		Level 4 NICUs can provide sophisticated types of respiratory support for very sick babies, including extracorporeal mechanical oxygenation, or ECMO. Level 4 NICUs also offer a wide variety of neonatal surgeries, including heart surgeries for babies born with congenital heart disease.
life- or limb-threatening emergency		Life- or limb-threatening emergency means any event that a prudent layperson would believe threatens his life or limb in such a manner that a need for immediate medical care is created to prevent death or serious impairment of health.
living will		A written statement detailing a person's desires regarding their medical treatment in circumstances in which they are no longer able to express informed consent, especially an advance directive.
Local Coverage Determination	LCD	A Local Coverage Determination (LCD) is a decision made by a Medicare Administrative Contractor (MAC) on whether a particular service or item is reasonable and necessary and, therefore, covered by Medicare within the specific jurisdiction (region) that the MAC oversees.
locked-in syndrome		Locked-in syndrome is a rare disorder of the nervous system. People with locked-in syndrome are • paralyzed except for the muscles that control eye movement, and • conscious (aware) and can think and reason but cannot move or speak, although they may be able to communicate with blinking eye movements.

		Locked-in syndrome may result from the following: ○ Traumatic brain injury (TBI) ○ Diseases of the circulatory system ○ Diseases that destroy the myelin sheath (a protective covering that surrounds nerve cells) ○ A medication overdose
long-term acute care hospital	LTACH	A long-term acute care hospital (LTACH) is a specialty hospital that is certified as an acute care hospital but focuses on patients who, on average, stay more than twenty-five days. Many of the patients in LTACHs are transferred there from an intensive or critical care unit. LTACHs specialize in treating patients who may have more than one serious condition but who may improve with time and care and return home or, if unable to go home, admitted to a skilled nursing facility (SNF).
long-term care insurance		Long-term care insurance is coverage that provides nursing home care, home health care, and personal or adult day care for individuals age sixty-five or older or with a chronic or disabling condition that needs constant supervision. Long-term care insurance offers more flexibility and options than many public assistance programs, such as Medicaid.
managed care organization		A term originally used to refer to prepaid health plans, generally health maintenance organizations (HMOs), that furnish care through a network of providers under a fixed budget and manage costs. It is a health care delivery system organized to manage cost, utilization, and quality. There are several types of managed care plans, but the most common are health maintenance organization (HMO),

		exclusive preferred organization (EPO), point of service (POS), and preferred provider organization (PPO). Managed care exists for persons who have not only private health care insurance but also Medicaid and Medicare.

maternal child health		Under the Social Security Act of 1935, Title V provided programs for maternity, infant, and child care, as well as a full range of medical services for children. Funds were allocated to states to pay for maternal and child health and crippled children services, including physicians, dentists, public health nurses, medical social workers, and nutritionists. Unlike other sections of the Social Security legislation, Title V was not an entitlement program. It consisted of four parts.
		
		    o maternal and child health services
		    o services for crippled children
		    o child welfare services
		    o vocational rehabilitation.
		
		Title V is the longest-standing public health legislation in American history, and it continues to work to improve the health of women and children. The maternal child portion is administered through the Health Resources and Services Administration (HRSA) with a focus on the following:
		
		    o Infant health
		    o Early childhood health
		    o Child and adolescent health
		    o Maternal health
		    o Mental and behavioral health
		    o Children and youth with special health care needs
		    o Building MCH leaders and the MCH workforce

medical necessity		Medical necessity refers to a decision by your health plan that your treatment, test, or procedure is necessary to maintain or restore your health or to treat a diagnosed medical problem. In order to be covered under the health plan, a service must be considered medically necessary. (Keep in mind that covered doesn't mean the health plan pays for it; you still have to pay your required cost-sharing—co-pay, deductible, or coinsurance—before the health plan starts to pay any of the cost, even for covered services.) Medicare and private insurers have varying criteria for determining whether a given procedure is medically necessary based on the patient's circumstances. Medicare uses National Coverage Determinations and private Medicare plans (i.e., Medicare Advantage) use Local Coverage Determinations in order to ensure that the criteria for medical necessity are met.
Medicare Administrative Contractor	MAC	The Centers for Medicare and Medicaid Services (CMS) once included fiscal intermediaries, but in 2003, CMS replaced the Part A fiscal intermediaries and Part B carriers with Medicare Administrative Contractors (MACs). MACs manage provider claims for payment and establish regional policy guidelines, called Local Coverage Determinations (LCDs). The MACs are the primary resource for audiologists and speech-language pathologists providing and billing for services to Medicare beneficiaries. A MAC is a "private health care insurer that has been awarded a geographic jurisdiction to process Medicare Part A and Part B medical claims or Durable Medical Equipment (DME) claims for Medicare Fee-For-Service (FFS) beneficiaries."

		CMS uses this network of MACs to serve as "the primary operational contact between the Medicare FFS program and the health care providers enrolled in the program." MACs are multistate, regional contractors responsible for administering both Medicare Part A and Medicare Part B claims. CMS says there are currently twelve Part A and Part B MACs and four durable medical equipment MACs in the program. The federal government contracts with a selection of MACs, or Medicare intermediaries, to administer its Medicare program in districts across the country.
		
		• As of December 2020, the approved Medicare intermediaries for Parts A and B claims and the states and territories they work in are the following:
		
		  o Noridian Healthcare Solutions LLC
		  o DME MAC Jurisdiction A (Connecticut, Delaware, District of Columbia, Maine, Maryland, Massachusetts, New Hampshire, New Jersey, New York, Pennsylvania, Rhode Island, Vermont)
		  o DME MAC Jurisdiction D (Alaska, Arizona, California, Hawaii, Idaho, Iowa, Kansas, Missouri, Montana, Nebraska, Nevada, North Dakota, Oregon, South Dakota, Utah, Washington, Wyoming, American Samoa, Guam, Northern Mariana Islands)
		  o MAC Jurisdiction E (California, Hawaii, Nevada, American Samoa, Guam, Northern Mariana Islands)

<table>
<tr><td></td><td></td><td>

    ○ MAC Jurisdiction F (Alaska, Arizona, Idaho, Montana, North Dakota, Oregon, South Dakota, Utah, Washington, Wyoming)

- CGS Administrators LLC

    ○ DME MAC Jurisdiction B (Illinois, Indiana, Kentucky, Michigan, Minnesota, Ohio, Wisconsin)

    ○ DME MAC Jurisdiction C (Alabama, Arkansas, Colorado, Florida, Georgia, Louisiana, Mississippi, New Mexico, North Carolina, Oklahoma, South Carolina, Tennessee, Texas, Virginia, West Virginia, Puerto Rico, U.S. Virgin Islands)

    ○ MAC Jurisdiction 15 (Kentucky, Ohio)

- Wisconsin Physicians Service Government Health Administrators

    ○ MAC Jurisdiction 5 (Iowa, Kansas, Missouri, Nebraska)

    ○ MAC Jurisdiction 8 (Indiana, Michigan)

- National Government Services Inc.

    ○ MAC Jurisdiction 6 (Illinois, Minnesota, Wisconsin)

    ○ MAC Jurisdiction K (Connecticut, New York, Maine, Massachusetts, New Hampshire, Rhode Island, Vermont)

</td></tr>
</table>

		• Novitas Solutions Inc.
		
		    ○ MAC Jurisdiction H (Arkansas, Colorado, New Mexico, Oklahoma, Texas, Louisiana, Mississippi)
		    ○ MAC Jurisdiction L (Delaware, District of Columbia, Maryland, New Jersey, Pennsylvania. Includes Part B for counties of Arlington and Fairfax in Virginia and the city of Alexandria in Virginia)
		
		• Palmetto GBA LLC
		
		    ○ MAC Jurisdiction J (Alabama, Georgia, Tennessee)
		    ○ MAC Jurisdiction M (North Carolina, South Carolina, Virginia, West Virginia. Excludes Part B for the counties of Arlington and Fairfax in Virginia and the city of Alexandria in Virginia)
		
		• First Coast Service Options Inc.
		
		    ○ MAC Jurisdiction N (Florida, Puerto Rico, U.S. Virgin Islands)

Medicare Administrator Contractor appeal process		If you or your loved one has traditional Medicare and choose to appeal a coverage decision from Medicare for any Part A or Part B claims denial, which includes any claim submitted by a home health (HH) agency or hospice agency (H) or durable medical equipment (DME), the regional MAC will be involved in the dispute, including holding a redetermination of coverage. MACs process these appeals claims and decide on that redetermination.

		These include Medicare Part D (prescription drug) appeals. If you disagree with Part D costs or coverage decisions, the MAC will work with CMS to determine appropriate coverage based on regional or national law. MACs that handle DME claims are fewer in number and oversee a larger region. They only work on DME issues, including DME claims for reimbursement and appeals.
Medicare Part A benefit period		Under original Medicare A benefit period, Part A begins the day you're admitted to the hospital and ends when you've been discharged for at least sixty days. If you've been out of the hospital for more than sixty days and are admitted again, a new benefit period begins. Each Medicare benefit period requires that you meet a deductible, which changes each year (for example for 2023, it is $1,600). After meeting your deductible, you pay nothing out of pocket for hospital costs for the first sixty days you are admitted. For stays beyond that, you can expect to pay coinsurance. For example, these are the following: • If you are in the hospital between sixty-one and ninety days during one benefit period, you will be charged a daily rate (for example, for 2023, each day will cost $400). • If you are unable to be discharged even after a stay of ninety days, each day you stay for more than the ninety days, you will be charged a daily rate (for example, for 2023, each day will cost $800).

		• Starting on day 91, you start tapping into your lifetime reserve days for Medicare Part A. You have sixty reserve days. Once they are used up and you encounter a long hospitalization, you are responsible for all costs starting with day 91 in the hospital. If you or your loved one can stay out of the hospital for sixty consecutive days, you can renew the benefit period, but any days used in the lifetime reserve days are not renewable.
Medicare Part B benefit period		Medicare Part B is an optional benefit beneficiaries must elect to enroll in. Part B helps to cover medical services like doctors' services, outpatient care, and other medical services that Part A doesn't cover. Part B helps pay for covered medical services and items when they are medically necessary. Part B also covers some preventive services like exams, lab tests, and screening shots to help prevent, find, or manage a medical problem.
Medicare Outpatient Observation Notice	MOON	Notice of Observation Treatment and Implication for Care Eligibility Act (NOTICE Act) requires hospitals and critical access hospitals (CAH) to provide written notification to individuals whose insurance is either the original Medicare or a Medicare managed care plan. The letter issued is termed the MOON letter (Medicare Outpatient Observation Notice). This letter is issued to inform Medicare beneficiaries (including health plan enrollees) that they are outpatients receiving observation services and are not inpatients of a hospital or critical access hospital.

Medicare Part D doughnut hole		Most plans with Medicare prescription drug coverage (Part D) have a coverage gap (called a doughnut hole). This means that after you and your drug plan have spent a certain amount of money for covered drugs, you have to pay all costs out of pocket for your prescriptions up to a yearly limit. Once you have spent up to the yearly limit, your coverage gap ends, and your drug plan helps pay for covered drugs again.
Medicare psychiatric benefit		*Inpatient services.* Medicare Part A covers inpatient mental health services in both general hospitals and psychiatric hospitals, but the latter is limited to 190 total days per beneficiary across their lifetime. Traditional Medicare beneficiaries pay a deductible and coinsurance for each benefit period, which, for hospital services, begins on the day of admission and ends after a beneficiary has had no inpatient care for 60 consecutive days. Cost-sharing requirements vary across plans for Medicare Advantage enrollees. *Outpatient services.* Medicare Part B covers outpatient mental health services delivered by psychiatrists or other physicians, clinical psychologists, clinical social workers, clinical nurse specialists, nurse practitioners, and physician assistants. The services covered include standard services, like psychiatric evaluation, individual and group therapy, and medication management. After paying their annual deductible, traditional Medicare beneficiaries pay 20 percent of the Medicare-approved amount for covered services. As with inpatient services, cost-sharing requirements vary across Medicare Advantage plans.

Medicare skilled nursing facility benefit period		Under the original Medicare plan, your loved one can receive care in a skilled nursing facility (SNF) for up to one hundred days if the care they require is skilled and remains skilled during the entire one hundred days. The SNF benefit period is divided into days one to twenty and days twenty-one to one hundred. The co-payments are as follows: • For days one to twenty, Medicare pays the full cost for covered services. You pay nothing. • For days twenty-one to one hundred, Medicare pays all but has a daily coinsurance for covered services. You pay a daily coinsurance, which is adjusted annually. For 2023, it is $200 per day. • For days beyond one hundred, Medicare pays nothing. You pay the full cost for covered services. If your loved one has a Medicare Supplement Insurance (Medigap) policy with original Medicare or has a Medicare Advantage Plan, your costs may be different, or you may have more coverage.
Medicare Supplement		A private medical expense insurance policy that provides reimbursement for out-of-pocket expenses, such as deductibles and coinsurance payments, or benefits for some medical expenses specifically excluded from Medicare coverage.
Medigap policy		Individual medical expense insurance policies sold by state-licensed private insurance companies. A term commonly used to describe Medicare supplemental insurance policies available from various companies. Medigap is private insurance that may be purchased by

		Medicare-eligible individuals to help pay the deductibles and co-payments required under Medicare. Medigap policies generally do not pay for services not covered by Medicare, such as level 1 nursing home care.
member		The insured person under a health plan.
mental health illness		Mental illnesses are disorders ranging from mild to severe that affect a person's thinking, mood, or behavior. According to the National Institute of Mental Health, nearly one in five adults live with a mental illness. Many factors contribute to mental health conditions, including the following: • Biological factors, such as genes or brain chemistry • Life experiences, such as trauma or abuse • Family history of mental health problems A serious mental illness (SMI) is a mental illness that interferes with a person's life and ability to function. Despite common misperceptions, having an SMI is not a choice, a weakness, or a character flaw. It is not something that just passes or can be snapped out of with willpower.
mental health parity		The Mental Health Parity and Addiction Equity Act of 2008 (MHPAEA) is a federal law that generally prevents group health plans and health insurance issuers that provide mental health and substance use disorder (MH/SUD) benefits from imposing less favorable benefit limitations on those benefits than on medical/surgical coverage.

		Mental health parity requirements predate the ACA (Affordable Care Act), although the ACA expanded the parity law to apply to individual market plans and employer-sponsored coverage. Under the parity requirement, a health plan cannot have more restrictive coverage limits for mental health treatment than it has for medical/surgical treatment.
Medical Orders for Life Sustaining Treatment		States vary with the name they use for developing a patient specific set of medical orders only appropriate for seriously ill people. The Medical Orders for Life Sustaining Treatment (MOLST) program may be known as POLST in other states. The form is designed to improve the quality of care seriously ill people receive at the end of life. MOLST is based on the patient's current health status, prognosis, and goals for care and is a form that is completed jointly between the treating physician and you or your loved one.
military treatment facility	MTF	Military hospitals and clinics are the core of the Military Health System. They are located on military installations around the world, and they furnish medical and dental care to eligible individuals.
Mobile Integrated Health-care and mobile health care providers	MIH	This is a program that was tested and proved successful by MedStar, an ambulance provider in the Fort Worth area, in 2009. In this program, MedStar worked with the local hospitals and providers to help reduce the number of unnecessary emergency room trips by patients identified as high utilizer groups (HUGs). This program was so successful that many communities have now followed and provide the same services. Under the program, MedStar's mobile health care providers (MHPs) conduct regular home visits, evaluate social determinants of health, connect the patients to available resources, and teach the patients how to better manage their own healthcare.

mobility		Mobility, the ability to move or walk freely and easily, is critical for functioning well and living independently.
National Provider Identifier number		A National Provider Identifier (NPI) number is a code given to all medical providers by Medicare and Medicaid. The code is ten digits and is unique for each entity, whether a person or organization. Anyone who practices medicine is given a number and so is included on an NPI registry for easy access.
network		The facilities, providers, and suppliers your health insurer or plan has contracted with to provide health care services.
Newborns' and Mothers' Health Protection Act	NMHPA	The Newborns' and Mothers' Health Protection Act of 1996 (NMHPA) is a federal law that affects the length of time a mother and newborn child are covered for a hospital stay in connection with childbirth.
Nonpreferred drugs or tier 3 drugs		FDA-approved brand-name prescription drugs. What this means for you: typically, these drugs will cost you the most, and there is often a lower-priced tier 1 or tier 2 alternative.
nonpreferred provider		A provider who does not have a contract with your health insurer or plan to provide services to you. You will pay more to see a nonpreferred provider. Check your policy to see if you can go to all providers who have contracted with your health insurance or plan or if your health insurance or plan has a tiered network, and you must pay extra to see some providers.
Notice of Medicare Non-Coverage	NOMNC	Informs beneficiaries of their discharge when a beneficiary is receiving care in a skilled nursing facility (SNF) or provided by a home health agency (HHA), hospice, or outpatient rehabilitation facility (CORF) provider; and their Medicare covered services are pending. This notice allows you to request an expedited appeal.

Nursing Home Compare		The Nursing Home Compare website features a quality rating system that gives each nursing home a rating of between one and five stars. Nursing homes with five stars are considered to have above-average quality, and nursing homes with one star are considered to have quality much below average. There is one overall five-star rating for each nursing home and separate ratings for health inspections, staffing, and quality measures.
obesity		A person is classified as having obesity (being overweight) and may be referred to as a bariatric patient when they have a body mass index (BMI) that is equal to or greater than thirty. BMI is used to measure weight in relation to height. Obesity classes are then determined by what range your BMI falls into.
observa-tion	OBS	An overnight stay for observation is not hospitalization but is basically outpatient care until the treating physician determines you need admission or can be discharged.
Office of Inspector General	OIG	Since its 1976 establishment, the Office of Inspector General (OIG) has been at the forefront of the nation's efforts to fight waste, fraud, and abuse and to improve the efficiency of Medicare, Medicaid, and more than one hundred other Department of Health and Human Services (HHS) programs.
off-label		It is important to know that before a drug can be approved, a company must submit clinical data and other information to FDA for review. The company must show that the drug is safe and effective for its intended uses. Safe does not mean that the drug has no side effects. Instead, it means the FDA has determined the benefits of using the drug for a particular use outweigh the potential risks.

When your loved one is prescribed a drug for its approved use, you can be sure of the following:

- That FDA has conducted a careful evaluation of its benefits and risks for that use.
- The decision to use the drug is supported by strong scientific data.
- There is approved drug labeling for health care providers on how to use the drug safely and effectively for that use. Once the FDA approves a drug, health care providers generally may prescribe the drug for an unapproved use when they judge that it is medically appropriate for your loved one.

Unapproved use of an approved drug is often called off-label use. This term can mean that the drug is:

- Used for a disease or medical condition that it is not approved to treat, such as when a chemotherapy is approved to treat one type of cancer, but health care providers use it to treat a different type of cancer.
- Given in a different way, such as when a drug is approved as a capsule, but it is given instead in an oral solution.
- Given in a different dose, such as when a drug is approved at a dose of one tablet every day, but a patient is told by their health care provider to take two tablets every day.

open enroll-ment		The time when you can choose to enroll in a health plan or reenroll in a health plan you are already in. You can usually do this without waiting periods or proof of insurance. If you are eligible for Medicare, the open enrollment period is the time of year you can enroll or make changes to your Medicare coverage. This is also known as annual enrollment period or annual election period.
ombuds-man		The ombudsman program is a public/government/community-supported program that advocates for the rights of long-term care residents. Volunteers visit local facilities weekly, monitor conditions of care, and try to resolve problems involving meals, finances, medication, therapy, placement, and communication with staff. To find the ombudsman office in your or your loved one's area, you can call the United Way 2-1-1 phone system. Or if your loved one is a facility, the facility is required to have this information posted for all to see.
Original Medicare		Original Medicare is a fee-for-service health plan that has two parts: Part A (hospital insurance) and Part B (medical insurance). After you pay a deductible, Medicare pays its share of the Medicare-approved amount, and you pay your share (coinsurance and deductibles). Medicare was incepted in 1965 under the Social Security Act and Title 18.
Orphan Drug		According to the US Food and Drug Administration (FDA), an orphan drug is defined as one "intended for the treatment, prevention or diagnosis of a rare disease or condition, which is one that affects less than 200,000 persons in the US" (which equates to approximately 6 cases per 10,000 population), "or meets cost recovery provisions of the act." The FDA has authority to grant orphan drug designation to a drug or biological product to prevent, diagnose, or treat a rare disease or condition.

orthotics		Orthotics can be defined as, "Devices that differ from a prosthetic device as rather than replace the body part it supports and/or rehabilitates an existing body part. Orthotics are rigid or semi-rigid devices called braces, which are applied to the outside of the body as a means of either support of a weak or deformed body part or to restrict or eliminate motion in a diseased or injured body part." Orthotics are generally customized for the individual and cannot be used by anyone else. Orthotic devices encompass all leg, arm, back and neck devices (braces), special corsets (i.e., sacroiliac, lumbosacral, or dorsolumbar corsets and belts), and special shoes when they are attached to a brace.
orthotist		An orthotist is a health care professional who makes and fits braces and splints (orthoses) for people who need added support for body parts that have been weakened by injury, disease, or disorders of the nerves, muscles, or bones. They work under a doctor's orders to adapt purchased braces or create custom-designed braces.
ostomy		An artificial opening in an organ of the body created during an operation, such as a tracheostomy, colostomy, ileostomy, or gastrostomy, or urostomy.
out of area	OOA	The health care providers (facilities, doctors, specialists, and suppliers) that are not contracted with your health insurer or plan to provide health care services. If you choose to receive out-of-network care, you may have higher costs. While some plans may cover out of network care, meaning they'll pay part of the costs, other plans do not cover any costs for going out-of-network.

out-of-pocket	OOP	The amount of money you will have to pay if your health plan does not cover 100 percent of the costs.
out-of-pocket maximum		Dollar amounts set by MCOs (managed care organizations) that limit the amount a member has to pay out of his own pocket for particular health care services during a particular time period. The most you could pay during a coverage period (usually one year) for your share of the costs of covered services. After you meet this limit, the plan will usually pay 100 percent of the allowed amount. This limit helps you plan for health care costs. This limit never includes your premium, balance-billed charges, or health care your health insurance or plan doesn't cover. Some health insurance or plans don't count all of your co-payments, deductibles, coinsurance payments, out-of-network payments, or other expenses toward this limit. Also known as out-of-pocket maximum or out-of-pocket threshold.
outpatient		Treatment that is provided to a patient who is able to return home after care without an overnight stay in a hospital or other inpatient facility.
over the counter	OTC	Over-the-counter medicine is also known as OTC or nonprescription medicine. All these terms refer to medicine that you can buy without a prescription. They are safe and effective when you follow the directions on the label and as directed by your health care professional.
palliative care		Palliative care is care given to improve the quality of life of patients who have a serious or life-threatening disease, such as cancer. Palliative care is an approach to care that addresses the person as a whole, not just their disease. The goal is to prevent or treat, as early as possible, the symptoms and side effects of the disease and its treatment in addition to

		any related psychological, social, and spiritual problems. Palliative care is specialized medical care for people living with a serious illness, such as cancer or heart failure. Patients in palliative care may receive medical care for their symptoms, or palliative care, along with treatment intended to cure their serious illness. Palliative care is meant to enhance a person's current care by focusing on quality of life for them and their family. Palliative care is a resource for anyone living with a serious illness, such as heart failure, chronic obstructive pulmonary disease, cancer, dementia, Parkinson's disease, and many others. Palliative care can be helpful at any stage of illness and is best provided soon after a person is diagnosed. In addition to improving quality of life and helping with symptoms, palliative care can help patients understand their choices for medical treatment. The organized services available through palliative care may be helpful to any older person having a lot of general discomfort and disability very late in life.
parenteral nutrition		Parenteral nutrition, often called total parenteral nutrition, is the medical term for infusing a specialized form of food through a vein (intravenously). The goal of the treatment is to correct or prevent malnutrition. Parenteral nutrition provides liquid nutrients, including carbohydrates, proteins, fats, vitamins, minerals, and electrolytes.
partial hospital-ization		A partial hospitalization program (PHP) is a structured mental health program and type of addiction treatment where clients participate in activities during the day and return home at night. These programs are available at inpatient or residential treatment facilities. PHPs provide structured, comprehensive care while still allowing people to live their lives

		outside treatment. They are sometimes called intensive outpatient programs (IOPs) or day programs because they don't require an overnight stay. Partial hospital programs are for people diagnosed with a substance use disorder (SUD), alcohol use disorder (AUD), mental health disorder, or dual diagnosis (a SUD and co-occurring mental health disorder). Someone in a partial hospitalization program is medically monitored during treatment. They participate in a variety of evidence-based therapies. While the name can seem intimidating, a partial hospitalization program is simply a special outpatient treatment program. It's for people who need a higher level of behavioral health care than standard outpatient programs can provide.
patient choice		New discharge planning requirements of the IMPACT Act addresses post-acute care transitions, patient choice, and patient access to medical information. Among other requirements, the rule mandates that hospitals share quality and resource use measures about skilled nursing facilities, home health agencies, inpatient rehabilitation facilities, and long-term care hospitals with patients as part of the discharge planning process to fulfill patient goals of care and treatment preferences and with the desired outcomes of increased transparency, patient empowerment, and quality care.
Patient Self-De-termina-tion Act	PDSA	Patient Self-Determination Act (PDSA) was an amendment proposed in 1990 and functions to amend titles XVIII and XIX of the Social Security Act (Medicare and Medicaid respectively). The PSDA mandates that hospitals, skilled nursing facilities, hospice organizations, home health organizations, and HMOs

		perform a number of specific actions and ensure that other certain conditions are met. Among those mentioned above, it is required that patients be informed of their right to be involved in making decisions with regard to the medical care they receive. It is also required that the patient is asked about advance directives and to document any wishes the patient might have with regard to the care they want or do not want. It required that no discrimination take place by any health care organization against any patient putting forth advance directives. It mandates that patient advance directives be implemented if necessary, assuming those wishes are legally valid and permissible by state law. It requires education programs, including advance directives, bioethics, patient wishes, and the concept of patient self-determination. The PDSA went further to instruct the secretary of the United States Department of Health and Human Services to coordinate an investigative study reviewing the implementation of advance directive decisions.
payer of last resort		A payer of last resort is an entity that pays after any other primary health plans have been billed. For instance, after a primary health plan, a secondary or even a third health plan payer can come in and pay the last of a bill.
payers		In health care, a payer is a person, organization, or entity that pays for the care services administered by a health care provider. This term most often refers to private insurance companies, which provide customers with health plans that offer cost coverage and reimbursements for medical treatment and care services. There are three different types of health care payers: commercial, private, and government/public. A commercial payer refers to publicly traded insurance companies,

| | | like UnitedHealth, Aetna, or Humana, while private payer refers to private insurance companies like, Blue Cross Blue Shield. A public payer refers to government-funded health insurance plans, like Medicare, Medicaid, and the Children's Health Insurance Program (CHIP).

Currently, the top five payer in the market are the following:

• UnitedHealth Group (49.5 million members)
• Anthem (40.2 million members)
• Aetna (merged with CVS; 22.2 million members)
• Cigna (15.9 million members)
• Humana (14 million members)

These top payers are part of private insurance plans while payers like Medicaid and Medicare are part of the public sector. |
| physician certification of medical necessity for nonemergent ambulance transport (NEAT) | NEAT | Your loved one's condition must require both the ambulance transportation itself and the level of service provided for the billed service to be considered medically necessary. In addition to the medical necessity requirements, the service must meet all other Medicare or health plan coverage and payment requirements. Thus, bed confinement is not the sole criterion in determining the medical necessity of ambulance transportation. To be considered bed-confined, the following criteria must be met: your loved one is unable to get up from bed without assistance or is unable to ambulate or is unable to sit in a chair or wheelchair. |

physician certification of medical necessity for nonemergent transportation (NEMT)	NEMT	When nonemergent transportation, such as a wheelchair van, is needed, as your loved one cannot be transported via a private vehicle. To help ensure coverage, your loved one's physician must complete the physician certification of medical necessity for nonemergent transportation form. If this is not filled out and signed, your claim, when submitted, will be denied.
prognosis		A medical term used to attempt to predict the likely or expected development of a disease, including whether the signs and symptoms will improve or worsen (and how quickly) or remain stable over time; expectations of quality of life, such as the ability to carry out daily activities; the potential for complications and associated health issues; and the likelihood of survival (including life expectancy). A prognosis is made on the basis of the normal course of the diagnosed disease, the individual's physical and mental condition, the available treatments, and additional factors. A complete prognosis includes the expected duration, function, and description of the course of the disease, such as progressive decline, intermittent crisis, or sudden, unpredictable crisis.
peritoneal dialysis		Peritoneal dialysis is a treatment for kidney failure that uses the lining of your abdomen, or belly, to filter your blood inside your body. Health care providers call this lining the peritoneum. There are two types of peritoneal dialysis: continuous ambulatory peritoneal dialysis (CAPD) and automated peritoneal dialysis. The main differences between the two types of peritoneal dialysis are the schedule of exchanges. One uses a machine, and the other is done by hand.

persistent vegetative state	PVS	The condition of patients with severe brain damage in whom coma has progressed to a state of wakefulness without detectable awareness. Such patients have sleep-wake cycles but no ascertainable cerebral cortical function and are unaware, and they no longer think know how to reason or recognize another, and they do not recognize or feel emotion of pain. Recovery of consciousness from a posttraumatic persistent vegetative state is unlikely after twelve months in adults and children. Recovery from a nontraumatic persistent vegetative state after three months is exceedingly rare in both adults and children. Patients with degenerative or metabolic disorders or congenital malformations who remain in a persistent vegetative state for several months are unlikely to recover consciousness. The life span of adults and children in such a state is substantially reduced. For most such patients, life expectancy ranges from two to five years; survival beyond ten years is unusual.
personnel health information	PHI	Information that relates to an individual's past, present, or future physical or mental health or condition or the past, present, or future payment for the provision of health care to an individual, including demographic information, received from or on behalf of a health care provider, health plan, clearinghouse, or employer, which either identifies the individual or could be reasonably used to identify the individual. It includes such information contained in any form or medium (electronic, paper, oral, etc.).

personal emergency response system	PERS	Personal emergency response systems, or medical alert, offer a fast and easy way to get help during an emergency, whether for a medical issue, a fall, a fire, or something else. Broadly, these systems (necklaces, buttons, and bracelets) all have a help button that dials up an emergency response center and connects you to a live agent.
placebo		A placebo is a pill, liquid, or powder that has no treatment value. It is often called a sugar pill. In clinical trials, experimental drugs are often compared with placebos to evaluate the treatment's effectiveness.
point of service	POS	POS organizations are essentially a hybrid of the HMO and PPO models. Enrollees have the flexibility to see providers that are in-network or out-of-network but pay a higher share of costs. POS plans may require you to see your primary care provider for a referral before seeking specialist care. POS plan enrollees pay more to see out-of-network providers unless their primary care provider makes a direct referral. POS plans seek to offer enrollees flexibility and choice in seeking care while controlling costs and utilization.
preferred provider	PPO	A type of medical plan in which coverage is provided to participants through a network of selected health care providers, such as hospitals and physicians. Enrollees may seek care outside the network but pay a greater percentage of the cost of coverage than within the network. PPOs offer more flexibility to enrollees and generally have larger provider networks, but may cost more. Enrollees in a PPO can seek care from both in-network and out-of-network providers. PPOs utilize a preferred provider network and offer in-network care at a lower price. Referrals from a primary care

		provider are not usually required to access specialty care. PPOs cover preventive care at 100 percent. Since beneficiaries have more flexibility in the providers they see, monthly premiums are likely to be higher than premiums for an HMO plan.
preventive health		Routine health care, including screenings, checkups, and patient counseling, to prevent or discover illness, disease, or other health problems.
principle or agent or attorney in fact		You, the person drawing up a document for use in your healthcare or for finances and you want to appoint an agent or attorney-in-fact. (In case you are wondering, your agent does not have to be an attorney). Your agent or attorney in fact can be a family member or friend – anyone you trust to carry out your wishes.
protected health information	PHI	Information that relates to an individual's past, present, or future physical or mental health or condition or the past, present, or future payment for the provision of health care to an individual, including demographic information, received from or on behalf of a health care provider, health plan, clearinghouse, or employer, which either identifies the individual or could be reasonably used to identify the individual. It includes such information contained in any form or medium (electronic, paper, oral, etc.).
physical medicine and rehabilitation	PM&R	Physical medicine and rehabilitation (PM&R), also known as physiatry, is a medical specialty that involves restoring function for a person who has been disabled as a result of a disease, disorder, or injury. Physiatry provides integrated, multidisciplinary care aimed at recovery of the whole person by addressing the individual.

physiatrist		A physical medicine and rehabilitation physician, also known as a PM&R physician, or a physiatrist treats a wide variety of medical conditions that affect the brain, spinal cord, bones, joints, ligaments, muscles, and tendons.
power of attorney		An important part of lifetime planning is the power of attorney. A power of attorney is accepted in all states, but the rules and requirements differ from state to state. A power of attorney gives one or more persons the power to act on your behalf as your agent. The person named in a power of attorney to act on your behalf is commonly referred to as your agent or attorney-in-fact. With a valid power of attorney, your agent can take any action permitted in the document. A power of attorney allows you to choose who will act for you and defines his or her authority and its limits, if any. In some instances, greater security against having a guardianship imposed on you may be achieved by you also creating a revocable living trust. Health Care Power of Attorney (HCPOA) The principal can sign a durable power of attorney for health care, or health care POA (HCPOA), if they want an agent to have the power to make health-related decisions. This document, also called a health care proxy, outlines the principal's consent to give the agent POA privileges in the event of an unfortunate medical condition. The POA for health care is legally bound to oversee medical care decisions on behalf of the principal. As such, it kicks in when the principal can no longer make health-related decisions on their own.

		Financial Power of Attorney
		The financial POA is a document that allows an agent to manage the business and financial affairs of the principal, such as signing checks, filing tax returns, mailing and depositing Social Security checks, and managing investment accounts when and if the latter becomes unable to understand or make decisions. The agent must carry out the principal's wishes to the best of their ability, at least to the extent of what the agreement spells out as the agent's responsibility. A financial POA gives that individual a wide range of power over one's bank account, including the ability to make deposits and withdrawals, sign checks, and make or change beneficiary designations. Financial POAs can be divided up into several different categories. These are the general power POA, limited power POA, and durable POA. • *General power POA.* This POA allows the agent to act on behalf of the principal in any matters, as allowed by state laws. The agent under such an agreement may be authorized to handle bank accounts, sign checks, sell property, manage assets, and file taxes for the principal. • *Limited POA.* A limited power of attorney gives the agent the power to act on behalf of the principal in specific matters or events. It might explicitly state that the agent is only allowed to manage the principal's retirement accounts. This type of POA may be in effect for a specific period. For example, if the principal will be out of the country for two years, the authorization might be effective only for that period.

<table>
<tr><td></td><td></td><td>

- *Durable power of attorney (DPOA).* The durable POA (DPOA) remains in control of certain legal, property, or financial matters specifically spelled out in the agreement, even after the principal becomes mentally incapacitated. While a DPOA can pay medical bills on behalf of the principal, the durable agent cannot make decisions related to the principal's health, such as taking the principal off life support. When the agent acts on behalf of the principal by making investment decisions through a broker, the broker would ask to see the DPOA.

The conditions for which a durable POA may become active are set up in a document called the springing power of attorney. A springing POA defines the kind of event or level of incapacitation that should occur before the DPOA springs into effect. A power of attorney can remain dormant until a negative health occurrence activates it to a DPOA. A springing power of attorney should be very carefully worded to avoid any problems in identifying precisely when and if the triggering event has happened. The following provisos apply generally nationwide, and everyone who needs to create a POA should be aware of them:

- There is no standard POA form for all fifty states; state law and procedures vary.
- All states accept some version of the durable power of attorney

</td></tr>
</table>

| Physician Orders for Life Sustaining Treatment | POLST | A POLST (Physician Orders for Life Sustaining Treatment) is basically a more detailed and specific DNR (do not resuscitate) order. Like a DNR, this form is filled out with your doctor and based on your end-of-life care decisions. Once signed, doctors, emergency medical professionals, and other health care professionals must honor the instructions on your POLST form no matter where you are (at a hospital, care facility, your own home, etc.). In an emergency situation, any procedures that are legally required of emergency personnel will be overridden. Depending on what state you live in, a POLST may go by one of the following names:

• MOST (Medical Orders for Scope of Treatment)
• MOLST (Medical Orders for Life Sustaining Treatment)
• POST (Physician Orders for Scope of Treatment)
• TPOPP (Transportable Physician Orders for Patient Preferences)

Helpful tip: POLST forms are often printed on brightly colored paper so that they're easy to see and find. The forms differ in name and structure depending on where you live but are conceptually the same across all states. If it is a POLST, it is available in several languages. To find the form used in your state or the one in which your loved one is getting care. |
| preadmission screening and annual resident review | PASARR | A process for determining whether a person being considered for admission has any mental illness or mental retardation. Federal law requires nursing homes that participate in Medicare or Medicaid to screen all individuals prior to admission. If an initial evaluation |

		reveals mental illness or mental retardation, a more in-depth evaluation is performed to determine whether the individual needs special services that cannot be provided in a nursing home. Individuals whose mental conditions change during their stay in the facility will be retested. This form is required for all patients entering a skilled nursing facility and is either completed by the hospital discharge planner or by the admissions coordinator at the facility.
precertification		A utilization management technique that requires a health care insurance plan member or the physician in charge of the member's care to notify the plan in advance of plans for a patient to undergo a course of care, such as a hospital admission or complex diagnostic test. Also known as prior authorization.
primary care physician		General medical care that is provided directly to a patient without referral from another physician. It is focused on preventive care and the treatment of routine injuries and illnesses.
prior authorization		Prior authorization is a process by which a medical provider must obtain approval from a patient's health plan or health entity (i.e., Medicaid or Children's Medical Services) before moving ahead with a particular treatment, procedure, or medication. Without prior approval, your health insurance plan or the health entity used may not pay for your treatment, leaving you responsible for the full bill. Prior authorization is also known as precertification, predetermination, and preapproval and different health plans and health entities have different rules in terms of when prior authorization is required. The name used to seek authorization can vary from health

		plan or agency providing the service and may be referred to as a service authorization request (SAR) or treatment authorization request (TAR), or it may be referred to as precertification, predetermination, or approval.
pro-spective payment		A method of reimbursement in which Medicare payment is made based on a predetermined, fixed amount. The payment amount for a particular service is derived based on the classification system of that service (see also resource utilization groups).
prosthesis		Prosthetic devices "are devices (other than dental) which replace all or part of an internal or external body organ, limb or part or replace all or part of the function of a permanently inoperative or malfunctioning internal or external body organ or part." Prosthetic devices include artificial limbs, terminal devices (i.e., hand or hook) and artificial eyes, parenteral or enteral nutrition, cardiac pacemakers, prosthetic lenses, and breast prosthesis (including surgical brassiere for post mastectomy patients, maxillofacial devices, and devices that replace all or part of the ear or nose). Refers to an artificial body part or artificial substitute for a missing part of the body. The artificial parts that are most commonly thought of as prostheses are those that replace lost arms and legs, but a prosthesis might be a bone, artery, and heart valve replacements; an artificial eye; and after a breast removal, a breast prosthesis might be ordered following a partial, full, or double mastectomy. A cranial prosthesis is a wig for medical patients who have permanent hair loss (such as alopecia areata, alopecia totalis, or trichotillomania) or temporary hair loss resulting from treatment for chemotherapy, radiation, or any other clinical disease.

		Prostheses have evolved from wooden legs and hooks that replaced hands to sophisticated plastic, fiberglass, and metal devices designed to fit limbs amputated at different points. They may have working joints and allow motion either by amplification of electric current generated by muscle contractions or by actual attachment to the muscles.
prosthetist		A prosthetist is a health care professional who makes and fits artificial limbs (prostheses) for people with disabilities. This includes artificial legs and arms for people who have had amputations due to conditions, such as cancer, diabetes, or injury.
psychiatric hold or 5150 or seventy-two-hour hold		A 5150 order and a psychiatric hold are two terms to describe the same legal process. As such, they both entail the same type of treatment. Typically, a 5150 order is granted when an individual is deemed harmful to themselves or others or is unable to adequately handle their own issues. The overarching idea is that this specific time frame mitigates the risk of excessively long detainment. Furthermore, many health experts believe that patients can be appropriately evaluated, monitored, and discharged within those three days. Regardless of the term used, all are commonly referred to as involuntary commitment. A psychiatric hold is a legally mandated stay at a psychiatric facility—in most states, seventy-two hours or less. The intent of such a hold is aimed at providing a safe space and professional care to those going through a mental health crisis. Holds occur both so individuals do not harm themselves or others, as well as to help them recognize their own need for continued mental health care.

		While each state has its own laws, seventy-two hours is the most common limit across the country (hence the standard phrase seventy-two-hour hold). This model also takes place in several other countries, including Canada, Australia, and France. The seventy-two-hour hold comes from the Lanterman–Petris–Short Act (LPS). This act was signed into California law in 1968. At the time, the intention was to end "inappropriate and indefinite involuntary commitment." In addition, the law initiated the right to engage in psychiatric evaluation and treatment. The law states that an eligible person can be held involuntarily for a maximum of seventy-two hours at a time. In other words, they may not be at the hospital for the full three days, but the hospital has the legal right to keep them there if deemed necessary.
pulmonary rehabilitation		Pulmonary rehabilitation is a supervised medical program that helps people who have lung diseases live and breathe better. You may need pulmonary rehabilitation if you have a lung disease, such as chronic obstructive pulmonary disease (COPD). During the program, you will learn exercises and breathing techniques. Pulmonary rehabilitation can help you gain strength, reduce symptoms of anxiety or depression, and make it easier to manage routine activities, work, and outings or social activities that you enjoy.
Qualified Medicare Beneficiary	QMB	The Qualified Medicare Beneficiary (QMB) Program is one of the four Medicare Savings Programs that allows you to get help from your state to pay your Medicare premiums. This program helps pay for Part A premiums, Part B premiums, and deductibles, coinsurance, and co-payments. In order to qualify

		for QMB benefits, you must meet the following income requirements, which can also be found on the Medicare Savings Programs page: • Individual monthly income limit: $1,060 • Married couple monthly income limit: $1,430 • Individual resource limit: $7,730 • Married couple resource limit: $11,600 Please note, these limits change from year to year, so please check the Medicare Savings Programs page for the most up-to-date income requirements. To apply, call your state Medicare program. For more information, please visit Medicare.gov or call 1-800-MEDICARE (1-800-633-4227). TTY users can call 1-877-486-2048. It's important to call or fill out an application if you think you could qualify for savings even if your income or resources are higher than the amounts listed in any written literature you may have.
Quality Improvement Organization	QIO	The QIO program, one of the largest federal programs dedicated to improving health quality for Medicare beneficiaries, is an integral part of the US Department of Health and Human Services national quality strategy for providing better care and better health at lower cost. By law, the mission of the QIO program is to improve the effectiveness, efficiency, economy, and quality of services delivered to Medicare beneficiaries. Based on this statutory charge and CMS's program experience, CMS identifies the core functions of the QIO program: • Improving quality of care for beneficiaries

<table>
<tr><td></td><td></td><td>

- Protecting the integrity of the Medicare Trust Fund by ensuring that Medicare pays only for services and goods that are reasonable and necessary and that are provided in the most appropriate setting
- Protecting beneficiaries by expeditiously addressing individual complaints, such as beneficiary complaints; provider-based notice appeals; violations of the Emergency Medical Treatment and Labor Act (EMTALA); and other related responsibilities as articulated in QIO-related law.

Medicare Quality Improvement (QIOs) organizations are Medicare's boots on the ground to drive and champion improvement in our nation's health care system. Working on behalf of the Centers for Medicare and Medicaid Services (CMS) since 1984, QIOs are an independent and objective voice to help improve health care delivery, safety, and efficiency in every US state and territory through a combination of

- improvement collaboratives with local health care providers and provider organizations;
- targeted assistance for individual health care providers;
- direct intervention with Medicare beneficiaries and the health care community; and
- serving as conveners

</td></tr>
</table>

quality of care complaints		If you are dissatisfied with the quality of care or services you or your loved one receives if the care was provided by a health plan, you can start the process by calling the health plan's Member Services number, which is on the back of the person's insurance card. People with Medicare and their representatives who have a complaint or quality of care concern can get help from their Beneficiary and Family Centered Care (BFCC)-QIO (BFCC-QIO). BFCC-QIOs manage all complaints and quality of care reviews, EMTALA, and other types of case review for people with Medicare and their representatives.
Railroad Retirement Program		The Railroad Retirement Program is similar to Social Security in terms of the benefits it offers. But there are several key differences between the two. First, railroad workers only pay money into the Railroad Retirement plan, not Social Security. The money railroad workers pay in taxes goes into funding the Railroad Retirement Program and the benefits it pays. You can't double-dip and receive full benefits from both railroad retirement and Social Security. Benefits are paid out to workers based on the number of months of service they have as railroad employees and their earnings credits. Employees receive one month of credit for every month they work for an eligible railroad employer, regardless of how many days of the month they actually worked. The RRB is responsible for administering retirement benefit payments. These benefits can't be paid until you end your railroad employment. You also have to reach a certain age threshold to apply for railroad retirement benefits. The earliest age that you could draw railroad retirement benefits is sixty, if you have

		thirty years of qualifying railroad service. You can receive your full railroad retirement benefit at this age if you meet the thirty years of service retirement. Otherwise, you can start drawing railroad retirement benefits at age sixty-two. But just like Social Security, your benefit amount is reduced for each year before full retirement age that you start drawing benefits. Spouses can also receive retirement benefits once they reach a certain age. The benefit amounts they're able to draw depends on how old their spouse is, the number of years of service they have as a railroad employee and when they retire. But generally, if you retire at age sixty with thirty years of railroad service your spouse would be able to begin receiving benefits once they turn sixty if they haven't already. The same rules apply for reducing benefit amounts when retirement benefits are taken before your spouse reaches their full retirement age.
range of motion	ROM	Range of motion (ROM) exercises are physical therapy exercises designed to increase movement and joint flexibility. As a health care caregiver, these exercises are needed for any person who sits or lies for a prolonged period of time. Range of motion exercises help improve a patient's joint stiffness, improve muscle strength and endurance, and reduce the risk of further injury. There are three main groups of ROM exercises, which are active, active-assistive, and passive. In active ROM exercises, patients move their joints themselves. On the contrary, in active-assistive ROM exercises, patients may require your help to complete the full motion. Finally, in passive ROM exercises, the health care provider or a device moves the joint, without the active participation of the patient.

readmission		A hospital readmission is an episode when a patient who had been discharged from a hospital is admitted again to that hospital or another within a specified time interval. Readmission to the hospital could be for any cause, such as worsening of disease or new conditions. Unplanned hospital readmission is not always related to the previous visit.
reasonable and necessary		Insurers only cover reasonable, customary, and necessary services. This means the care or services are safe and effective for the treatment of an illness or injury and not experimental or investigational. It also includes the duration and frequency of services to be rendered, and it is appropriate for the item or service(s). It also is to ensure the service or item is furnished in accordance with accepted standards of medical practice for the diagnosis or treatment of the patient's condition or to improve the function of a malformed body member. It must also be furnished in an appropriate medical setting to meet the patient's medical need(s) and condition(s). Many plans will exclude cover for treatment charges deemed outside the insurer's reasonable and customary range. A charge is considered reasonable and customary if it aligns with the average costs for that service within your geographical area. This means that if your loved one's doctor charges above this level, then he may have to pay the difference. If you are unsure about whether the treatment cost meets this criterion, you can check with your loved one's provider. Another way to prevent being caught off guard and paying a different cost is by seeking treatment at a medical provider within your loved one's insurer's network or by seeking treatment preauthorization in advance.

Rehabilitation Act of 1973		The Rehabilitation Act of 1973 is a federal law prohibiting discrimination against people with disabilities by federal agencies, federal contractors, or programs receiving federal funds and it protects persons using public areas.
residential treatment facilities		Residential treatment facilities house and provide therapy for patients with drug and alcohol addictions, emotional or behavioral problems, or mental illness. They are clinically focused and offer treatments such as psycho-analytic therapy, behavioral management, group counseling, family therapy, and medication management. Residents have usually been unsuccessful with outpatient treatments but are not appropriate for an inpatient psychiatric unit.
Resource Utilization Group	RUG	RUGs are a set of fifty-three categories that make up the resident classification system used by the Medicare program and a skilled nursing facility to adjust the payment rate a skilled nursing facility receives (see also prospective payment system).
respite care		Respite care offers relief for home caregivers by providing services to individuals unable to care for themselves. Respite services can be furnished on a short-term basis in a home or institutional setting, like a nursing facility or assisted care living facility. Most insurances will cover a short-term period of respite in a long-term care facility, as this can help prevent caregiver burnout and an unnecessary hospitalization. Thus, check with your loved one's health plan to see if such coverage is allowed and what documentation might be needed for a prior authorization can be obtained.
retrospective review		Retrospective review is the process used by health plans and insurers of determining coverage after treatment has been given.

room and board	R&B	Means just that—the person entering such a home gets a room for payment, and no personal care or meals or other services are provided.
second opinion		A second opinion means that you choose to see another doctor or specialist after you've received an initial diagnosis or treatment plan for a medical condition. The second doctor reviews your medical history and gives their interpretation of your health. If you do not get the second opinion within your health plan's provider network, these expenses will be excluded by most private health insurance plans and you must pay the cost of the visit.
self-inject-ables		Means you as the caregiver must give your loved one the medication using a syringe and needle to put the medication into your loved one's body. An injectable might be referred to as a shot. Injectables are given in a large muscle, such as the arm or thigh or buttocks, and this is called an intramuscular injection, as the needles goes deeper into a muscle). Or the medicine might be injected into tissue (such as your tummy), and this means the needle only penetrates the skin or fat tissues. If you must give an injection, it is imperative that you have been trained, and a health care provider has taught you about the medication and any preparatory steps specific to that medication. Simply reading the instructions or a how-to is not sufficient. You must first learn how to do so and what syringe and needle you should use by getting educated by the health care provider who is prescribing the medication to be injected. It is also imperative when you are taught the one teaching you doesn't just show you what to do, but you actually get to practice how to do all steps to be used. This method of teaching is called teach-back.

self-insured		A self-insured health plan (also known as a self-funded health plan) is coverage offered by an employer or association in which the employer (or association) takes on the risk involved with providing coverage instead of purchasing coverage from an insurance company. According to a 2021 Kaiser Family Foundation analysis, 64 percent of covered workers are in plans that are either fully or partially self-funded plans, including 82 percent of covered workers at large companies. So if you have employer-sponsored health insurance and particularly if you work for a large employer, it's likely that your coverage is self-insured. Self-insured health plans are not subject to state insurance regulations. Instead, they're regulated at the federal level, under ERISASelf-insured plans are also not subject to state laws designed to protect consumers from surprise balance billing.
service area		A geographic area where a health insurance plan accepts members if it limits membership based on where people live. For plans that limit which doctors and hospitals you may use, it's also generally the area where you can get routine (nonemergency) services. The plan may end your coverage if you move out of the plan's service area.

services for individuals aged sixty-five or older in an institution for mental diseases and under age twenty-one		This service is often referred to as IMD over sixty-five. It is an option that most states have chosen to offer in their Medicaid program. Services may be provided either in a hospital or in a nursing facility that is considered an institution for mental diseases (IMD), meaning that the facility meets the federal and state requirements of a hospital or nursing facility but is also considered an IMD. Ordinarily states are responsible for the costs of IMDs; the federal Medicaid program specifically excludes reimbursement for residents of an IMD. The two exceptions are individuals over age sixty-five who receive this service and younger individuals who receive the psych under twenty-one service. Individuals in either type of IMD who are between the ages of twenty-two and sixty-four may not receive Medicaid reimbursement. Individuals applying to or receiving this service in a nursing facility are subject to the preadmission screening and resident review (PASRR) process.
skilled nursing care or services		Skilled care is nursing and rehabilitation therapy care that can only be safely and effectively performed by or under the supervision of professionals or technical personnel. It's health care given when you need skilled nursing or skilled therapy to treat, manage, and observe your condition and evaluate your care. Skilled care services require they be delivered by a licensed professional, such as a registered nurse or physical therapist, occupational therapist, speech pathologist, or social worker.

skilled nursing facility	SNF	A facility licensed by a state to provide nursing or rehabilitation care and services. It is health care given when you need short-term skilled nursing or skilled therapy on a daily basis to treat, manage, and observe your condition and evaluate your care. Health plans or Medicare-covered services in a skilled nursing facility include but aren't limited to the following: • A semiprivate room (a room you share with other patients) • Meals • Skilled nursing care • Physical therapy (if needed to meet your health goal) • Occupational therapy (if needed to meet your health goal) • Speech-language pathology services (if they're needed to meet your health goal) • Medical social services • Medications • Medical supplies and equipment used in the facility • Ambulance transportation (when other transportation endangers your health) to the nearest supplier of needed services that aren't available at the SNF • Dietary counseling SNF's offer twenty-four-hour skilled nursing and personal care. They also have rehabilitation services. Patients must be medically stable to qualify for SNF level of care. They must also have a need that must be performed by a skilled, licensed professional on a daily basis.

		Examples are complex wound care and rehabilitation when a patient cannot tolerate three hours of therapy a day. SNFs are sometimes called nursing homes, rehabilitation centers, or convalescent hospitals. All mean the same, as these facilities provide nursing care for chronically ill or short-term and long-term residents of all ages.
skilled nursing facility advance beneficiary notice		This is a written notice issued in order to transfer financial liability to beneficiaries before the SNF provides an item or service that is usually paid for by Medicare but may not be paid for in this particular instance because it is not medically reasonable and necessary or is custodial in nature.
social determinants of health	SDH	The social determinants of health (SDH) are the conditions in which people are born, grow, work, live, and age and the wider set of forces and systems shaping the conditions of daily life. Social determinants of health (SDOH) have a major impact on people's health, well-being, and quality of life. Examples of SDOH include safe housing, transportation, and neighborhoods; racism, discrimination, and violence; education, job opportunities, and income; access to nutritious foods and physical activity opportunities; polluted air and water; and language and literacy skills.
Social Security	SS	Social Security is a program run by the federal government. The program works by using taxes paid into a trust fund to provide benefits to people who are eligible.

Social Security Administration	SSA	The Social Security Administration assigns Social Security numbers and administers the Social Security retirement, survivors, and disability insurance programs. They also administer the Supplemental Security Income program for the aged, blind, and disabled. You can find the nearest Social Security office by calling the national number at 1-800-772-1213 by visiting the Social Security website.
social services		Local social service agencies are ones you may want to explore for help with a variety of topics and at times possibly help with location of a caregiver. To find a social service agency in your area, this website has a link where you can type in your state, and it will bring up the services within your state.
speech therapy		Speech therapy assesses and treats speech disorders and communication problems. It helps people develop skills like comprehension, clarity, voice, fluency, and sound production. Speech therapy can treat childhood speech disorders or adult speech impairments caused by stroke, brain injury, or other conditions.
special health care need		The health care and related needs of children who have chronic physical, developmental, behavioral, or emotional conditions. Such needs are of a type or amount beyond that required by children generally.
specialist		A physician who focuses on a specific area of medicine or a group of patients to diagnose, manage, prevent, or treat certain types of symptoms and conditions.

spinal cord injury	SCI	A spinal cord injury (SCI) is damage to the tight bundle of cells and nerves that sends and receives signals from the brain to and from the rest of the body. The spinal cord extends from the lower part of the brain down through the lower back. SCI can be caused by direct injury to the spinal cord itself or from damage to the tissue and bones (vertebrae) that surround the spinal cord. This damage can cause temporary or permanent changes in sensation, movement, strength, and body functions below the site of injury.

The extent of disability depends on where along the spinal cord the injury occurs and the severity of the injury. An injury higher on the spinal cord can cause paralysis in most of your body and affect all limbs (tetraplegia or quadriplegia). Quadriplegia, also known as tetraplegia, is a form of paralysis that affects all four limbs plus the torso (*quad* originates from the Latin word for *four*). Most people with tetraplegia have significant paralysis below the neck, and many are completely unable to move.

A lower injury to the spinal cord may cause paralysis affecting your legs and lower body (paraplegia). This paralysis affects all or part of the trunk, legs, and pelvic organs. A spinal cord injury can be classified by two types: complete or incomplete.

1. An incomplete injury means the spinal cord is still able to transmit some messages to or from the brain. People with incomplete injuries retain some sensory function and may have some control of muscle activity below the injury site.
2. A complete injury means that there is no nerve communication below the injury site; sensory and motor function below this site is lost.

standard of care		A standard of care refers to informal or formal guidelines that are generally accepted in the medical community for the treatment of a disease or condition, and it includes a diagnostic and treatment process that a clinician should follow for a certain type of patient, illness, or clinical circumstance. In legal terms, the level at which the average, prudent provider in a given community would practice. It is how similarly qualified practitioners would have managed the patient's care under the same or similar circumstances. Evidence-based standards of care might be developed by a specialist society or organization and the title of standard of care awarded at their own discretion.
Supplemental Nutrition Assistance Program		The Supplemental Nutrition Assistance Program (SNAP) is a federal program that provides nutrition benefits to low-income individuals and families that are used at stores to purchase food. The program is administered by state and local agencies. SNAP also refers to food stamps. By using the FDA website, you can click on your state to find the local office and its application. The local office where you apply might be called Social Services, Public Assistance, or Human Services.
surrogate		A surrogate decision maker, also known as a health care proxy or as agents, is an advocate for incompetent patients. If a patient is unable to make decisions for themselves about personal care, some agent must make decisions for them. If there is a durable power of attorney for health care, the agent appointed by that document is authorized to make health care decisions within the scope of authority granted by the document. If people have court-appointed guardians with authority to make health care decisions, the guardian is the authorized surrogate. If a person can appoint and use a surrogate even if they have decision- making capacity.

		The hierarchy of health care surrogates may vary according to the law of the specific state, but an example order of priority is listed here. 1. The patient's guardian 2. The patient's spouse 3. Any adult son or daughter of the patient 4. Either parent of the patient 5. Any adult brother or sister of the patient 6. Any adult grandchild of the patient or an adult relative who has exhibited special care and concern, who has maintained close contact, and who is familiar with the patient's activities, health, and religious or moral beliefs.
substance abuse versus addiction		Substance abuse differs from addiction. Many people with substance abuse problems are able to quit or can change their unhealthy behavior. Addiction, on the other hand, is a disease. It means you can't stop using even when your condition causes you harm. Substance abuse is not limited to illegal drugs and alcohol but can be from use of prescription and over-the-counter medications. These can be just as dangerous and addictive as illegal drugs. You can abuse medicine if you do the following: • Take medicine prescribed for someone else. • Take extra doses or use a drug other than the way it's supposed to be taken. • Take the drug for a nonmedical reason.

		These are the types of prescription drugs that are most often abused. • Opioid pain relievers • Stimulant medications used to treat attention deficit hyperactivity disorder • Anxiety and sleep medicines The most commonly abused OTC drugs are cough and cold medicine that have dextromethorphan, which in high doses can make you feel drunk or intoxicated.
Tax Identification Number	TIN	A Tax Identification Number (TIN) is a nine-digit number used as a tracking number by the Internal Revenue Service (IRS).
teach-back		Teach-back is a technique for health care providers to ensure that they have explained medical information clearly so that patients and their families understand what is communicated to them. Regardless of a patient's health literacy level, it is important that staff ensure that patients understand the information they have been given. The teach-back method is a way of checking understanding by asking patients to not only state in their own words what they need to know or do about what is being taught, but if the teaching also included techniques on how to administer care, the patient or family is also given opportunities until they have managed the technique, and they can demonstrate back what was taught.
telehealth		Telehealth, sometimes called telemedicine, lets your health care provider care for you or your loved one without an in-person office visit. Telehealth is done primarily online with Internet access on your computer, tablet,

or smartphone. You can get a variety of specialized care through telehealth. Telehealth is especially helpful to monitor and improve ongoing health issues, such as medication changes or chronic health conditions.

There are several options for telehealth care.

- Talk to your health care provider live over the phone or video chat.
- Use remote monitoring so your health care provider can check on you at home. For example, you might use a device to gather vital signs to help your health care provider stay informed on your progress.
- It can also be used to

    - obtain lab or X-ray results;
    - provide online mental health treatments, counseling, and medication management;
    - provide online medical health treatments for migraines and management of urinary tract infections, skin conditions, and wounds and minor colds and stomachaches;
    - help with medication management;
    - remotely monitor certain chronic medical conditions, such as but not limited to diabetes, high blood pressure, HIV, kidney disease, or asthma;

		○ remotely monitor your vital signs, health goals, blood pressure, cholesterol, blood sugar, oxygen levels, and if pregnant or postpartum, to reduce the frequency of in-office prenatal visits, obtain breastfeeding help and lactation services quickly, receive birth control counseling, and prescriptions; ○ remotely monitor such services as physical and occupational therapy or nutritional counseling; and ○ remotely monitor such mental treatments such as management of stress, anxiety, depression, and other conditions virtually or to receive mental health treatment, including online therapy, counseling, and medication management and treatment of follow up for such conditions as attention deficit disorder (ADD) and attention deficit hyperactivity disorder (ADHD).
the five-star quality rating system for providers		The Social Security Act mandates the establishment of minimum health and safety and standards that must be met by providers and suppliers participating in the Medicare and Medicaid programs. Thus, the Centers for Medicare and Medicaid Services (CMS) created a tool to help consumers, their families, and their caregivers to compare health care providers more easily and to help identify areas about which you may want to ask questions. The tool allows a rating for any health care provider, such as any patient care institutions,

		such as hospitals, critical access hospitals, hospices, nursing homes, and home health agencies. It also covers suppliers that provide for diagnosis and therapy rather than sustained patient care, such as laboratories, clinics, and ambulatory surgery centers. The star rating is from one to five and is based not only from on-site surveys but also from consumer surveys and other sources where a provider is evaluated for the care and services it provides.
The Joint Commission	JC	Founded in 1951, the Joint Commission is the nation's oldest and largest standards-setting and accrediting body in health care. As an independent, not-for-profit organization, the Joint Commission seeks to continuously improve health care for the public, in collaboration with other stakeholders, by evaluating health care organizations and inspiring them to excel in providing safe and effective care of the highest quality and value.
tertiary care		Highly specialized medical care that involves advanced, complex, and comprehensive care, procedures, treatments, techniques, and methods of therapy and diagnosis involving equipment and personnel not economically feasible in a smaller institution because of underutilization (not using enough).
third-party administrator	TPA	A third-party administrator is a company that provides operational services, such as claims processing and employee benefits management under contract to another company. Insurance companies and self-insured companies often outsource their claims processing, and many of their administrative functions, such as premium billing, customer enrollment, and other day-to-day operations, are often handled this way.

third-party payer	TPP	Insurers routinely coordinate benefits by determining whether a third party is liable for payment of a particular service provided to a covered member and then denying payment up front, as the claim is the obligation of another insurer. That insurer might be if you or your loved one is injured in an auto accident or fall in a business or public place or someone's residence; it is that insurance that is responsible for payments for the services rendered for the injury.
tracheostomy		A tracheotomy or a tracheostomy is an opening surgically created through the neck into the trachea (windpipe) to allow direct access to the breathing tube and is commonly done in an operating room under general anesthesia. A tube is usually placed through this opening to provide an airway and to remove secretions from the lungs.
traumatic brain injury	TBI	Traumatic brain injury (TBI) happens when a sudden external, physical assault damages the brain. It is one of the most common causes of disability and death in adults. TBI is a broad term that describes a vast array of injuries that happen to the brain. The damage can be focal (confined to one area of the brain) or diffused (happens in more than one area of the brain). The severity of a brain injury can range from a mild concussion to a severe injury that results in coma or even death.
treatment or service authorization request	SAR	Certain procedures and services are subject to authorization by Medicaid before reimbursement can be approved. Authorization requests are made with a treatment authorization request (TAR) or a service authorization request. Authorization requirements are based on federal and state law.

teletype-writer	TTY	A TTY (teletypewriter) is a communication device used by people who are deaf, hard of hearing, or have severe speech impairment. People who don't have a TTY can communicate with a TTY user through a message relay center (MRC). An MRC has TTY operators available to send and interpret TTY messages.
types of admissions		There are generally three types of admissions. • Elective hospital admissions make up most admissions, as you or your loved one requires the care, treatment, or surgery that can only be provided by a hospital. • Direct admission would occur after the patient has seen or spoken to their doctor, who feels they must be admitted for immediate medical care. The doctor may arrange an ambulance to take you or your loved one to the hospital or request that you or your loved one go directly to the hospital. • Emergency admissions go through the hospital's emergency department. A medical emergency is any serious injury, condition, or symptom posing an immediate risk to someone's life or health. If after stabilization and an admission is required, you or your loved one will be admitted to a medical or surgical bed or a specialized unit with the admission status listed as an emergency admission.

		Note: If you or your loved one is placed in observation, this is not an admission. While you or your loved one may be in a hospital bed and stay for many days and nights and undergo any sort of nursing care, diagnostic tests, treatments, medications, and food, identical to that of inpatients, this does not mean you or your loved one's status is considered an admission. You or your loved one is getting care and services as an outpatient until it can be determined by the ordering physician should an admission occur as more tests and treatment are needed or a discharge can occur.
Urban Indian Health Programs		Health programs available to American Indians and Alaska Natives living in urban areas. Urban health programs serve the following: • Members or descendants of federally recognized tribes, bands, or other organized groups of Indians, including those tribes, bands, or groups terminated since 1940 • Members or descendants (in the first or second degree) of state recognized tribes • Eskimos, Aleuts, other Alaska Natives, or their descendants
urgent care	UC	Urgent care clinics provide immediate medical attention for minor medical conditions that are not life or limb threatening, and they do not require treatment at a hospital emergency room. You can expect to receive the same quality and compassionate care you receive from your primary care physician. If you have a non-life-threatening illness or injury and you want to avoid the long waits and expensive costs of the emergency department.

urgent care clinic		It is a type of walk-in clinic focused on the delivery of urgent ambulatory care in a dedicated medical facility outside a traditional emergency department located within a hospital. Urgent care centers primarily treat injuries or illnesses requiring immediate care but not serious enough to require an ED visit or your medical condition is life threatening.
US Library of Congress		The Library of Congress provides Congress with objective research to inform the legislative process, administers the national copyright system, and manages the largest collection of books, recordings, photographs, maps, and manuscripts in the world. In it is the national center for library service to the blind and physically handicapped, and it offers many concerts, lectures, and exhibitions for the general public. Those outside the Washington, DC, area have access to the library's growing electronic resources through the Library of Congress.
US Preventive Services Task Force	USPSTF	The United States Preventive Services Task Force (USPSTF) was first formed in 1984 to assist physicians in making decisions about which preventive services to offer patients. It is a type of walk-in clinic focused on the delivery of urgent ambulatory care in a dedicated medical facility outside a traditional emergency department located within a hospital. Urgent care centers primarily treat injuries or illnesses requiring immediate care but not serious enough to require an ED visit, or your medical condition is not life threatening. The US Preventive Services Task Force is an independent volunteer panel of national experts in disease prevention and evidence-based medicine. The task force works to improve the health of people nationwide by making evidence-based recommendations about clinical preventive services.

Veterans Affairs	VA	The Department of Veterans Affairs runs programs benefiting veterans and members of their families. It offers education opportunities and rehabilitation services and provides compensation payments for disabilities or death related to military service, home loan guaranties, pensions, burials, and health care that includes the services of nursing homes, clinics, and medical centers.
veterans benefit information		Veterans can continue to get information about benefits or file a claim for benefits by visiting the VA website at www.va.gov. Veterans with claims specific or other questions may request information via Inquiry Routing & Information System (IRIS) or telephone at 1-800-827-1000. You can explore the benefits offered by the VA for you or your loved one as well as forms you might need to apply for care or services by going to the benefits. VA.gov website.
Veterans Health Administration	VHA	The Veterans Health Administration is America's largest integrated health care system, providing care at 1,298 health care facilities, including 171 medical centers and 1,113 outpatient sites of care of varying complexity (VHA outpatient clinics), serving 9 million enrolled veterans each year. On the VA.gov website, you can explore the VA centers near you and your loved one.
well-baby care		Routine doctor visits for comprehensive preventive health services that occur when a baby is young and annual visits until a child reaches age twenty-one. Services include physical exam and measurements, vision and hearing screening, and oral health risk assessments.

wellness program		A program intended to improve and promote health and fitness that's usually offered through the workplace, although insurance plans can offer them directly to their enrollees. The program allows your employer or plan to offer you premium discounts, cash rewards, gym memberships, and other incentives to participate. Some examples of wellness programs include programs to help you stop smoking, diabetes management programs, weight loss programs, and preventative health screenings.
workers' compensation	WC	Workers' compensation insurance, also called workers' comp insurance, helps cover medical expenses and lost wages for small business owners if an employee is injured or becomes sick. This coverage can include rehabilitation services and death benefits too. An employee can only receive benefits if their injury or illness relates to their job duties or employment. Workers' comp insurance could cover injuries caused by lifting heavy equipment, slipping on a wet or oily surface, or sustaining injury due to fires or explosions. If an employee isn't acting within the scope of their employment and becomes injured, such as playing football with friends on a day off, workers' compensation insurance won't cover them. These medical costs are to be assumed by your private health plan. Each state has its own unique set of workers' compensation laws that employers must follow. These regulations help ensure that employers provide coverage for the cost of work-related injuries or occupational diseases, regardless of employee negligence. You can find your state's workers' compensation official on their website.

About the Author

PEGGY ROSSI HAS been a nurse for over sixty-two years, entering Sacramento State College as one of the first schools in the US to allow a student to graduate with a Bachelor of Science in Nursing degree. To further her education, she graduated from Golden Gate University in 1985 with a master's in public administration. She was very active in the field of discharge planning from the time of its inception of Medicare and Medicaid in 1965, and she has then been active in the field of case management since the early 1980s, when she was hired to be a medical case manager for a major commercial insurer. In addition to her Registered nursing license, she was licensed as a public health nurse.

From these areas, she found her true career love, serving primarily over the years as director of discharge planning and case management for health plans, medical groups, and two major tertiary hospitals in the greater Sacramento area. Two of her biggest accomplishments have been the following:

1. Writing in its entirety for Foundation Health and its Department of Defense contracts for the CRI (CHAMPUS Reform Initiative, now TRICARE), the entire case management program (programs, policies, and procedures; job descriptions; and all the training material needed to teach new nurses in all regions covered by the contract between Foundation Health and DoD). She also did all the writing regarding the benefit of case management as Foundation Health applied for other DOD contracts for other regions of the US. Once the program was up and running, she then

served as a consultant for any region when difficult case management problems arose.

2. Writing again in its entirety the medical management program for a startup new HMO: Western Health Advantage (WHA). This included, as was done for Foundation Health, all documents required for the medical management program (UM, CM, and QM).

Due to a leg injury, she had to resign as the director of case management for a large tertiary hospital but was immediately hired by the Center for Case Management. In this position, she worked as both a consultant and interim director over discharge planning or case management departments of many hospitals across the US. Prior to her retirement in 2021, she served as a nurse consultant for one of California's twenty-one regional centers, contracted with the CA: Department of Developmental Services. In this role, she worked closely with the physician advisers, the case manager assigned to clients and their families. During this period of employment, the Coronavirus pandemic hit, and her role quickly changed. She then was to follow that any client admitted to the hospital had a safe discharge in place, and they were placed at the right level of care.

Her motto over the years has been, "Learn and never quit," and with this philosophy, she does exactly that. As such and to keep current on discharge planning and case management issues and any laws and regulations that may impact case management and the continuum of care, she reads many professional journals and websites.

She also possesses a great passion to teach others about discharge planning and case management and the benefits it offers. Over the years, she has written articles for both professionals and the lay public. At one point during her employment with Foundation Health, she wrote a monthly article for the lay public on finding community, state, or federal resources, especially for children with special needs. During and after the publication of her last text on case management, she was a contributing author to HCPro's *Case Management Monthly*, writing articles of key importance to case managers. This column was entitled "From the Director's Desk."

Her greatest accomplishments include not only writing program plans and other key documents for many of her employers but also writing three textbooks for case management. Her first two texts are *Case Management in Healthcare: A Practical Guide* (WB Saunders 1999) and *Case Management in Healthcare 2nd Edition* (WB Saunders 2003). It was this later text that won the *American Journal of Nursing* award for best nursing management text in 2003. Over the years, these two texts have been used in multiple schools of nursing for both their upper and lower division for nurses. Her third text is to assist hospitals as they train new staff to the role, and it is entitled *The Hospital Case Management Orientation Manual* (HCPro 2014).

Because of her love for case management, she knows how important it is to be certified, and that certification attests to the fact the professional has met the gold standards for his profession. As such, her first certification was in utilization management, and then she was in the first group of candidates who sought case management certification (CCM) in the early nineties. Subsequently, she was later certified by the American Case Management Association as a registered nurse (ACM-RN) and then **case management** administrator certification (CMAC).

Over the years, she has remained active in both the national and local chapter of CMSA, serving as president in the early nineties. She has participated in the chapter's educational committee and the programs it has presented. Additionally, she has been a speaker for several of the local CMSA events, as well as for other professional medical groups, always with the topic centering on case management.

It is from her love of nursing and teaching, and she has seen the struggles loved ones go through as they perform caregiving, so she wanted to share her expertise with others. Thus, this book, *Caregiver, a Role We Least Expected*, was written.